# ANNALS OF THE NEW YORK ACADEMY OF SCIENCES

*Volume 1059*

# TUMOR PROGRESSION AND THERAPEUTIC RESISTANCE

ANNALS OF THE NEW YORK ACADEMY OF SCIENCES
*Volume 1059*

# TUMOR PROGRESSION AND THERAPEUTIC RESISTANCE

*Edited by Wafik S. El-Deiry*

*The New York Academy of Sciences*
*New York, New York*
*2005*

**Library of Congress Cataloging-in-Publication Data**

Tumor progression and therapeutic resistance / edited by Wafik S. El-Deiry.
p. ; cm. — (Annals of the New York Academy of Sciences ; v. 1059)
This volume is the result of an international conference, held on November 8–9, 2004, in Philadelphia, Pennsylvania.
Includes bibliographical references and index.
ISBN 1-57331-543-5 (cloth : alk. paper) — ISBN 1-57331-544-3 (pbk. : alk. paper)
1. Cancer invasiveness—Congresses. 2. Metastasis—Congresses. 3. Drug resistance in cancer cells—Congresses. 4. Cancer Cells—Congresses. 5. Cell transformation--Congresses. I. El-Deiry, Wafik S. II. Series.
[DNLM: 1. Cell Transformation, Neoplastic—genetics—Congresses. 2. Disease Progression--Congresses. 3. Drug Resistance, Neoplasm—Congresses. 4. Genes, Tumor Suppressor—Congresses. 5. Neoplasms, Experimental—therapy—Congresses. 6. Signal Transduction—Congresses. W1 AN626YL v.1059 2005 / QZ 202 T9245 2005]
Q11.N5 vol. 1059
[RC269]
500 s—dc22
[616.99'407]

2005029003

GYAT/PCP

*Printed in the United States of America*

**ISBN 1-57331-543-5** (cloth)
**ISBN 1-57331-544-3** (paper)
**ISSN 0077-8923**

ANNALS OF THE NEW YORK ACADEMY OF SCIENCES

*Volume 1059*
*November 2005*

# TUMOR PROGRESSION AND THERAPEUTIC RESISTANCE

*Editor*
WAFIK S. EL-DEIRY

This volume is the result of the conference on **Tumor Progression and Therapeutic Resistance**, held November 8–9, 2004, in Philadelphia, Pennsylvania.

CONTENTS

**Financial assistance was received from:**

- ABRAMSON CANCER CENTER AT THE UNIVERSITY OF PENNSYLVANIA
- GLOBAL TECHNOLOGY COMMUNITY LLC
- PFIZER INC.
- THE FELS INSTITUTE FOR CANCER RESEARCH
- THE KIMMEL CANCER CENTER AT THOMAS JEFFERSON UNIVERSITY
- THE WISTAR INSTITUTE

# Tumor Progression and Therapeutic Resistance

## An Overview

LINDA HOTCHKISS MEHTA

*New York Academy of Sciences, New York, New York 10016, USA*

This volume contains highlights of a meeting that spanned the entire breadth of translational cancer research emanating from both academic laboratories and industry. It is the expectation of the editor that this effort will encourage further such interactions and accelerate progress in the field.

Advances are occurring on multiple fronts, and the reports provided here include the discovery of molecular targets and pathways (oncogene, cell survival, tumor suppression, cell death), host–neoplasm interactions (cell adhesion, matrix proteases), early detection, and monitoring progression. The progress in our understanding of tumor progression and metastasis is presented, along with further information on immune surveillance, *in vivo* molecular imaging, animal models, and drug discovery and chemistry, high-throughput assays, mechanism determination, target validation, therapeutic window, and some progress in clinical trials for more advanced agents and targets.

Patrick Everley and Bruce Zetter begin the volume with their report on the use of the techniques of proteomics and how this approach has been applied to the analysis of proteins in cancer, including the identification of temporal changes in protein levels as tumors develop and metastasize.

For normal biological function to occur in cells, the temporal and spatial expression of proteins must be precisely regulated and coordinated. Shuttling between the nucleus and the cytoplasm by means of cellular signaling pathways mediated by protein kinases regulates the function of certain proteins. Shao-Chun Wang and Mien-Chie Hung summarize findings that indicate a role for molecular localization in cancer.

The incidence of melanoma is increasing rapidly: in just 40 years, the rate in the population has gone from 3 to 13 per 100,000. Activating mutations in BRAF have been identified in over 60% of melanomas, and Keiran Smalley and Meenhard Herlyn report on a therapeutic intervention involving the RAF inhibitor BAY 43-9006 and chemotherapy and the promise offered in research using small molecule inhibitors for targeting signaling cascades.

Mark Nelson *et al.* address advances and setbacks in colorectal cancer, which is the third most fatal malignant neoplasm in the United States. The setbacks include the recall of cyclooxygenase-2 inhibitors from clinical trials, but these authors report on promising work using selenium compounds and further discuss the biochemical and molecular mechanisms for the anticancer effects of selenomethionine.

Address for correpondence: Linda Hotchkiss Mehta, New York Academy of Sciences, 2 East 63rd Street, New York, NY 10016. Voice: 212-880-2913; fax: 1-212-880-2089.
lmehta@nyas.org

**Ann. N.Y. Acad. Sci. 1: ix–xi (2005). © 2005 New York Academy of Sciences.**
**doi: 10.1196/annals.1339.050**

Prostate tumorigenesis in transgenic mouse models has revealed roles for the transcription factors Nkx3.1, a homeodomain protein, and Egr 1, a zinc finger protein. Sarki Abdulkadir provides evidence that these proteins regulate gene programs involved in prostate tumorigenesis.

Sulindac sulfone has the ability to inhibit tumorigenesis in both animals and patients with familial adenomatous polyposis, but the mechanisms of action have not been fully elucidated. Wen-Chi Chang *et al.*, in a paper presented at the conference by Margie Clapper, provide data that demonstrate sulindac sulfone's actions in modulating the APC/β-catenin pathway *in vitro.*

Bin-Bing Zhou reports that ADAMs (a combination of a disintegrin and metalloproteases), which are zinc-dependent transmembrane metalloproteases, act as "sheddases" or multiple ErbB ligands in ErbB signaling pathways. Dr. Zhou's group has identified a selective small molecule inhibitor of ADAM proteases that block this action. The ErbB pathway has been a target for anticancer drugs, and their approach will soon be tested in the clinic.

Combination treatments have become standard practice in cancer chemotherapy, but they present a challenge for clinical testing. Shannon Decker and Edward Sausville point out that it is not feasible to test all possible drug combinations before introducing them as treatments and that another method for preclinical assessment of promising combinations is needed. They propose modeling approaches that take into consideration a biologic rationale, *in vitro* results in more than one tumor type, *in vivo* pharmacology, and selectivity of primary tumor cell activity.

Trastuzumab has demonstrated antitumor actions, but many patients are resistant to its effects when it is used as a single agent and a few suffer from severe side effects. Keng-Hsueh Lan, Chien-Hsing Lu, and Dihua Yu present recent progress in understanding the mechanisms of trastuzumab function and those cellular defects that lead to resistance to its effects.

The structural and functional features of Par-4 (prostate apoptosis response-4) are presented by Padhma Ranganathan and Vivek Rangnekar in their contribution to this volume. Par-4's regulation of apoptosis occurs on multiple levels, all of which have the potential to be developed into targeted cancer therapies.

Nicholas Nicolaides *et al.* describe the use of morphogenics in identifying targets and drug development, which makes use of mutations in DNA mismatch repair (MMR) genes. Germline MMR mutations have been linked to genetic predisposition to a number of malignancies. *Morphogenics* uses a dominant negative MMR gene to create genetic diversity within cellular systems. This genetic diversity produces a wide range of phenotypes that can be used in the development of better pharmaceutical approaches to treatment as well as in the discovery of pharmaceutical targets.

One target that shows promise in the prevention and treatment of colon cancer is the adenomatous polyposis coli (APC) tumor suppressor gene. Most somatic cells in colorectal polyps and cancers contain APC mutations or deletions. Eugene Gerner *et al.* report that loss of APC function in turn leads to changes in other genes, including ornithine decarboxylase (OCS), the first enzyme in polyamine synthesis. Difluoromethylornithine (DFMO) is a selective inhibitor of ODC and shows promise as a colorectal cancer chemopreventive agent. As DFMO is regulated by the c-Myc oncogene, which is itself influenced by APC, it appears that APC and APC-dependent genes will be useful genetic markers of risk and possible targets for therapies.

Xiaobing Tian *et al.* stress the urgent need for better early detection of breast and pancreatic cancers in their chapter. Human breast cancer cells (estrogen receptor–positive) display elevated levels of Myc protein, cyclin D1 protein, and insulin-like growth factor 1 receptor (IGF1R). Likewise, pancreatic cancer cells show elevated levels of *KRAS* mRNA and IGF1R. Tian *et al.* report on employing scintigraphic imaging or positron emission tomography (PET) to detect these elevations.

The c-Myc transcription factor's role in neoplastic transformation led Duonan Yu *et al.* to look at its target genes, because which of these genes is most implicated in tumorigenesis has been unclear. In their contribution, they identify IL10R and Mcy11 as potential targets for therapeutic interventions.

The proteasome inhibitor bortezomib dramatically sensitizes some human cancer cell lines to the apoptotic effects of Apo2L/TRAIL, particularly certain renal, colon, or breast tumor cells. Alan Brooks *et al.* found that neither p53 nor Bax were necessary for this sensitization, and the search for the molecular basis of the sensitization effect continues. Nevertheless, they suggest that the Apo2L/TRAIL combination has a more powerful apoptotic effect.

Magdalena Karbowniczek and Elizabeth Petri Henske investigated the role of tuberin in cellular differentiation. Tuberous sclerosis complex (TSC) is a syndrome that can feature seizures, mental retardation, autism, and tumors in brain, retina, kidney, heart, and skin. They report here on the genetic and biochemical basis of the renal and pulmonary manifestations of TSC, angiomyolipomas, and lymphangiomyomatosis. Their results suggest that tuberin and hamartin are involved in regulation of cellular migration and differentiation, and they hypothesize that abnormalities may be the result of aberrant B-Raf activity.

Ching Ching Leow *et al.* report on research capitalizing on the downregulation of *Hath1* in colon adenocarcinomas. In mice, the *Hath1* orthologue, *Math1*, has been found to be necessary for cell fate determination of intestinal secretory cell, including goblet cells, which are found to be greatly reduced in colon adenocarcinomas. Leow *et al.* have discovered that *Hath1* inhibits proliferation and tumorigenesis of colon cancer cells and suggest that the molecular mechanism may be through *Hath1* regulation of MUC2 expression and repression of *Hath1* following the activation of the Wnt signaling pathway.

Solid tumors often feature hypoxia, which is associated with genetic instability and tumor progression. Ranjit Bindra *et al.* show evidence in their contribution that the expression of RAD51 is repressed by hypoxia in cell lines from many tissues and that this repression persists during the post-hypoxia period. They also found that reduced Rad51 expression was correlated with functional impairments in homologous recombination (HR) repair in these cells. They therefore are proposing a novel mechanism of hypoxia-induced genetic instability via suppression of the HR pathway in cancer cells.

The potential for developing therapeutic interventions through the mechanisms and pathways described here increases with each advance in our knowledge about the molecular and cellular events accompanying malignant tumor progression. This meeting and the research reported on in this volume represent the forefront of this effort.

# Proteomics in Tumor Progression and Metastasis

PATRICK A. EVERLEY AND BRUCE R. ZETTER

*Departments of Surgery and Cell Biology, Children's Hospital / Harvard Medical School, Boston, Massachusetts 02115, USA*

**ABSTRACT: With the ultimate goal of systematically identifying and characterizing proteins within an organism, the field of proteomics has generated much excitement in the past few years. Coupled with mass spectrometry, various quantitative and functional techniques are now available that allow for large-scale analyses of proteins implicated in cancer. New techniques are just now being applied to identifying the temporal changes in protein levels associated with tumor development. This review will focus on the use and promise of proteomic technologies as they apply to the study of tumor progression and metastasis.**

**KEYWORDS: quantitative proteomics; functional proteomics; SILAC; ICAT; electrophoresis; tumor progression and metastasis; mass spectrometry; ABPP**

## INTRODUCTION

Proteomics, simply defined, is the systematic study of proteins. With the completion of the human genome,[1,2] much attention has been focused on determining how cells use their encoded genome to carry out essential functions. Applications of proteomics include identification and quantification of proteins, analysis of protein structures, and the characterization of protein–protein interactions to elucidate important physiological pathways. Recent advances in the development of new tools for proteomics research have pushed this field to the forefront of biological research.

In contrast to genomics—the study of genes at the DNA and mRNA levels—the field of proteomics claims several advantages. For example, proteins carry out the majority of functional processes in the cell, making the study of DNA and mRNA less relevant in characterizing protein–protein interactions. Evidence from a number of laboratories has shown a relatively poor correlation between the levels of mRNA and protein,[3,4] suggesting that post-transcriptional mechanisms play an important role in regulating protein expression. Detection of these changes can be difficult unless researchers are looking directly at protein levels. On the other hand, while it is predicted that there are approximately 30,000 genes in human cells, many scientists expect the total number of protein isoforms expressed to be over 100,000 as a result of alternative splicing and the vast array of post-translational modifications (PTMs).

Address for correspondence: Bruce R. Zetter, Children's Hospital, Karp Family Research Building, 11th floor, Vascular Biology Program, 300 Longwood Avenue, Boston, MA 02115. Voice: 617- 919-2320; fax: 617-730-0268.

bruce.zetter@childrens.harvard.edu

**Ann. N.Y. Acad. Sci. 1059: 1–10 (2005). © 2005 New York Academy of Sciences.**
**doi: 10.1196/annals.1339.001**

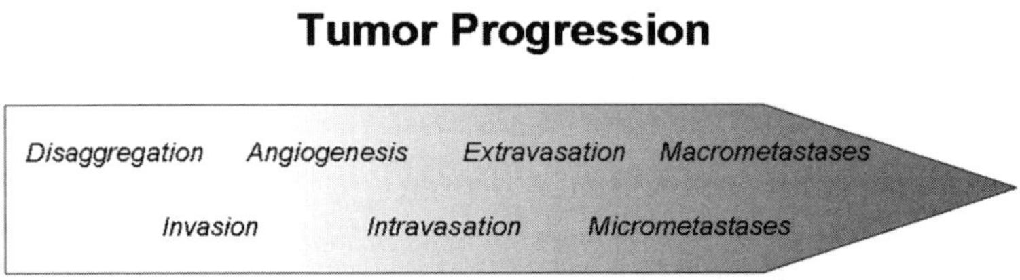


**FIGURE 1.** Elements of tumor progression.

These PTMs can influence protein function by altering the stability, activity, localization, and/or structural conformation. This creates challenges in proteomics, both in the size of potential analyses and the development of technologies used to study the many classes of proteins.

As discussed throughout this volume, cancer cells acquire properties required to form metastatic colonies, a process known as tumor progression (FIG. 1). This process can be rapid or may require years or decades to provide detectable metastasis. Properties attained by tumor cells during metastatic progression may include (a) disaggregation of cells in the primary tumor; (b) increased motility of primary tumor cells; (c) enhanced degradation of extracellular matrix; (d) induction of new blood vessels (angiogenesis); (e) entry of tumor cells into the circulation; (f) exit of tumor cells into tissue in distant organs; (g) formation of micrometastases; and (h) conversion of micrometastases to macrometastases. The mechanisms underlying progression include both genetic (mutational) and epigenetic changes that result in the alteration of protein profiles in cancer cells over time. The identification of these profiles and of the individual proteins that compose them is the topic of this review.

## MASS SPECTROMETRY IN PROTEOMICS

One such technology that has been particularly useful for proteomic studies is mass spectrometry (MS). In use for nearly 100 years for small molecule studies, MS has more recently been applied to large-scale protein analyses. Protein identification using MS was difficult prior to the inventions of matrix-assisted laser desorption/ionization (MALDI) and electrospray ionization (ESI) in the 1980s, for which the 2002 Nobel Prize in chemistry was shared.[5] MALDI and ESI permit the ionization of peptides and their subsequent analysis by MS. Today, most MS-based technologies developed to study proteins rely on MALDI, ESI, or similar ionization methods.

The use of MS in proteomics relies on its ability to provide data for protein identification and quantification, and is dependent upon the type of MS instrumentation used. For example, ESI is commonly coupled to ion-trap instruments, which can yield peptide sequence data from their ability to fragment peptides along their amino acid backbones (FIG. 2). To accomplish this task, protein samples are typically digested with trypsin, with the resulting peptides loaded onto an HPLC column and eluted with an increasing organic modifier. Since analysis by mass spectrometry is

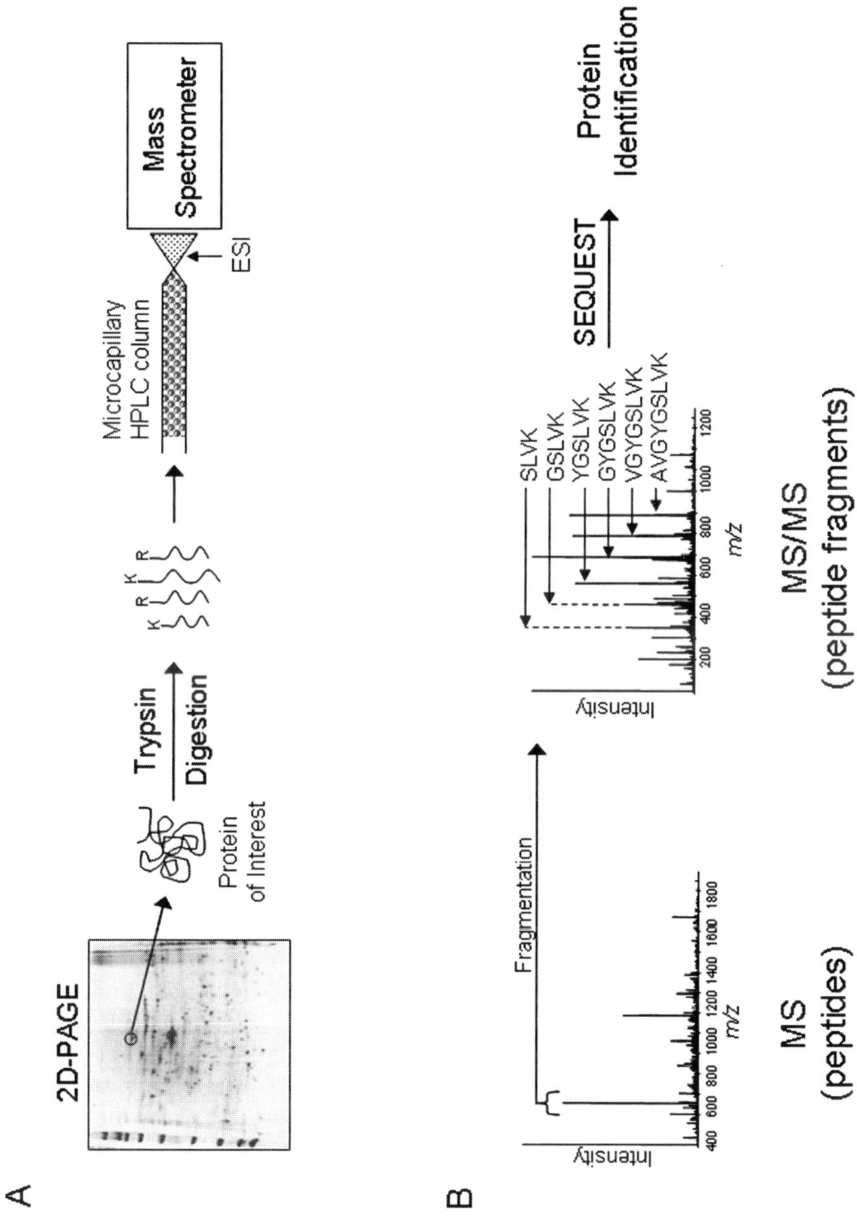


**FIGURE 2.** *See following page for legend.*

dependent on the peptide acquiring a charge and its entry into the gas phase, a voltage is applied between the HPLC column and the instrument. This electric field promotes peptide charge acquisition as they enter the gas phase, such that each peptide ion will have an associated mass-to-charge (*m/z*) ratio. Upon entering the mass spectrometer, peptide ions are detected by their *m/z* ratio in the precursor ion spectrum (MS). Peptides of sufficient intensity are individually selected and further subjected to fragmentation (collision-induced dissociation, or CID), with the product ion spectrum (MS/MS) providing the sequence information for peptides. An algorithm such as SEQUEST [6] is then used to correlate experimental MS/MS data with theoretical spectra from a protein database, thus providing a peptide sequence and therefore protein identification. Applications of MS as it pertains to cancer research are discussed throughout this review.

## PROTEOMIC TOOLS APPLIED TO CANCER RESEARCH

One of the first proteomic methods applied to cancer research was two-dimensional polyacrylamide gel electrophoresis (2D-PAGE).[7] Protein samples from cell lines or tissue specimens are separated by their isolectric points (pI) in the first dimension and by molecular weight in the second. As compared to one-dimensional gels, initial separation by protein pI with 2D-PAGE allows for increased resolution of proteins and can provide information about protein degradation or PTMs. After staining the gel with Coomassie blue or silver for visualization, individual protein spots representing differences between samples are then excised and processed for Edman degradation or MS, thereby providing protein identification. Alternatively, the gels can be studied using software to assess differences in intensity between the two samples, with the goal of classifying cancers based on their staining profiles.

The utility of this method as a tool for cancer studies has been obvious since the mid-1970s when Subramanian *et al.* used 2D-PAGE to compare ribosomal proteins in neoplastic vs. non-neoplastic cells.[8] In the early 1980s, this method was applied to the analysis of human samples from prostate cancer patients.[9] More recently, 2D-PAGE has been valuable for the analysis of tumor cell lines possessing pathologically distinct phenotypes. Many labs have proven its effectiveness for studying protein differences in ovarian,[10] leukemia,[11] breast,[12] and prostate[13] cancer cell lines.

The analyses of tumor vs. normal samples often reveal interesting changes at the protein level. However, 2D gels are limited in several aspects. Interesting spots resolved by 2D-PAGE must be excised individually and processed for MS identification, a process that can prove tedious when many proteins are to be analyzed. Poor solubility presents a problem for the study of extremely hydrophobic proteins, such

**FIGURE 2.** Identification of a protein by ESI-MS/MS. (**A**) Protein samples are resolved by 2D-PAGE and a spot of interest is excised and digested with trypsin. Peptides are loaded onto a microcapillary HPLC column and eluted with an organic gradient. Peptides are ionized into the gas phase and acquire one or more protons prior to entering the mass spectrometer, conferring a specific *m/z* ratio for each peptide. (**B**) MS scan separates peptide ions by *m/z* ratio, with most intense peaks selected for fragmentation (CID) and further analysis. MS/MS data is searched against a sequence database using an algorithm such as SEQUEST to determine peptide sequence and therefore protein identification.

as those embedded in cellular membranes, which may not solubilize prior to analysis in gel-based methods. Furthermore, quantifications based on staining intensity may be inaccurate for proteins of relatively low abundance due to a limitation in dynamic range.

## QUANTITATIVE PROTEOMICS IN CANCER

Although 2D-PAGE provided some of the first quantitative studies in proteomics, the recent use of fluorescence and stable isotopes allows for a more extensive comparison of protein levels among different samples. The ability to accurately quantify proteins between tumor samples has obvious benefits. Indeed, a protein that is highly expressed in tumors compared to normal controls may serve as a useful diagnostic biomarker. One example is prostate-specific antigen, the serum levels of which are used to help clinicians diagnose prostate cancer and monitor tumor recurrence.[14] In addition, many cancer drugs currently in development are targeted against proteins with high expression levels in tumor samples. Identifying additional proteins vital for cancer progression could lead to new diagnostic and prognostic markers as well as new therapeutic targets.

While there are several quantitative methods available, one well-characterized technology is 2D differential in-gel electrophoresis (2D-DIGE). In this approach, two distinct samples are individually labeled with different fluorescent tags (such as Cy3 and Cy5), mixed, and separated by 2D-PAGE.[15] The mixing and analysis on the same 2D gel ensures that the samples are subjected to the same conditions, thereby limiting experimental variation. The gel is then scanned, first at the wavelength corresponding to Cy3, and then at the wavelength excitable for Cy5. A comparison of these two fluorescent signals provides information on the relative abundance of specific proteins in the two samples. Spots can then be excised and processed for protein identification via MS. By comparing proteins obtained from tumor vs. normal cells, Zhou *et al.* used 2D-DIGE to uncover a significant number of proteins differentially expressed in esophageal cancer.[15] Their studies resulted in the identification of over 160 proteins dysregulated by at least threefold. Additional experiments were performed with clinical patient samples to discern differences among varying stages of breast cancer.[16] While these studies show the power of this technology for cancer research, some major hurdles to overcome for 2D-PAGE also hold true for 2D-DIGE, such as relatively low throughput and a limited utility for the analysis of membrane proteins.

Perhaps the most accurate way of quantifying protein expression is through the use of stable isotope incorporation followed by MS. This can be accomplished by replacing isotopic variants of the same atom, such as substituting deuterium for hydrogen or $^{13}C$ for $^{12}C$. Labeling cells or tissues with isotopic variants (e.g., $^{12}C$ vs. $^{13}C$) will give rise to "light" and "heavy" populations. Protein from different samples can then be mixed at equal amounts (light:heavy) and enzymatically digested, thereby providing a single sample containing peptides from both cellular conditions. Peptides with the same amino acid sequence in the light and heavy samples, differing only in isotopic label, are essentially identical in their chemical properties and will therefore co-elute during chromatographic separation. While changing a few atoms may seem insignificant, these differences are easily resolved by a mass spectrometer. Relative quantitative data are obtained by comparing the peak intensities between light and heavy peptides in the MS scan, and the additional information provided by MS/MS will yield protein identification.

The two most common ways of incorporating stable isotopes into biological samples for proteomics experiments are through the use of isotope-coded affinity tags (ICAT) and stable isotope labeling with amino acids in cell culture (SILAC). The first of these techniques, ICAT, relies on the quantification of peptides resulting from the selective isotopic labeling of cysteine residues *in vitro*.[17–19] An ICAT tag utilizes three elements: an iodoacetamide group to react with cysteine, a linker region substituted with either nine $^{13}C$ (heavy tag) or $^{12}C$ (light tag) atoms, and biotin to selectively isolate the ICAT-labeled peptides prior to MS. Protein from two different cellular states is harvested and isotopically labeled with either the light or heavy ICAT tag. Proteins are then mixed together, digested, and avidin-purified to capture only labeled peptides. This results in a significant reduction in mixture complexity because only cysteine-containing peptides are retained. Analysis of the samples by MS then provides protein identification and relative quantification. This technology has recently been applied to the study of tumor progression in prostate cancer[20] and p53-mediated apoptosis in colorectal cancer.[21] Even though the chemical labeling steps of ICAT can reduce overall sensitivity, the greatest advantage of ICAT is that the protein labeling is performed post-extraction, suggesting that ICAT could be applied to the analysis of human patient specimens. To date, however, there has not been any publication on the use of ICAT in clinical samples.

SILAC, like ICAT, offers a means of introducing stable isotopes into biological samples for quantitative studies.[22–24] However, instead of labeling after protein extraction, cells are cultured in the presence of either $^{12}C$- or $^{13}C$-containing amino acids (FIG. 3). Following protein collection, samples are combined, digested, and analyzed

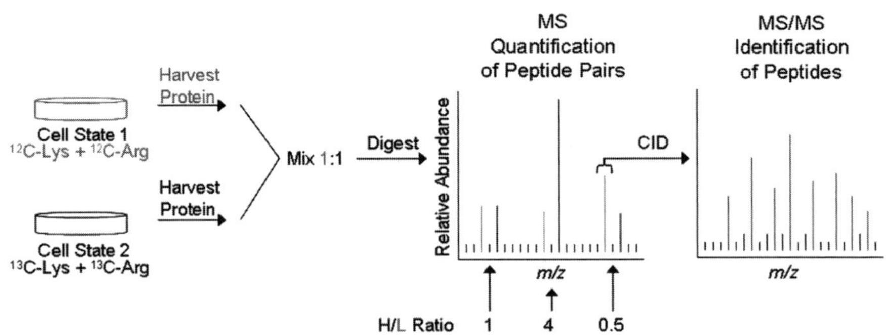


**FIGURE 3.** Schematic diagram of the SILAC procedure. Cells representing two separate conditions, such as low and high metastatic potential, are cultured in the presence of $^{12}C$ or $^{13}C$ lysine and arginine, giving rise to "light"(——) and "heavy" (——) populations. Protein is collected from each, mixed at a 1:1 ratio based on protein concentration, and proteolytically digested with trypsin. Upon analysis by mass spectrometry, co-eluting heavy (——) and light (——) peptides are quantified (H/L ratio) using intensity information provided by the MS scans. Abundant peptides are further selected for CID, yielding MS/MS data to be used for protein identifications.

by MS. Our group has recently applied SILAC to the study of prostate cancer progression, resulting in the identification and relative quantification of over 440 proteins,[25] with validation of many of these proteins currently in progress. The major advantage of this metabolic incorporation is that no chemical labeling steps are involved, which increases sensitivity. Furthermore, the use of essential amino acids as SILAC "reagents" ensures improved proteome coverage. This allows for the identification and quantification of peptides that may have otherwise been missed by using the cysteine-specific nature of ICAT. However, since SILAC is dependent upon metabolism for isotopic incorporation, its main disadvantage is that it is most applicable to cell culture as opposed to animal studies or human samples.

In the past few years, surfaced-enhanced laser desorption/ionization (SELDI) has been applied to the discovery of cancer biomarkers. This technique allows complex clinical samples such as serum to be spotted on a protein chip and directly analyzed by MS, with the prospect of diagnosing cancer based upon the proteomic signature patterns obtained. SELDI has already been applied to the study of ovarian[26] and prostate[27, 28] cancers, among others. SELDI is primarily used to generate patterns of protein expression without easily identifying the altered proteins. Although SELDI has generated much excitement, it has also been the topic of intense scrutiny and debate within the proteomics community. Some of its current limitations include poor instrument resolution, protein chip variability, and an inability to identify biomarkers already in use by clinicians.[29] While this technique is being improved, it should be stressed that these obstacles must be overcome if SELDI is to be routinely used for clinical diagnostic purposes.

## FUNCTIONAL PROTEOMICS IN CANCER

As discussed, the purpose of quantitative proteomics is to develop and apply methods that will provide information about changes in protein levels resulting from different biological phenomena. While these approaches are effective in revealing relative protein abundances, functional protein levels are often difficult to evaluate due to numerous post-translational modifications. This is particularly true for many enzymes, whose functions result from selective peptide cleavages following protein translation. With the goal of better understanding protein activities, functional proteomics encompass methods that include but are not limited to the analysis of protein–protein interactions and the use of chemical probes to selectively isolate and characterize enzyme activity levels.

Mapping protein–protein interactions is useful for several reasons. First, the discovery of novel binding interactions can lead to the identification of proteins previously unknown to be implicated in cancer. Second, it allows for categorizing the already increasing amount of existing data on proteomics. For example, simply identifying and quantifying large numbers of proteins in cancer samples is of little value without knowledge of how these proteins are involved in pathways important for tumor progression and maintenance. Finally, with a significant amount of pathway overlap in cancer, it can help provide an understanding of how various signaling pathways intersect.

Walensky *et al.* have recently applied a novel chemical strategy to study protein–protein interactions in cancer.[30] They designed "stapled" peptides to interact with

BCL-2 family members, thereby activating apoptosis. Such peptides maintain their secondary helical structure, are resistant to protease degradation, and are able to penetrate cellular membranes, making them a potentially valuable alternative to other less effective therapies. The stapled BCL-2 interacting peptides used in this study were shown to inhibit the growth of leukemia xenographs *in vivo*, suggesting a new approach to anti-tumor therapy.

Activity-based proteomics is a rather new field that seeks to study proteins on the basis of their functional output. Pioneered by the Cravatt laboratory,[31] activity-based protein profiling (ABPP) holds considerable promise as a tool for cancer-based studies. ABPP makes use of a multifunctional chemical probe—one end of the probe contains a fluorophosphonate (FP) group that will covalently bind to the active site of serine hydrolases; the other end carries a fluorescent tag to permit functional readout. Complex protein samples are first incubated with the probe to allow enzyme derivatization. Samples are then separated on a one-dimensional gel and imaged using a fluorescent scanner. Since probes will only bind to active serine hydrolases, the observed gel band intensities reflect the relative amount of active enzyme present in the sample. The resulting enzyme profiles have been used to classify cells on their state of invasiveness and also to distinguish melanoma from breast cancer cell lines.[32] More recently, ABPP has been applied to the study of *in vivo* breast tumor xenographs,[33] providing one of the first applications of this technique beyond cell culture.

## CONCLUSIONS

Throughout the late 1990s, genomics generated considerable excitement as it attempted to understand how the regulation of genes contributed to diseases such as cancer. Additional work showed that PTMs and other post-transcriptional mechanisms are critical for controlling gene expression. Accordingly, many efforts were refocused on proteins because they carry out the vast majority of functions within the cell and serve as the most common drug targets. The term "proteomics" was coined to describe research directed toward the discovery and characterization of proteins encoded by an organism's genome. Initially, gel-based studies provided the first efforts to explain how cancer functions at the protein level. Whether interested in clinical samples or cells growing in culture, 2D-PAGE and, more recently, 2D-DIGE, allow for large-scale comparisons of protein expression and serve as useful techniques for biomarker discovery.

The field of proteomics has experienced a rapid expansion in recent years, fueled mainly by the development of MS as a protein identification and quantification tool. What once took hours by Edman degradation to identify proteins could now be performed in a matter of seconds. This has in turn resulted in increased cancer studies that attempt to identify novel biomarkers of disease. MS has added advantages, such as compatibility with complex mixtures and the ability to analyze very small quantities of protein. Furthermore, stable isotope-labeling methods, such as ICAT and SILAC, are easily coupled to MS and provide relative quantitative information for proteins, which can then be exploited to evaluate potential markers or drug targets in cancer.

Improvements in proteomics technology such as those outlined in this review hold great promise for the study of tumor progression and metastasis. With appropriate clinical samples, we will be able to determine the protein changes that specify different stages of the metastatic cascade. These proteins can then be studied for their specific contribution to tumor progression, developed as cancer biomarkers, or be utilized as new therapeutic targets. Continued improvements in mass spectrometry techniques will only accelerate the pace of discovery in the field.

## ACKNOWLEDGMENTS

This work was supported by Grant CA-37393 from the National Institutes of Health. We also thank S. Gygi for helpful discussions during manuscript preparation.

## REFERENCES

1. LANDER, E.S. *et al.* 2001. Initial sequencing and analysis of the human genome. Nature **409:** 860–921.
2. VENTER, J.C. *et al.* 2001. The sequence of the human genome. Science **291:** 1304–1351.
3. AHRAM, M. *et al.* 2002. Proteomic analysis of human prostate cancer. Mol. Carcinog. **33:** 9–15.
4. GYGI, S.P. *et al.* 1999. Correlation between protein and mRNA abundance in yeast. Mol. Cell. Biol. **19:** 1720–1730.
5. CHO, A. & D. NORMILE. 2002. Nobel Prize in chemistry. Mastering macromolecules. Science **298:** 527–528.
6. ENG, J.K., A L. MCCORMACK & J.R. YATES III. 1994. An approach to correlate tandem mass spectral data of peptides with amino acid sequences in a protein database. J. Am. Soc. Mass Spectrometry **5:** 976–989.
7. O'FARRELL, P.H. 1975. High resolution two-dimensional electrophoresis of proteins. J. Biol. Chem. **250:** 4007–4021.
8. SUBRAMANIAN, A.R., J.M. GILBERT & A. KUMAR. 1975. Comparison of ribosomal proteins from neoplastic and non-neoplastic cells. Resolution by two-dimensional gel electrophoresis. Biochim .Biophys. Acta **383:** 93–96.
9. EDWARDS, J.J. *et al.* 1982. Proteins of human urine. II. Identification by two-dimensional electrophoresis of a new candidate marker for prostatic cancer. Clin. Chem. **28:** 160–163.
10. SMITH-BECKERMAN, D.M. *et al.* 2005. Proteome changes in ovarian epithelial cells derived from women with BRCA-1 mutations and family histories of cancer. Mol. Cell. Proteomics.**4:** 156–168
11. KAVALLARIS, M. *et al.* 2001. Multiple microtubule alterations are associated with Vinca alkaloid resistance in human leukemia cells. Cancer Res. **61:** 5803–5809.
12. O'NEIL, K.A. *et al.* 2003. Profiling the progression of cancer: separation of microsomal proteins in MCF10 breast epithelial cell lines using nonporous chromatophoresis. Proteomics **3:** 1256–1269.
13. LIU, J.W. *et al.* 2003. Annexin II expression is reduced or lost in prostate cancer cells and its re-expression inhibits prostate cancer cell migration. Oncogene **22:** 1475–1485.
14. BARRY, M.J. 2001. Clinical practice. Prostate-specific-antigen testing for early diagnosis of prostate cancer. N. Engl. J. Med. **344:** 1373–1377.
15. ZHOU, G. *et al.* 2002. 2D differential in-gel electrophoresis for the identification of esophageal scans cell cancer-specific protein markers. Mol. Cell. Proteomics **1:** 117–124.
16. SOMIARI, R.I. *et al.* 2003. High-throughput proteomic analysis of human infiltrating ductal carcinoma of the breast. Proteomics **3:** 1863–1873.
17. LI, J., H. STEEN & S.P. GYGI. 2003. Protein profiling with cleavable isotope-coded affinity tag (cICAT) reagents: the yeast salinity stress response. Mol. Cell. Proteomics **2:** 1198–1204.

18. YI, E.C. *et al.* 2005. Increased quantitative proteome coverage with (13)C/(12)C-based, acid-cleavable isotope-coded affinity tag reagent and modified data acquisition scheme. Proteomics **5:** 380–387.
19. GYGI, S.P. *et al.* 1999. Quantitative analysis of complex protein mixtures using isotope-coded affinity tags. Nat. Biotechnol. **17:** 994–999.
20. MEEHAN, K.L. & M.D. SADAR. 2004. Quantitative profiling of LNCaP prostate cancer cells using isotope-coded affinity tags and mass spectrometry. Proteomics **4:** 1116–1134.
21. GU, S. *et al.* 2004. Global investigation of p53-induced apoptosis through quantitative proteomic profiling using comparative amino acid-coded tagging. Mol. Cell. Proteomics **3:** 998–1008.
22. ONG, S.E. *et al.* 2002. Stable isotope labeling by amino acids in cell culture, SILAC, as a simple and accurate approach to expression proteomics. Mol. Cell. Proteomics **1:** 376–386.
23. BLAGOEV, B. *et al.* 2003. A proteomics strategy to elucidate functional protein-protein interactions applied to EGF signaling. Nat. Biotechnol. **21:** 315–318.
24. ONG, S.E., I. KRATCHMAROVA & M. MANN. 2003. Properties of 13C-substituted arginine in stable isotope labeling by amino acids in cell culture (SILAC). J. Proteome Res. **2:** 173–181.
25. EVERLEY, P.A. *et al.* 2004. Quantitative cancer proteomics: stable isotope labeling with amino acids in cell culture (SILAC) as a tool for prostate cancer research. Mol. Cell. Proteomics **3:** 729–735.
26. PETRICOIN, E.F. *et al.* 2002. Use of proteomic patterns in serum to identify ovarian cancer. Lancet **359:** 572–577.
27. ADAM, B.L. *et al.* 2002. Serum protein fingerprinting coupled with a pattern-matching algorithm distinguishes prostate cancer from benign prostate hyperplasia and healthy men. Cancer Res. **62:** 3609–3614.
28. PETRICOIN, E.F., III, *et al.* 2002. Serum proteomic patterns for detection of prostate cancer. J. Natl. Cancer Inst. **94:** 1576–1578.
29. DIAMANDIS, E.P. 2004. Mass spectrometry as a diagnostic and a cancer biomarker discovery tool: opportunities and potential limitations. Mol. Cell. Proteomics **3:** 367–378.
30. WALENSKY, L.D. *et al.* 2004. Activation of apoptosis in vivo by a hydrocarbon-stapled BH3 helix. Science **305:** 1466–1470.
31. LIU, Y., M.P. PATRICELLI & B.F. CRAVATT. 1999. Activity-based protein profiling: the serine hydrolases. Proc. Natl. Acad. Sci. USA **96:** 14694–14699.
32. JESSANI, N. *et al.* 2002. Enzyme activity profiles of the secreted and membrane proteome that depict cancer cell invasiveness. Proc. Natl. Acad. Sci. USA **99:** 10335–10340.
33. JESSANI, N. *et al.* 2004. Carcinoma and stromal enzyme activity profiles associated with breast tumor growth in vivo. Proc. Natl. Acad. Sci. USA **101:** 13756–13761.

# Cytoplasmic/Nuclear Shuttling and Tumor Progression

SHAO-CHUN WANG AND MIEN-CHIE HUNG

*Department of Molecular and Cellular Oncology, The University of Texas M.D. Anderson Cancer Center, Houston, Texas 77030, USA*

ABSTRACT: **Protein localization is a highly dynamic biological process. To ensure a proper cellular function, the spatial distribution of different proteins needs to be delicately regulated and coordinated. In cancer, this process is tightly correlated with the outcome of cell proliferation and the response to apoptotic stress. Here we summarize our recent studies regarding the role of subcellular trafficking on cancer cell growth through an AKT-independent regulation of the forkhead transcription factor and, on cancer metastasis, through the regulated localization and subsequent protein degradation of the Snail protein, a key transcription factor involved in epithelial-mesenchymal transition (EMT). In both cases, cellular signaling pathways mediated by distinct protein kinases modulate the appropriate protein localization and functioning. Finally, we address a novel translocation pathway for tyrosine kinase receptors between the cell membrane and the nucleus. We demonstrate that the ErbB family proteins are also expressed in the nucleus and can function as transcriptional regulators. Using a genomic approach, we have identified a number of the target genes regulated by this pathway that are closely related to cancer cell proliferation and metastasis. Our findings, together with the seminal discoveries by other groups, highlight the importance of protein localization in cancer biology and its potential to be a therapeutic target for cancer.**

KEYWORDS: **cytoplasmic; nuclear; IKK; forkhead; FKHRL1; FOXO3a; AKT; Snail; GSK3β; β-TrCP; EMT; ErbB; COX-2**

## IKKβ AND TUMOR PROGRESSION

Cancer development poses a rigorous threat to the organism when the tumor progresses, which is underlined by unrestrained cell growth and metastasis. While intensive studies have been devoted to these areas in the past decades, the mechanism and the development of strategies for cancer targeting remain to be further explored. It is now a well-accepted concept that the delicately controlled temporal and spatial expression of proteins is critical for cell function. As shown in the studies conducted by others and our group, shuttling between the nucleus and the cytoplasm regulates the function of particular proteins. Here we summarize the recent findings initiated in our group and demonstrate that, in addition to normal cells, molecular localization is also a critical regulatory point in cancer.

Address for correspondence: M.-C. Hung, The University of Texas, M.D. Anderson Cancer Center, Department of Molecular and Cellular Oncology, Unit 108, 1515 Holcombe Blvd., Houston, TX 77030. Voice: 713-792-3668; fax: 713-794-0209.
mhung@mdanderson.org

**Ann. N.Y. Acad. Sci. 1059: 11–15 (2005).** 
**doi: 10.1196/annals.1339.002**

One well-known example is the forkhead transcription factor. As shown in the seminal finding by Dr. Michael Greenberg's laboratory, the survival-promoting serine/threonine kinase AKT/PKB negatively regulates the forkhead transcription factors including FKHRL1, also known as FOXO3a, by phosphorylating them at three conserved serine/threonine residues, which leads to retention of FKHRL1 in the cytoplasm by association with the 14-3-3 sequester protein. It is known that AKT is a survival-promoting factor, especially in cancer cells. Phosphorylation of FKHRL1 by AKT prevents it from entering the nucleus to trigger the apoptotic mechanism, thus contributing to the anti-apoptotic activity of AKT.[1] This observation can also be extended to human breast cancer tumor tissues, in which FKHRL1 cytoplasmic expression is significantly correlated with activated AKT in the same tumor tissues.[2] Interestingly, in the same study, we also found that in some tumor samples that lacked activated AKT, the FKHRL1 protein was still retained in the cytoplasm. This observation suggests that, in addition to AKT, there are other AKT-independent mechanisms for cytoplasmic sequestration of the forkhead transcription factors. Using immunohistochemical staining of archived human breast cancer tumor tissues, we found that the level of nuclear FKHRL1 inversely correlates with expression of the IKKβ (see below). Consistent with the pro-apoptotic function of FKHRL1, nuclear FKHRL1 expression is positively correlated with the survival rate of breast cancer patients. Further analysis of the FKHRL1 protein sequence revealed several sites sharing the consensus signature for phosphorylation by IKKβ. One of the sites, serine 644, was later confirmed to be the major residue phosphorylated by IKKβ. IKKβ physically interacts with FKHRL1 and inhibits FKHRL1's transactivation activity and prevents its nuclear translocation. Phosphorylation of FKHRL1 by IKK causes proteolysis of FKHRL1 through a ubiquitin-dependent proteasome pathway. It appears that this IKK-mediated downregulation pathway of FKHRL1 is independent from that of AKT reported previously. In tumor tissues, cytoplasmic FKHRL1 correlates with the expression of IKKβ or activated AKT and associates with poor survival in breast cancer.

The IκB kinase (IKK) complex is the most crucial enzyme in the NF-κB signaling pathway.[3] IKK phosphorylates the NF-κB–associated inhibitor IκB and targets the IκB to ubiquitination and degradation. This allows the NF-κB dimmers to translocate to the nucleus where they function as transactivators to turn on a repertoire of anti-apoptotic, angiogenic, and oncogenic genes. Consistent with this note, the activity of IKK is often activated constitutively in breast cancer, which results in the sustained activation of NF-κB during the development of breast carcinoma. In our study, we demonstrate the second arm of the IKK oncogenic function through the downregulation of FKHRL1.[2] Expression of constitutively active IKK enhances cell proliferation *in vitro* and tumorigenesis *in vivo*. More importantly, this enhancement in tumor formation can be overridden by overexpression of FKHRL1, indicating the IKK–FKHRL1 pathway is a critical pathway regulating cell growth and survival and the IKK complex is a potential target for cancer intervention.

## GSK3β AND EMT

As mentioned earlier, the other key negative regulator of the forkhead transcription factor is the AKT kinase. We previously showed that AKT phosphorylation of the Cdk inhibitor p21 can sequester this cell cycle regulator in the cytoplasm.[4] A similar observation was also made by others for the p27 protein.[5–7] These studies show that the AKT pathway can regulate the subcellular localization of multiple molecules through a direct substrate-kinase mechanism. However, an indirect mechanism is also possible. It has been demonstrated by others that AKT phosphorylates and inhibits the activity of the glycogen synthase kinase-3 (GSK3).[8] In our recent study, we further identify that GSK3β phosphorylates the transcription factor Snail and suppresses metastasis.[9] Snail, and its family member Slug, contain zinc-fingers and function as transcription repressors. They recognize the CAGGTG binding site that was identified first in Drosophila and then in other mammals and humans.[10,11] Through negative regulation of the target genes, such as E-cadherin, these repressors enhance epithelial–mesenchymal transition (EMT), which is a critical phenotypic switch during development and cancer metastasis.[12–14] Epithelial cells are normally polarized and display keratin filaments and membrane junctions, such as adherens and desmosomes. After EMT induction, they lose the specific features for their epithelial origin and acquire mesenchymal characteristics as marked by elevated vimentin expression and a flattened morphology. In cancers, dramatic phenotype changes occur when cells leave an organized epithelial layer and acquire invasive phenotype and initiate metastasis.

In our study, it was noted that the Snail protein is highly unstable in most cell line systems tested, with a half-life of about 25 min.[9] This short half-life can be significantly prolonged by co-treatment with proteosome inhibitors plus inhibitors of the GSK3β, suggesting a potential role of GSK3β in post-translational modification of Snail. Indeed, GSK3β associates with Snail and phosphorylates the transcription factor at two distinct consensus motifs for GSK3β phosphorylation. Phosphorylation at one of the motifs creates a recognition site for the ubiquitin E3 ligase, β-TrCP, which is also involved in the IKK-forkhead pathway as described above, leading to Snail degradation; hence, this result explains the observed high instability of Snail. On the other hand, phosphorylation at the second motif, which is next to the first site at the C-terminal side, reveals a distinct level of regulation of Snail by GSK3β. We show that phosphorylation at this motif results in sustained Snail cytoplasmic accumulation and prevents it from functioning in the nucleus as a transcription factor. Thus, this study establishes a dual regulation model of GSK3β on Snail, namely, subcellular localization and protein degradation. It is known that the phosphorylation pattern by GSK3β is usually a sequential event, with the most C-terminal target motif phosphorylated first and then the next N-terminal one.[15] Therefore, a scenario can be proposed that GSK3β phosphorylates the C-terminal motif of Snail first, resulting in cytoplasmic translocation of Snail, and the second phosphorylation by GSK3 subjects Snail to the β-TrCP-powered degron. Consistent with these results, a Snail variant (Snail-6SA), which abolishes the known phosphorylation sites by GSK3β, is stabilized and the protein expression exclusively occurs in the nucleus. More importantly, this variant of Snail readily downregulates E-cadherin expression and induces EMT in non-motile breast epithelial cells *in vivo,*[9] which can be a very valuable tool for further study for cell phenotype transition during metastasis. This study presents an example of an indirect mode of AKT regulation, in which AKT regulates functions of downstream proteins through an intermediate signaling molecule. AKT is a molecule at center stage of cell signaling. In addition to GSK3β/Snail, it has been shown that the Cdk inhibitor p21 and the E3 ligase MDM2 that negatively controls p53 turnover are also on the list for which the subcellular localization controls their functional consequences.[4,16] Together with the story of IKK and FKHRL1 mentioned earlier, molecular trafficking between the nucleus and the cytoplasm plays an essential role in cancer development, for which a more integrated understanding may eventually lead to a specific targeting strategy for cancer therapy.

## NUCLEAR LOCALIZATION OF TKR AND TUMOR PROGRESSION

All the above-mentioned trafficking is between the cytoplasm and the nucleus. Our recent studies also highlight the significant role of membrane tyrosine kinase receptors (TKR) in the regulation of nuclear activity through translocation of the membrane proteins to the nucleus. The TKRs of the ErbB family are frequently found to be associated with breast cancer development because they are significantly involved in cell proliferation, invasion, anti-apoptosis, and resistance to certain anticancer therapies.[17] However, besides the well-known traditional signaling pathways by the TKRs on the cell membrane, many TKRs have also been found in the nucleus. The ever-growing list includes virtually every member in the ErbB family, including the epithelial growth factor receptor (EGFR),[18] ErbB-2/*neu,*[19] ErbB-3,[20] ErbB-4,[21] fibroblast growth factor receptors (FGFR), and vascular endothelial growth factor receptor (VEGFR).[22] Nuclear localization of these receptors, such as EGFR, preferentially occurred in highly proliferating cells. However, due to the lack of efficient strategies to identify their nuclear targets, the functions of these nuclear TKRs in breast cancer remain elusive.[22] The C-terminal intracellular region of EGFR, ErbB-2/*neu*, ErbB-4, and FGFR is associated with a transactivation activity,[22] suggesting a transcriptional function of these receptors *in vivo*. Indeed, our previous findings show that the EGFR receptor complex binds to an AT-rich consensus sequence and transactivates transcription from the sequence. This sequence can be found on the cyclin D1 promoter, which is further confirmed by using chromatin immunoprecipitation assays. EGFR therefore functions as a transcription factor to activate a gene required for cell proliferation.[18]

To further facilitate the understanding of nuclear TKRs' functionality, we have recently developed a cloning strategy employing chromatin immunoprecipitation (ChIP) to identify the potential target genes of nuclear ErbB-2. Using this approach, multiple genomic regions (one of them is the *COX-2* gene promoter) are found to interact with ErbB-2 protein *in vivo.*[19] ErbB-2 forms a complex at a specific nucleotide sequence of the *COX-2* promoter and is able to stimulate its transcription. This association occurs not only in the cell culture, but is also observed in fresh human breast cancer tumor tissues by ChIP assay. Blocking COX-2 activity in ErbB-2-overexpressing breast cancer cells significantly suppressed the invasion activity. This study provides physiological evidence for the interaction between ErbB-2 nuclear function and COX-2 expression, and is of biomedical importance to warrant a more systematic searching of other TKR nuclear targets using similar pan-genomic strategies.

The next important biological question is how the protein functions are regulated in different cellular locations. Is it the intrinsic autonomous property of the protein or the shuffling of different binding partners in different locations, or both? It should not be difficult now to envision a molecular network in the cells which is heavily involved in this process. All these studies have positioned us at the beginning of the road, and a new field derived from these studies is about to unfold in the near future.

## REFERENCES

1. BRUNET, A. *et al.* 1999. Akt promotes cell survival by phosphorylating and inhibiting a Forkhead transcription factor. Cell **96:** 857–868.
2. HU, M.C. *et al.* 2004. IkappaB kinase promotes tumorigenesis through inhibition of forkhead FOXO3a. Cell **117:** 225–237.
3. KARIN, M., Y. CAO, F.R. GRETEN & Z.W. LI. 2002. NF-kappaB in cancer: from innocent bystander to major culprit. Nat. Rev. Cancer **2:** 301–310.
4. ZHOU, B.P. *et al.* 2001. Cytoplasmic localization of p21Cip1/WAF1 by Akt-induced phosphorylation in HER-2/neu-overexpressing cells. Nat. Cell. Biol. **3:** 245–252.
5. VIGLIETTO, G. *et al.* 2002. Cytoplasmic relocalization and inhibition of the cyclin-dependent kinase inhibitor p27(Kip1) by PKB/Akt-mediated phosphorylation in breast cancer. Nat. Med. **8:** 1136–1144 .
6. SHIN, I. *et al.* 2002. PKB/Akt mediates cell-cycle progression by phosphorylation of p27(Kip1) at threonine 157 and modulation of its cellular localization. Nat. Med. **8:** 1145–1152.
7. LIANG, J. *et al.* 2002. PKB/Akt phosphorylates p27, impairs nuclear import of p27 and opposes p27-mediated G1 arrest. Nat. Med. **8:** 1153–1160.
8. CROSS, D.A., D.R. ALESSI, P. COHEN, *et al.* 1995. Inhibition of glycogen synthase kinase-3 by insulin mediated by protein kinase B. Nature **378:** 785–789.
9. ZHOU, B.P. *et al.* 2004. Dual regulation of Snail by GSK-3beta-mediated phosphorylation in control of epithelial-mesenchymal transition. Nat. Cell. Biol. **6:** 931–940.
10. INUKAI, T. *et al.* 1999. SLUG, a ces-1-related zinc finger transcription factor gene with antiapoptotic activity, is a downstream target of the E2A-HLF oncoprotein. Mol. Cell **4:** 343–352.
11. MAUHIN, V., Y. LUTZ, C. DENNEFELD & A. ALBERGA. 1993. Definition of the DNA-binding site repertoire for the Drosophila transcription factor SNAIL. Nucleic Acids Res. **21:** 3951–3957.
12. SAVAGNER, P. 2001. Leaving the neighborhood: molecular mechanisms involved during epithelial-mesenchymal transition. Bioessays **23:** 912–923.
13. THIERY, J.P. 2003. Epithelial-mesenchymal transitions in development and pathologies. Curr. Opin. Cell. Biol. **15:** 740–746.
14. THIERY, J.P. 2002. Epithelial-mesenchymal transitions in tumour progression. Nat. Rev. Cancer **2:** 442–454.
15. COHEN, P. & S. FRAME. 2001. The renaissance of GSK3. Nat. Rev. Mol. Cell. Biol. **2:** 769–776.
16. ZHOU, B.P. *et al.* 2001. HER-2/neu induces p53 ubiquitination via Akt-mediated MDM2 phosphorylation. Nat. Cell. Biol. **3:** 973–982.
17. YARDEN, Y. & M.X. SLIWKOWSKI. 2001. Untangling the ErbB signalling network. Nat. Rev. Mol. Cell. Biol. **2:** 127–137.
18. LIN, S.Y. *et al.* 2001. Nuclear localization of EGF receptor and its potential new role as a transcription factor. Nat. Cell. Biol. **3:** 802–808.
19. WANG, S.-C. *et al.* 2004. Binding at and transactivation of the COX-2 promoter by nuclear tyrosine kinase receptor ErbB-2. Cancer Cell **6:** 251–261.
20. OFFTERDINGER, M., C. SCHOFER, K. WEIPOLTSHAMMER & T.W. GRUNT. 2002. c-erbB-3: a nuclear protein in mammary epithelial cells. J. Cell Biol. **157:** 929–940.
21. NI, C.-Y., M.P. MURPHY, T.E. GOLDE & G. CARPENTER. 2001. gamma-Secretase cleavage and nuclear localization of ErbB-4 receptor tyrosine kinase. Science **294:** 2179–2181.
22. CARPENTER, G. 2003. Nuclear localization and possible functions of receptor tyrosine kinases. Curr. Opin. Cell Biol. **15:** 143–148.

# Targeting Intracellular Signaling Pathways as a Novel Strategy in Melanoma Therapeutics

KEIRAN S.M. SMALLEY AND MEENHARD HERLYN

*The Wistar Institute, 3601 Spruce Street, Philadelphia, Pennsylvania 19104, USA*

**ABSTRACT: Melanoma has been one of the fastest rising malignancies in the last four decades with cases increasing from below 3 per 100,000 people to above 13. Despite worldwide efforts in prevention, diagnosis, and treatment, cases of melanoma continue to rise at an alarming rate of 2.5% annually in the United States. Although early primary melanomas are curable through surgery, treatment of advanced disease remains difficult and the strategies employed in the last 30 years have not significantly improved cure rates, which are less than 5%. The recent identification of activating mutations in BRAF in over 60% of cases of melanoma has caused much excitement in the melanoma community and may offer the first opportunity for a rational treatment program. Combination therapy using the RAF inhibitor, BAY 43-9006, and chemotherapy has led to impressive responses in some melanoma patients and provides a new paradigm for therapeutic intervention in this intractable disease. Besides activating mutations in BRAF, melanomas have constitutive activity in a number of other signaling pathways implicated in oncogenesis, including PI3 kinase/Akt, NFB, Src, and STAT3. With more and more selective small molecule inhibitors becoming available, there are good prospects for treating advanced melanoma using new combinations of signal transduction inhibitors and chemotherapy. In the current review, we discuss the role for these signaling pathways in melanoma and discuss the rationale for targeting signaling cascades using small molecule inhibitors.**

**KEYWORDS: melanoma; therapy; BRAF; Akt; NFkB; Src**

## INTRODUCTION

Despite attempts to treat melanoma using a wide variety of therapies, including immuno-, radio-, and chemotherapy, survival from disseminated disease remains very poor. Most standard chemotherapy drugs have failed in large-scale clinical trials for melanoma. To date, the only drug approved by the FDA for treatment of metastatic melanoma is the alkylating agent dacarbazine (DTIC), which, when given as a single agent, results in clinical responses of 5–10% of cases.[1] Part of the reason for this treatment failure is the notorious chemoresistance of melanoma. Unlike other cancers, drug resistance in melanoma is not acquired selectively following drug therapy, suggesting that chemoresistance in melanoma is intrinsic.

Address for correspondence: Meenhard Herlyn, The Wistar Institute, 3601 Spruce Street, Philadelphia, PA 19104. Voice: +1-215-898-3950; fax: +1-215-898-0980.
herlynm@wistar.upenn.edu

**Ann. N.Y. Acad. Sci. 1059: 16–25 (2005). © 2005 New York Academy of Sciences.
doi: 10.1196/annals.1339.005**

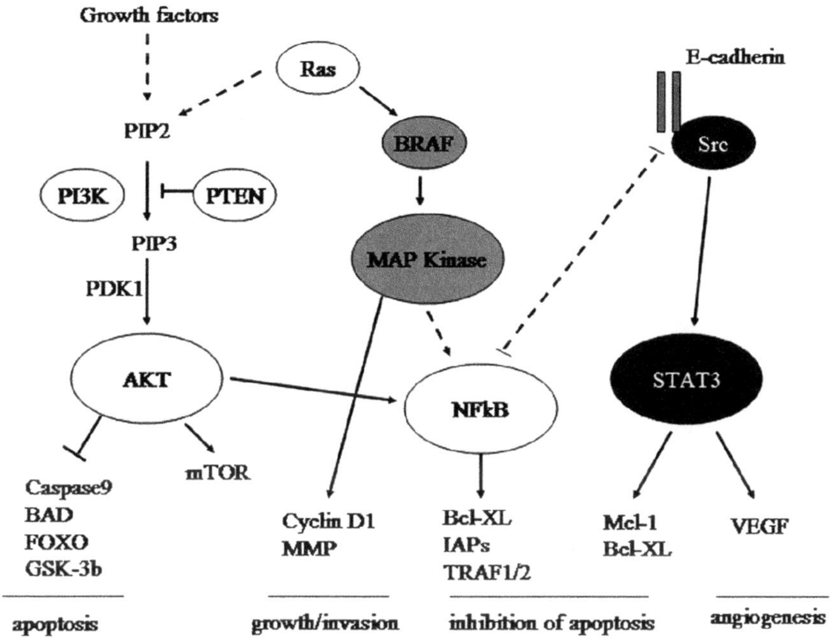


**FIGURE 1.** Scheme showing signaling pathways known to be constitutively active in melanoma.

During the oncogenic process, cancer cells must overcome inherent and microenvironmental control mechanisms that govern cell proliferation and the ability of a cell to survive outside of its immediate niche. Often these mechanisms, which are the same as those required for reduced apoptosis and drug resistance, convey survival advantages upon the cells. The past few years have seen a great increase in our understanding of which pathways are responsible for apoptosis resistance in cancer cells. Melanoma cells are known to have constitutive activity in many of these signaling pathways (Fig. 1). There is an emerging idea that inactivating these survival/apoptosis resistance pathways in combination with standard anticancer treatments may reverse the inherent chemoresistance of melanoma—leading to dramatically improved patient responses.

## BRAF: THE PARADIGM FOR TARGETED MELANOMA THERAPY

A genomewide screen of the ongoing Cancer Genome project at the Sanger Centre identified the V600E-activating mutation of BRAF in 66% of human melanomas.[2] The identification of this mutation has reinvigorated the melanoma research community and has provided a paradigm for the development of targeted melanoma therapies.

Biochemically, the effects of constitutive RAF activity are well described. BRAF is a key player in the Ras/Raf/MEK/ERK mitogen-activated protein (MAP) kinase pathway whose activation is implicated in a wide range of diverse cancers through its effects upon cell proliferation, invasion, and enhanced survival.[3] Subsequent structural biology studies showed that the V600E mutation, which accounts for 80% of the reported mutations in BRAF, works by destabilizing the inactive conformation of BRAF, shifting the equilibrium toward the active form of the kinase.[4] *In vitro* studies have shown that BRAF is an oncogene in immortalized mouse melanocytes[5] and that selective downregulation of BRAF V600E using RNAi causes cell death and reversal of the melanoma phenotype.[6]

Although the *in vitro* data are convincing, there is still some discussion in the melanoma community over the role of BRAF mutations in melanoma pathogenesis and progression. Studies have shown the presence of BRAF V600E mutations in unsuspicious benign nevi.[7] Other groups have reported a lack of BRAF mutations in early stage (radial growth phase, RGP) melanomas, and the reappearance of BRAF mutations at later stages, such as the vertical growth phase (VGP).[8] This possibly suggests that BRAF may be more important in melanoma progression than initiation.[8] Early clinical trials using the RAF kinase inhibitor BAY 43-9006 have been encouraging. Although BAY 43-9006 has little activity as a single agent, robust responses were seen when the RAF kinase inhibitor was used in combination with carboplatin and Taxol. At this stage, it is not clear whether these clinical responses are due to the inhibition of BRAF activity alone, because BAY 43-9006 may also have activity against other receptor tyrosine kinases, such as VEGFR. Although the BRAF story is still unfolding, it is the first positive example of how targeted therapy can work in melanoma. It also provides the rationale to look at other related signaling pathways that may play more important roles in resistance to apoptosis.

## TARGETING APOPTOSIS RESISTANCE: THE PI3-KINASE/AKT PATHWAY

The phosphoinositide 3 kinase (PI3K)/Akt pathway is a key regulator of survival of cancer cells and has been shown to be constitutively active in many cancers, including melanoma.[9] Activation of this pathway occurs through either paracrine/autocrine activation of growth factor receptors or loss of negative regulators of the pathway. In particular, the insulin-like growth factor (IGF)-I is known to aid the growth of early-stage melanoma cells, at least partly through activition of PI3-kinase/Akt.[10] The most commonly activated form of PI3K in cancer is type 1a PI3K, which is a heterodimer consisting of a p85 regulatory and a p110 catalytic subunit. PI3K is recruited to the membrane through activation of receptor tyrosine kinases and associated adaptor proteins binding to the SH2 domain of the p85 subunit. The p110 domain can also be recruited and activated through the activity of the small GTPase Ras. Following membrane recruitment and activation, PI3K then phosphorylates the phosphatidylinositol-4,5,bisphosphate ring (PIP2) at the 3′ position, converting PIP2 to PIP3. Once generated, PIP3 recruits and activates downstream serine-threonine kinases PDK1 and Akt (also known as protein kinase B). One of the most critical regulators of Akt is the phosphatase and tensin homologue (PTEN), which degrades the products of PI3K, thereby preventing the activation of Akt.[11] Studies have revealed that PTEN is lost in up to 30% of melanoma cell lines[12–14] but in only 10% of human tumor material.[15–16]

Akt is the central player in PI3K/Akt-mediated oncogenic behavior and phosphorylates a number of important downstream targets involved in the control of apoptosis. The Akt family consists of three members, Akt1–3,[17] which exhibit different expression patterns depending upon cell type. Although activating mutants of Akt have not been identified in melanoma cells,[18] they are known to have constitutive Akt activity. Of these, 43–50% of melanomas have selective constitutive activity in Akt3.[19] Inhibition of Akt in melanoma, using either PI3-kinase inhibitors or selective RNAi to Akt3, both reduce growth and induce apoptosis.[19–20] Not all of the downstream Akt-mediated phosphorylations lead to substrate activation. FOXO family members are known to induce apoptosis by activating genes such as Fas ligand and BIM. Phosphorylation of FOXO proteins by Akt results in their inactivation and cytoplasmic sequestration.[21] Similarly, Akt can phosphorylate the pro-apoptotic Bad family member, Bcl-2, also leading to its cytoplasmic sequestration.[22] The PI3-kinase/Akt pathway also plays a role in regulating cell proliferation through controlling entry into the cell cycle at the G1-checkpoint, via the inactivation of GSK3β, which regulates the degradation of both cyclin D1 and myc.[23–24] Another downstream target of Akt, linked to enhanced proliferation, is the mammalian target of rapamycin (mTOR). mTOR enhances cell growth through the dual activation of ribosomal S6 kinase (S6K1) and inhibition of the elongation-initiation factor 4E binding protein.

There are a number of reasons for targeting the PI3-kinase/Akt pathway in melanoma. Many of the downstream targets of Akt negatively regulate potentially "anti-oncogenic" proteins. The central role of Akt in the suppression of apoptosis in melanoma makes inhibitors of this pathway ideal for overcoming drug resistance. Indeed, there is evidence that aberrant activation of Akt is involved in the resistance of tumors to therapy. In breast cancer, loss of PTEN—leading to upregulated Akt activity—predicts resistance to the humanized ErbB2 antibody, herceptin.[25] Thus far, attempts to target Akt using pharmacological inhibitors have been hampered by poor drug selectivity. However, due to the central role of Akt in oncogenesis, it is expected that major efforts for the development of selective inhibitors are under way. One recently described Akt inhibitor, API-2, has high selectivity and an impressive *in vitro* profile against a wide range of cancer cell lines.[26]

## SRC AND STAT3

The Src family of non-receptor tyrosine kinases were among some of the first oncogenes to be identified. Members of this kinase family, which also include Fyn, Yes, and Lck, are known to be involved in tumor growth, dissemination, angiogenesis, and invasion.[27] Many of the downstream effects of Src are mediated through recruitment and activation of focal adhesion kinase (FAK), which in turn modulates paxillin and p190RhoGAP. To date, the role of Src activity in melanoma has been little studied. We recently investigated the effects of a novel Src kinase inhibitor, SU6656, on a range of melanoma cell lines corresponding to different tumor stages (RGP, VGP, and metastatic). Previous studies have shown that Src-transformed cells have altered morphology characterized by reduced numbers of bundled actin filaments and cellular contacts.[27] Our own studies revealed that prolonged treatment of melanoma cells using SU6656 (2 μM, 48 h) led to altered morphology in melanoma cells (FIG. 2A, B). It has also been demonstrated that Src is involved in the endocytosis of E-cadherin through the activation of Hakai, a Cbl-like E3 ubiquitin ligase involved.[28] In agreement with this finding, we demonstrated that SU6656 treatment upregulated expression of E-cadherin in RGP-stage melanoma cells (data not shown). Further investigation revealed that although E-cadherin was upregulated it was confined to the cytoplasm and therefore not functionally active. This suggested that although Src activity seems to downregulate E-cadherin expression levels there are other mechanisms responsible for its constitutive internalization. In contrast, SU6656 treatment was unable to restore E-cadherin expression in any of the VGP/ metastatic melanoma lines tested.

Src also coordinates the changing cell shape with the control of cell proliferation. Src-transformed fibroblasts have increased expression of key components of the cell-cycle machinery, such as cyclin D, cyclin A, and cyclin-dependent kinase 2, as well as constitutively hyperphosphorylated retinoblastoma protein. All of these pathways and molecules interact to drive the cells through the G1 checkpoint into S-phase. We found that inhibiting Src pharmacologically reduced the growth of three early-stage RGP-melanoma cell lines, but had little effect upon either VGP or metastatic lines (FIG. 2C). The ability of SU6656 to block cancer-cell invasion was investigated using a novel collagen-implanted melanoma spheroid assay. Src inhibition blocked the invasion of RGP- and VGP-derived cell lines into the surrounding collagen, but not that of metastatic melanoma (FIG. 2D). Assessment of spheroid viability showed that SU6656 increased the proportion of dead cells in RGP and VGP melanoma lines, but had little effect upon the viability of metastatic melanoma lines. It therefore seems that constitutive Src activity is involved in the growth and invasion of RGP melanoma cells. During melanoma progression to the VGP and metastatic stages, Src activity becomes redundant as constitutive activity is acquired in other signaling pathways.

Some of the downstream effects of Src are mediated by members of another signaling family, the signal transducers and activator of transcription (STAT). Constitutive STAT3 activation is found in both human melanoma cell lines and tissue samples.[29] Our own studies showed that melanoma cells expressed phospho-STAT3 in the nucleus and at focal adhesions. Furthermore, treatment of these same cells with a Src inhibitor leads to the loss of phospho-STAT3 from both the nucleus and focal adhesions, demonstrating that STAT3 is downstream of Src (unpublished data). STAT3 contributes to cell cycle control through regulation of transcription of genes such as cyclin D, cyclin E, p21, and Myc.[30–31] It may also play some role in angiogenesis, via upregulation of VEGF expression.[29] Disruption of Src and STAT3 signaling in melanoma cells led to downregulation of the anti-apoptotic proteins Bcl-XL and Mcl-1.[29] This suggests that STAT3 activity in melanoma cells promotes growth at least in part through the increased expression of anti-apoptotic genes.[29] The ability of Src and STAT3 to regulate cell survival and apoptosis in melanoma makes these pathways attractive to target in combination with established anticancer drugs.

## NFκB: SIGNALING AT THE CROSSROADS

Nuclear factor kappa B (NFκB) is a heterodimeric transcription factor that is mostly composed of 65 and 50 kDa subunits of the Rel protein family. In quiescent

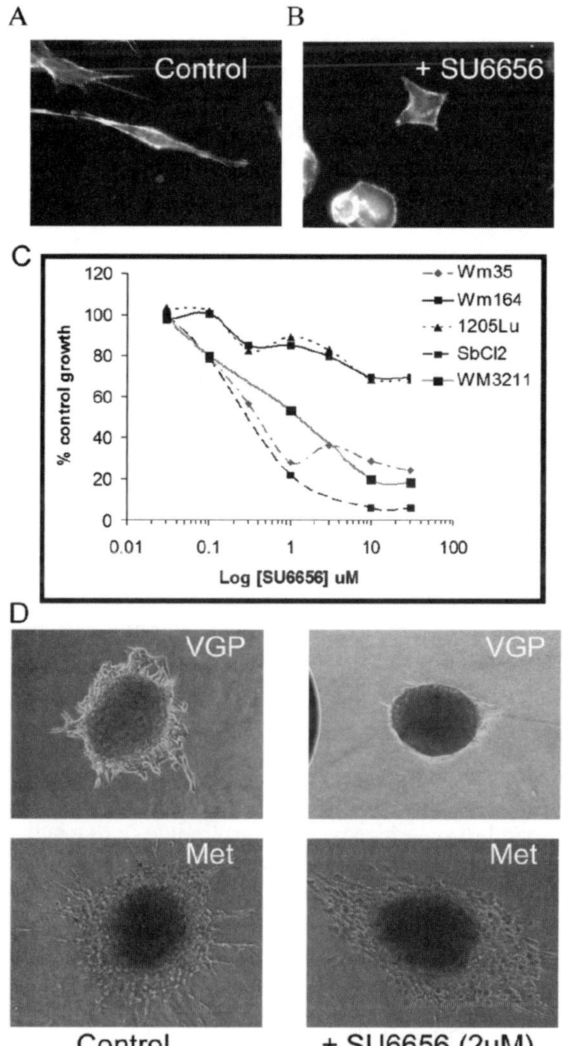


**FIGURE 2.** Effects of the Src inhibitor SU6656 upon melanoma behavior. Inhibition of Src activity in WM35 melanoma cells leads to altered cell morphology. (**A**) Control WM35 cells. (**B**) WM35 cells treated with 2 μM SU6656 for 48 h. Cells were fixed and permeabilized, and the actin cytoskeleton was stained using Texas-Red-Phalloidin, ×60. (**C**) Reduction of RGP-stage melanoma growth following treatment with pharmacological Src inhibition. RGP (WM35, SbCl2, and WM3211), VGP (WM164), and metastatic (1205Lu) melanoma cells were treated with increasing concentrations of SU6656 (0.1–30 μM) for 72 h, after which cell numbers were counted. Figure shows mean of three independent experiments. (**D**) Inhibition of Src blocks the collagen invasion of RGP and VGP, but not metastatic melanoma cells. Melanoma cells were grown as 3-D spheroids using the liquid overlay metho, after which they were imbedded in bovine collagen and left to invade for 72 h. Both the control VGP (WM 793) and metastatic (1205Lu) cells were found to invade into the collagen. Treatment with the Src inhibitor SU6656 (2 μM) only blocked the invasion of the RGP (WM35, not shown) and VGP melanoma cells. Panels are representative of three independent experiments.

cells, NFκB is located in the cytoplasm through the suppressive effects of a family of inhibitory proteins called IκB. Following stimulation by cytokines, such as TNF-α, IL-1, or LPS, the $NH_2$ terminus of IκB is phosphorylated leading to its ubiquination and degradation by the 26 S proteosome. Once released, the NFκB is free to enter the nucleus, where it activates gene transcription. NFκB is of great interest to cancer biologists because it occupies a pivotal position in the regulation of cell survival, controlling the expression of genes involved in the regulation of apoptotsis.[32] In addition to this, NFκB also regulates genes involved in angiogenesis, cell cycle control, adhesion, and migration.[32] Increased activity in the NFκB pathway arises through upregulation of the p50 and Rel A subunits[33, 34] or the downregulation of the inhibitor IκB.[35] NFκB can also be activated through either the PI3K/Akt or the MEK/ERK pathways. In melanoma, NFκB is constitutively active and linked to increased expression of cyclin D1, the anti-apoptotic factor TRAF2, Mel-CAM, and the pro-angiogenic cytokine GRO.[36] The role of increased NFκB activity in metastatic melanoma is demonstrated by studies showing that transfection of IκBα reduces subcutaneous tumor growth and metastatic spread of human melanoma in nude mice.[37]

Recent studies have demonstrated that in melanoma, loss of E-cadherin expression is linked to upregulation of NFκB activity,[38]which may implicate NFκB in the early stages of melanoma development. The cadherin switch, whereby E-cadherin expression is lost and N-cadherin expression upregulated, is one of the critical events whereby malignant melanocytes escape from local keratinocyte control.[39] The central role that NFκB occupies in many signaling pathways makes it a therapeutic ideal target. Currently, there are no selective small molecule inhibitors for the NFκB pathway. Instead attempts have been made to target it indirectly through inhibition of the 26 S proteosome, leading to increased levels of the IκB inhibitory subunit. One recent study has demonstrated that inhibiting NFκB activity, using the protesome inhibitor bortezomib, reduced melanoma cell growth *in vitro.*[40] More interestingly, bortezomib was found to synergize with temozolomide (a more soluble analogue of DTIC), leading to complete remission of melanoma xenografts in a murine model. Other studies have shown that NFκB activity is upregulated in melanoma cells following doxorubicin treatment, suggesting that it may be also involved in drug resistance.[41]

## A MORE PROMISING FUTURE: TOWARD RATIONAL THERAPY OF DISSEMINATED MELANOMA

The past 30 years have seen little improvement in melanoma therapy. Current survival for metastatic melanoma patients is 6–10 months, and there is much scope for improvement. The past few years have seen great leaps in our understanding of the mechanisms of drug resistance and cell survival in melanoma. As we have outlined, there are many pathways that are involved in suppressing apoptosis in melanoma. Many of these pathways are interlinked (FIG. 1). Careful experimentation is required to determine which of these pathways are the most important for regulating apoptosis in melanoma, and whether multiple pathways need to be inhibited for maximal effect. A more thorough understanding of these pathways, coupled with the development of newer, more selective, small molecule signal transduction inhibitors, offers a real chance to break the therapeutic deadlock. It is likely, as with the RAF inhibitor, BAY 43-9006, that signal transduction inhibitors will not work well as single agents. However, through the careful testing of these inhibitors with established cytotoxic treatments there is reason to believe that the tide is turning and that metastatic melanoma may one day become a manageable disease.

## ACKNOWLEDGMENTS

This work was supported by grants from the National Institutes of Health (CA 76674, CA 25874, CA 10815, CA 93372, CA 47159, CA 80999, CA 098101) and by funds from the Commonwealth Universal Research Enhancement Program, Pennsylvania Department of Health.

## REFERENCES

1. SERRONE, L., M. ZEULI, F.M. SEGA & F. COGNETTI. 2000. Dacarbazine-based chemotherapy for metastatic melanoma: thirty-year experience overview. J. Exp. Clin. Cancer Res. **19:** 21–34.
2. DAVIES, H., G.R. BIGNELL, C. COX, *et al.* 2002. Mutations of the BRAF gene in human cancer. Nature **417:** 949–954.
3. SMALLEY, K.S.M. 2003. A pivotal role for ERK in malignant melanoma? Int. J. Cancer **104:** 527–532.
4. WAN, P.T., M.J. GARNETT, S.M. ROE, *et al.* 2004. Mechanism of activation of the RAF-ERK signaling pathway by oncogenic mutations of B-RAF. Cell **116:** 855–867.
5. WELLBROCK, C., L. OGILVIE & D. HEDLEY. 2004. V599E B-RAF is an oncogene in melanocytes. Cancer Res. **64:** 2338–2342.
6. HINGORANI, S.R., M.A. JACOBETZ, G.P. ROBERTSON, *et al.* 2003. Suppression of BRAF(V599E) in human melanoma abrogates transformation. Cancer Res. **63:** 5198–5202.
7. POLLOCK, P.M., U.L. HARPER, K.S. HANSEN, *et al.* 2003. High frequency of BRAF mutations in nevi. Nat. Genet. **33:** 19–20.
8. DONG, J., R.G. PHELPS, R. QIAO, *et al.* 2003. BRAF oncogenic mutations correlate with progression rather than initiation of human melanoma. Cancer Res. **63:** 3883–3885.
9. LUO, J., B.D. MANNING & L.C. CANTLEY. 2003. Targeting the PI3K-Akt pathway in human cancer: rationale and promise. Cancer Cell **4:** 257–262.
10. SATYAMOORTHY, K., G. LI, B. VAIDYA, *et al.* 2001. Insulin-like growth factor-1 induces survival and growth of biologically early melanoma cells through both the mitogen-activated protein kinase and beta-catenin pathways. Cancer Res. **61:** 7318–7324.
11. SIMPSON, L. & R. PARSONS. 2001. PTEN: life as a tumor suppressor. Exp. Cell. Res. **264:** 29–41.
12. LI, J., C. YEN, D. LIAW, *et al.* 1997. PTEN, a putative protein tyrosine phosphatase gene mutated in human brain, breast, and prostate cancer. Science **275:** 1943–1947.
13. STECK, P.A., M.A. PERSHOUSE, S.A. JASSER, *et al.* 1997. Identification of a candidate tumour suppressor gene, MMAC1, at chromosome 10q23.3 that is mutated in multiple advanced cancers. Nat. Genet. **15:** 356–362.
14. TSAO, H., X. ZHANG, K. FOWLKES & F.G. HALUSKA. 2000. Relative reciprocity of NRAS and PTEN/MMAC1 alterations in cutaneous melanoma cell lines. Cancer Res. **60:** 1800–1804.
15. GULDBERG, P., P. THOR STRATEN, A. BIRCK, *et al.* 1997. Disruption of the MMAC1/PTEN gene by deletion or mutation is a frequent event in malignant melanoma. Cancer Res. **57:** 3660–3663.
16. TENG, D.H., R. HU, H. LIN, *et al.* 1997. MMAC1/PTEN mutations in primary tumor specimens and tumor cell lines. Cancer Res. **57:** 5221–5225.

17. Brazil, D.P., J. Park & D.A. Hemmings. 2002. PKB binding proteins. Getting in on the Akt. Cell **111:** 293–303.
18. Waldmann, V., J. Wacker & M. Deichmann. 2001. Mutations of the activation-associated phosphorylation sites at codons 308 and 473 of protein kinase B are absent in human melanoma. Arch. Dermatol. Res. **293:** 368–372.
19. Stahl, J.M., A. Sharma, M. Cheung, *et al.* 2004. Deregulated Akt3 activity promotes development of malignant melanoma. Cancer Res. **64:** 7002–7010.
20. Krasilnikov, M., V. Adler & S.Y. Fuchs. 1999. Contribution of phosphatidylinositol 3-kinase to radiation resistance in human melanoma cells. Mol. Carcinog. **24:** 64–69.
21. Burgering, B.M. & R.H. Medema. 2003. Decisions on life and death: FOXO Forkhead transcription factors are in command when PKB/Akt is off duty. J. Leukoc. Biol. **73:** 689–701.
22. Datta, S.R., A. Brunet & M.E. Greenberg. 1999. Cellular survival: a play in three Akts. Genes Dev. **13:** 2905–2927.
23. Diehl, J.A., M. Cheng, M.F. Roussel, *et al.* 1998. Glycogen synthase kinase-3beta regulates cyclin D1 proteolysis and subcellular localization. Genes Dev. **12:** 3499–3511.
24. Sears, R., F. Nuckolls, E. Haura, *et al.* 2000. Multiple Ras-dependent phosphorylation pathways regulate Myc protein stability. Genes Dev. **14:** 2501–2514.
25. Nagata, Y., K.H. Lan, X. Zhou, *et al.* 2004. PTEN activation contributes to tumor inhibition by trastuzumab, and loss of PTEN predicts trastuzumab resistance in patients. Cancer Cell **6:** 117–127.
26. Yang, L., H.C. Dan, M. Sun, *et al.* 2004. Akt/protein kinase B signaling inhibitor-2, a selective small molecule inhibitor of Akt signaling with antitumor activity in cancer cells overexpressing Akt. Cancer Res. **64:** 4394–4399.
27. Frame, M.C. 2004. Newest findings on the oldest oncogene; how activated src does it. J. Cell. Sci. **117:** 989–998.
28. Fujita, Y., G. Krause, M. Scheffner, *et al.* 2002. Hakai, a c-Cbl-like protein, ubiquitinates and induces endocytosis of the E-cadherin complex. Nat. Cell. Biol. **4:** 222–231.
29. Niu, G., T. Bowman, M. Huang, *et al.* 2002. Roles of activated Src and Stat3 signaling in melanoma tumor cell growth. Oncogene **21:** 7001–7010.
30. Odajima, J., I. Matsumura, J. Sonoyama, *et al.* 2000. Full oncogenic activities of v-Src are mediated by multiple signaling pathways. Ras as an essential mediator for cell survival. J. Biol. Chem. **275:** 24096–24105.
31. Sinibaldi, D., W. Wharton, J. Turkson, *et al.* 2000. Induction of p21WAF1/CIP1 and cyclin D1 expression by the Src oncoprotein in mouse fibroblasts: role of activated STAT3 signaling. Oncogene **19:** 5419–5427.
32. Karin, M. & A. Lin. 2002. NF-kappaB at the crossroads of life and death. Nat. Immunol. **3:** 221–227.
33. Meyskens, F.L., J.A. Buckmeier, S.E. McNulty, *et al.* 1999. Activation of nuclear factor-kappa B in human metastatic melanoma cells and the effect of oxidative stress. Clin. Cancer Res. **5:** 1197–1202.
34. McNulty, S.E., N.B. Tohidian & F.L. Meyskens. 2001. RelA, p50 and inhibitor of kappa B alpha are elevated in human metastatic melanoma cells and respond aberrantly to ultraviolet light B. Pigm. Cell Res. **14:** 456–465.
35. Yang, J. & A. Richmond. 2001. Constitutive IkappaB kinase activity correlates with nuclear factor-kappaB activation in human melanoma cells. Cancer Res. **61:** 4901–4909.
36. Baldwin, A.S. 2001. Control of oncogenesis and cancer therapy resistance by the transcription factor NF-kappaB. J. Clin. Invest. **107:** 241–246.
37. Huang, S., A. DeGuzman, C.D. Bucana, *et al.* 2000. Nuclear factor-kappaB activity correlates with growth, angiogenesis, and metastasis of human melanoma cells in nude mice. Clin. Cancer Res. **6:** 2573–2581.
38. Kuphal, S., I. Poser, C. Jobin, *et al.* 2004. Loss of E-cadherin leads to upregulation of NFkappaB activity in malignant melanoma. Oncogene **23:** 8509–8519.
39. Haass, N.K., K.S. Smalley & M. Herlyn. 2004. The role of altered cell-cell communication in melanoma progression. J. Mol. Histol. **35:** 309–318.

40. AMIRI, K.I., L.W. HORTON, B.J. LAFLEUR, *et al.* 2004. Augmenting chemosensitivity of malignant melanoma tumors via proteasome inhibition: implication for bortezomib (VELCADE, PS-341) as a therapeutic agent for malignant melanoma. Cancer Res. **64:** 4912–4918.
41. ROMANO, M.F., R. AVELLINO, A. PETRELLA, *et al.* 2004. Rapamycin inhibits doxorubicin-induced NF-kappaB/Rel nuclear activity and enhances the apoptosis of melanoma cells. Eur. J. Cancer **40:** 2829–2936.

# Studies into the Anticancer Effects of Selenomethionine against Human Colon Cancer

MARK A. NELSON, ANNE-CHRISTINE GOULET, ELIZABETH T. JACOBS, AND PETER LANCE

*Department of Pathology, Arizona Cancer Center, University of Arizona, Tucson, Arizona 85724, USA*

**ABSTRACT: Colorectal cancer is the third most frequent fatal malignant neoplasm in the United States and is expected to cause significant morbidity and mortality. The recent recall of cyclooxygenase-2 inhibitors from clinical trials highlights the need to develop other agents for cancer chemoprevention trials. Intervention strategies with selenium compounds represent a viable option to reduce colon cancer. Here we discuss epidemiologic studies and ongoing clinical trials with selenium. In addition, we discuss preclinical mechanistic studies that provide insights into the biochemical and molecular bases for the anticancer effects of selenomethionine.**

**KEYWORDS: colon cancer; selenomethionine; cancer chemoprevention; ERK; histone H3**

## COLON CANCER AND CANCER CHEMOPREVENTION

Adenocarcinomas of the colon and rectum (colorectal cancer, CRC) are epithelial tumors. According to the American Cancer Society, CRC is the third most common cancer in the United States, with an estimated 104,950 new cases of colon cancer, 40,340 new cases of rectal cancer, and 56,290 deaths from the disease in 2005. Almost all CRCs develop from benign neoplasms termed adenomas (adenomatous polyps) through the adenoma-carcinoma sequence in a process that is thought usually to take at least 10 years. Strategies to reduce CRC morbidity and mortality include improved detection of early-stage disease, better adjuvant therapy for advanced disease, and safe and affordable preventive therapy. Colonoscopic screening of asymptomatic individuals aged 50 years and older to diagnose adenomas and early CRC has become part of routine clinical practice. Adenomas are removed (by polypectomy) during the procedure in 10–20% of screening colonoscopies. Much research effort is currently directed toward development of safe and affordable long-term therapeutic agents that will prevent (chemoprevention) adenoma recurrence after

Address for correspondence: Mark A. Nelson, Ph.D., Department of Pathology, University of Arizona, 1501 N. Campbell Avenue, Tucson, AZ 85725. Voice: 520-626-1489; fax: 520-626-8864.

mnelson@azcc.arizona.edu

**Ann. N.Y. Acad. Sci. 1059: 26–32 (2005).** 
**doi: 10.1196/annals.1339.016**

polypectomy. Insights into the anticancer effects of selenium (Se) are based, in part, on epidemiological studies.

## EPIDEMIOLOGICAL STUDIES OF SELENIUM AND COLON CANCER

There is a limited amount of data regarding the associations between Se and colorectal adenomas or cancer, and these results have been mixed, inconclusive, and based predominantly on small studies. Several epidemiological investigations have shown an inverse association between Se and colorectal neoplasias,[1–6] cancer stage,[3] and survival,[5] while others have reported null results.[7,8] As mentioned above, the equivocal results in the studies of colorectal neoplasia may be due in part to the fact that the sample sizes tended to be relatively small,[4,6,7] resulting in a lack of precision of the association estimates.

The strongest support for a possible protective effect of Se intake came from a large, randomized controlled trial of Se in preventing non-melanoma skin cancer.[9] To date, this is the only clinical trial of Se on cancer risk that has been completed. The Se intervention did not reduce the rate of non-melanoma skin cancer, the primary end point of the trial. However, there was a statistically significant reduction of colorectal cancer as a secondary end point (relative risk [RR] = 0.58, 95% confidence interval [CI] = 0.18 to 0.95), which was slightly attenuated after longer follow-up (RR = 0.45, 95% CI = 0.19 to 1.08).[10] A marginally statistically significant overall reduction in colorectal adenomas, which became stronger in association with the lowest tertile of baseline Se, was also observed as a secondary end point in the trial.[11]

A more recent study provides insights into the relationship between Se and colorectal neoplasia. Jacobs *et al.* report their pooled analysis of three randomized clinical trials of dietary or nutrient interventions in preventing colorectal adenomas.[12] Individual-level data from each of the Wheat Bran Fiber (WBF) Trial,[13] the Polyp Prevention Trial (PPT),[14] and the Polyp Prevention Study (PPS)[15] were statistically reanalyzed to provide a more precise estimate of the association between blood Se concentration and adenoma risk than would be possible from any of the three studies alone. None of the trials tested Se as an intervention. Blood was collected at enrollment for PPT and PPS and one year after randomization for WBF and analyzed for Se levels. This pooled analysis, the largest epidemiologic investigation of the role of Se in preventing colorectal neoplasia, indicates that individuals in the highest quartile of blood Se concentration (median 150 ng/mL) had 34% lower odds (OR = 0.66, 95% CI = 0.50 to 0.87, $P_{trend}$ = .006) of developing a new adenoma throughout the follow-up, compared with those in the lowest quartile of plasma Se (median 113 ng/mL). This study reinforces the earlier secondary clinical data regarding Se in the colon-rectum[9,10] and should intensify interest in ongoing or planned prospective translational trials of Se, either alone or combined with other promising agents, in preventing colorectal adenomas.

Currently, the only clinical trial specifically designed to test whether Se can decrease the risk of colorectal adenoma recurrence is the Selenium Clinical Trial being conducted by Drs. Peter Lance and David Alberts at the Arizona Cancer Center. This trial originally had a 2 × 2 factorial design to test the effect of cyclooxygenase-2 (COX-2) inhibitor Celebrex and Se on adenoma recurrence. As a result of an excess

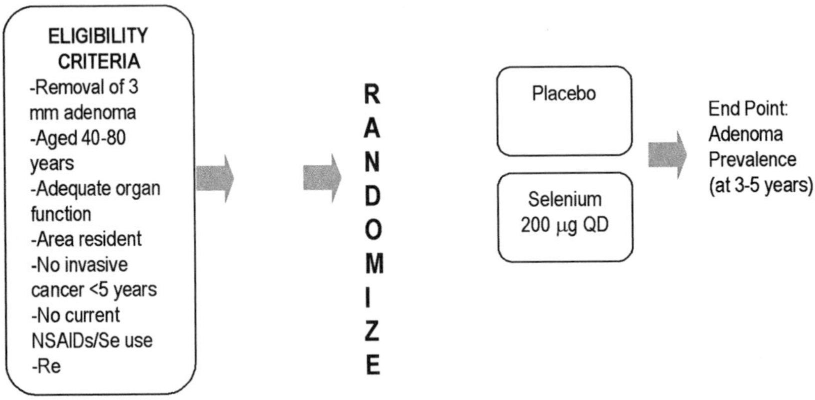


**FIGURE 1.** Protocol for the clinical evaluation of selenium as a cancer chemopreventive agent against human colon adenoma recurrence.

of cardiovascular adverse events associated with COX-2 inhibitors (rofecoxib and celecoxib) in other adenoma recurrence trials, the celecoxib component of the trial was closed in December 2004. The design of the study was such that the integrity of the Se component was maintained (FIG. 1). Randomization for the trial is expected to be complete in 2006. The primary objectives of the trial are to investigate the effect of Se supplementation on the rate of adenoma recurrence and to evaluate the safety of Se supplementation for chemoprevention.

## ANALYSIS OF SELENIUM COMPOUNDS IN SELENIUM-CONTAINING YEAST

The anticancer effects of high Se-containing yeast may be due in large part to L-selenomethionine (SeMet). SeMet represents an organic form of Se and is more bioavailable than an inorganic form such as $Na_2SeO_3$.[16] Substitution of methionine by SeMet represents a mechanism for nonspecific incorporation of Se into proteins *in vivo*. SeMet is metabolized primarily in the liver to a monomethylated intermediate for the expression of its anticancer activity, and epithelial tissues typically retain a low capacity to generate a monomethylated Se-metabolite form SeMet.

In the Selenium Clinical Trial described above, the Se supplement is formulated as high Se-containing yeast. Selenized yeast was chosen for the intervention because it was the agent used in the clinical trial by Clark *et al.*[9] where a reduction in colorectal cancer incidence was observed. Analytical speciation studies showed that the bulk of the Se in selenized-yeast is in the form of SeMet (85%);[16] however, other organic Se compounds can also be present in Se-yeast.[17,18] In regard to prostate cancer and the SELECT trial (selenium and vitamin E), SeMet is the form of Se being evaluated. Therefore, it is important to understand the biochemical and molecular bases for the anticancer effects of SeMet.

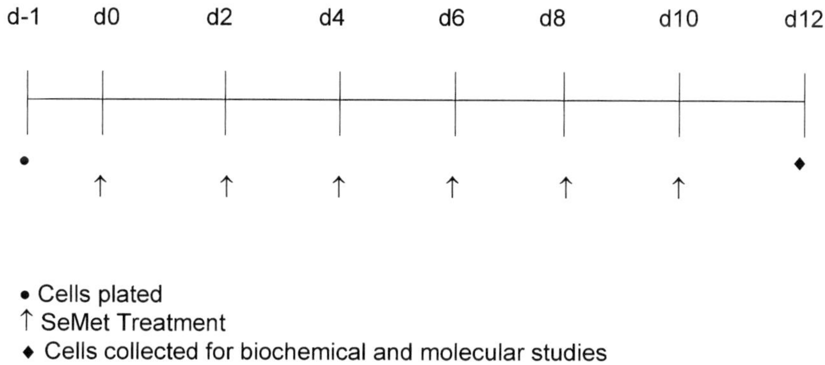


**FIGURE 2.** Experimental design for studying the anticancer effects of selenomethionine. Protocol for treating tumor cells with selenomethionine in cell culture.

## SELENIUM METABOLISM IN MAMMALIAN CELLS

Selenium exists both in organic and inorganic forms in natural diet and has been implicated as an essential micronutrient for human health. Organic Se is present mainly in the form of selenomethionine, selenocysteine, and Se-methylselenocysteine, whereas inorganic Se occurs either as selenite or selenate. Among organic forms, selenomethionine is the predominant form of Se in most Se rich diets.[19] Both chemical forms of Se have been under intense study as a promising chemopreventive agent for different Se of cancer. The varying degree of anticarcinogenic activity of different chemical forms of Se may be related to their metabolism *in vivo*.

It has been postulated that the conversion of SeMet to methylselenol ($CH_3SeH$) is important for its anticancer effects.[16–18] In animals, the liver and kidney are the major organs for Se metabolism; the conversion of SeMet to the monomethylated intermediate requires at least five steps. Epithelial cells located in the colon and prostate appear to have a low capacity to metabolize to produce monomethylated Se metabolite from SeMet.[16–18] There is a plethora of studies that utilize inorganic Se to address the anticancer effects of organic Se or use SeMet at concentrations 20–100 times above the physiological levels. However, high concentrations of SeMet in *in vitro* studies may not be relevant to the anticancer effects of SeMet at physiological relevant concentrations in humans. This prompted us to develop a multitreatment protocol to treat tumor cells in culture to investigate the anticancer effects of SeMet (FIG. 2).

## MOLECULAR STUDIES ON THE ANTICANCER EFFECTS OF SELENOMETHIONINE

Recent studies by our group provide evidence that SeMet can induce cell-growth arrest and that the growth inhibition is associated with S–$G_2$/M cell-cycle arrest.[20] Coincidental with the cell-cycle arrest, we observed an increase in cyclin B expression as well as phosphorylation of the cyclin-dependent kinase Cdc2. Since sustained activation of the mitogen-activated protein kinase (MAPK) cascade has been associated with cell-cycle arrest and growth inhibition, we evaluated whether MAP kinases could be activated by SeMet. We did not see activation of JNK or p38 in these studies. However, we found that SeMet induced phosphorylation of extracellular signal-regulated kinase (ERK) in a dose-dependent manner at physiologically relevant concentrations (i.e., 5–22 μM SeMet). We also demonstrated phosphorylation of the ribosomal S6 kinase (p90RSK) by SeMet. In addition, we observed phosphorylation of histone H3 on serine 10 in a concentration-dependent manner. Furthermore, the phosphorylation of p90RSK and histone H3 were both antagonized by the MEK inhibitor U0126, implying that SeMet-induced phosphorylation of p90RSK and histone H3 are at least in part ERK pathway dependent.[20] Based on these results, we propose that SeMet-induced growth arrest and phosphorylation of histone H3 are mediated by persistent ERK and p90RSK activation (FIG. 3). These new data provide valuable insights into the biological effects of SeMet at clinically relevant concentrations. Undoubtedly, other important relevant mechanisms, such as gene promoter methylation alterations in polyunsaturated fatty acid metabolism and modulation of DNA repair responses, could also play a role in the anticancer effects of SeMet. Future studies should also be directed at determining whether relevant mechanisms of growth inhibition occur *in vivo*.

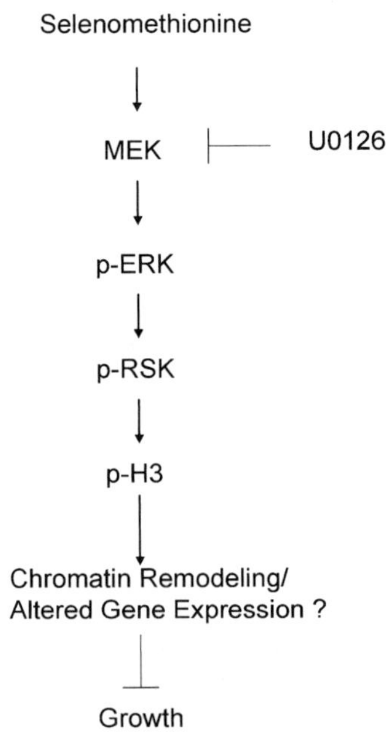


**FIGURE 3.** Hypothesis of mechanisms of persistent ERK-phosphorylation-mediated growth inhibition induced by selenomethionine.

## CONCLUSION

There may not be a more extensive body of evidence for a cancer prevention potential of a dietary component nutrient than there is for Se. The recall of COX-2 inhibitors from clinical trials has highlighted the need to identify effective, nontoxic chemopreventive agents. Even though there are gaps in our present understanding, in regard to the exact molecular and biochemical bases for the anticancer effects of various forms of Se, it is clear from epidemiological evidence, preclinical studies, and recent intervention trials that it is plausible to consider Se compounds as a potential cancer chemoprevention agent against colon cancer. Ongoing clinical trials and preclinical studies with Se alone and in combination with other compounds may lead to new effective strategies to combat human colon cancer.

## ACKNOWLEDGMENTS

This work is in memory of the late Dr. Larry Clark. We also thank Marianne Chigbrow, Claire Redman, Ph.D., and Peter Frisk, Ph.D., for their contributions. The work was supported by the American Institute for Cancer Research and the National Institutes of Health (Grant CA702008).

### REFERENCES

1. Willett, W.C. *et al.* 1983. Prediagnostic serum selenium and risk of cancer. Lancet **2:** 130–134.
2. Clark, L.C. *et al.* 1993. Plasma selenium concentration predicts the prevalence of colorectal adenomatous polyps. Cancer Epidemiol. Biomarkers Prev. **2:** 41–46.
3. Dworkin, B.M. *et al.* 1988. Selenium status and the polyp-cancer sequence: a colonoscopically controlled study. Am. J. Gastroenterol. **83:** 748–751.
4. Russo, M.W. *et al.* 1997. Plasma selenium levels and the risk of colorectal adenomas. Nutr. Cancer **28:** 125–129.
5. Psathakis, D. *et al.* 1998. Blood selenium and glutathione peroxidase status in patients with colorectal cancer. Dis. Colon Rectum **41:** 328–335.
6. Fernandez-Banares, F. *et al.* 2002. Serum selenium and risk of large size colorectal adenomas in a geographical area with a low selenium status. Am. J. Gastroenterol. **97:** 2103–2108.
7. Early, D.S. *et al.* 2002. Selenoprotein levels in patients with colorectal adenomas and cancer. Am. J. Gastroenterol. **97:** 745–748.
8. Nelson, R.L. *et al.* 1995. Serum selenium and colonic neoplastic risk. Dis. Colon Rectum **38:** 1306–1310.
9. Clark, L.C. *et al.* 1996. Effects of selenium supplementation for cancer prevention in patients with carcinoma of the skin. A randomized controlled trial. Nutritional Prevention of Cancer Study Group. JAMA **276:** 1957–1963.
10. Duffield-Lillico, A.J. *et al.* 2002. Baseline characteristics and the effect of selenium supplementation on cancer incidence in a randomized clinical trial: a summary report of the Nutritional Prevention of Cancer Trial. Cancer Epidemiol. Biomarkers Prev. **11:** 630–639.
11. Reid, M.E. *et al.* 2003. Selenium supplementation and colorectal adenomas: an extended analysis of the Nutritional Prevention of Cancer Trial. Second Annual AACR International Conference, Frontiers in Cancer Prevention. Phoenix, Arizona. p98.
12. Jacobs, E.T. *et al.* 2004. Selenium and colorectal adenoma: results of a pooled analysis. J. Natl. Cancer Inst. **96:** 1669–1675.

13. ALBERTS, D.S. *et al.* 2000. Lack of effect of a high-fiber cereal supplement on the recurrence of colorectal adenomas. Phoenix Colon Cancer Prevention Physicians' Network. N. Engl. J. Med. **342:** 1156–1162.
14. SCHATZKIN, A. *et al.* 1996. The polyp prevention trial I: rationale, design, recruitment, and baseline participant characteristics. Cancer Epidemiol. Biomarkers Prev. **5:** 375–383.
15. GREENBERG, E.R. *et al.* 1994. A clinical trial of antioxidant vitamins to prevent colorectal adenoma. Polyp Prevention Study Group. N. Engl. J. Med. **331:** 141–147.
16. IP, C. *et al.* 2000. Chemical speciation influences comparative activity of selenium-enriched garlic and yeast in mammary cancer prevention. J. Agric. Food Chem. **48:** 4452.
17. IP, C., D.J. LISK & H.E. GANTHER. 1998. Activities of structurally-related lipophilic selenium compounds as cancer chemopreventive agents. Anticancer Res. **18:** 4019–4025.
18. IP, C. 1998. Lessons from basic research in selenium and cancer prevention. J. Nutr. **128:** 1845–1854.
19. YANG, X. *et al.* 1997. Determination of the selenomethionine content in grain and human blood[from the Chinese]. Wei Sheng Yan Jiu **26:** 113–116.
20. GOULET, A.C. *et al.* 2005. Selenomethionine induces sustained ERK phosphorylation leading to cell-cycle arrest in human colon cancer cells. Carcinogenesis **26:** 109–117.

# Mechanisms of Prostate Tumorigenesis: Roles for Transcription Factors Nkx3.1 and Egr1

SARKI A. ABDULKADIR

*Department of Pathology, The University of Alabama at Birmingham, Birmingham, Alabama 35294, USA*

**ABSTRACT: Recent developments in the generation and analysis of transgenic mouse models have improved our understanding of the early stages of prostate tumorigenesis. Analysis of models based on the homeodomain protein Nkx3.1 and the zinc finger protein Egr1 suggests that these transcription factors play distinct roles in the initiation and progression of precursor prostatic intraepithelial neoplasia (PIN) lesions, respectively. *Nkx3.1* is a candidate prostate tumor suppressor gene (TSG) that demonstrates haploinsufficiency. Disruption of one or both copies of the murine *Nkx3.1* gene leads to the development of epithelial hyperplasia and PIN. This appears to be a consequence of delayed exit from the cell cycle by differentiating prostate luminal epithelial cells in *Nkx3.1* mutant mice. Gene expression profiling has provided additional insight into the basis of haploinsufficiency in Nkx3.1 mutant mice. A reduction in *Nkx3.1* dosage leads to dramatic alterations in the expression of a subset of genes by altering the probability of a target gene existing in the "on" or "off" state. The immediate early gene Egr1, on the other hand, is overexpressed in human and mouse prostate tumors and PIN lesions and regulates the expression of several genes implicated in prostate tumor progression, including platelet-derived growth factor and insulin-like growth factor II. Prostate cancer-prone mice lacking *Egr1* exhibit a significant delay in tumor progression. Specifically, *Egr1* deficiency impairs the transition from PIN to invasive carcinoma. Thus, Nkx3.1 and Egr1 regulate gene programs involved in distinct aspects of prostate tumorigenesis.**

**KEYWORDS: prostate cancer; transgenic mice; tumor suppressor; haploinsufficiency; Nkx3.1; Egr1; PIN; invasion; stochastic gene regulation**

## INTRODUCTION

Prostate cancer is a leading cause of cancer-related morbidity and mortality worldwide. Recent studies have elucidated some of the common genetic and epigenetic alterations with the development of prostate cancer. Accumulation of alterations in tumor-related genes is thought to result in the transformation of benign

Present address for correspondence: Sarki A. Abdulkadir, Vanderbilt University Medical Center, Tumor Biology Research Laboratories, Rm. 4918A The Vanderbilt Clinic, 23rd Avenue S. at Pierce Street, Nashville, TN 37232. Voice: 615-322-9668; fax: 615-343-9563. Sarki.abdulkadir@vanderbilt.edu

**Ann. N.Y. Acad. Sci. 1059: 33–40 (2005). © 2005 New York Academy of Sciences. doi: 10.1196/annals.1339.018**

prostatic epithelium to precursor lesions, such as prostatic intraepithelial neoplasia (PIN), with progression to invasive carcinoma and ultimately to metastatic disease. Although most prostate cancers are initially responsive to androgen ablation, tumors commonly recur as androgen-independent prostate cancer after treatment. A lot of effort is being expended on elucidating the determinants of metastatic and androgen-independent prostate cancer with a goal to enhancing therapeutic options. In addition, understanding the molecular pathways that lead to the initiation, maintenance, and progression of precursor lesions such as PIN is likely to have a significant impact on strategies aimed at prevention of prostate cancer. A reduction in the PIN burden will be expected to have tangible benefits in reducing cancer risk. Recent advances in molecular genetics as well as mouse modeling have shed new light on the processes involved in the initiation and progression of PIN lesions. Here, the roles of two prostate tumor-related genes (Nkx3.1 and Egr1) involved in the development and progression of PIN lesions are discussed.

## NKx3.1 AND PROSTATE TUMOR INITIATION

One of the most frequent chromosomal aberrations observed in prostate cancer involves loss of chromosomal region 8p12-22.[1,2] In some studies, up to 85% of prostate tumors are shown to have sustained chromosomal deletions at this locus.[3] Mutations in this area may constitute an initiating event in the development of prostate cancer because loss-of-heterozygosity a this region also occurs in 63% of preinvasive PIN foci.[4] One candidate for a prostate tumor suppressor located in this region is the homeobox protein NKX3.1.[5] *NKX3.1* encodes a homeodomain transcription factor whose expression is androgen-dependent and is largely restricted to the luminal epithelial cells of the prostates.[6] During embryogenesis, Nkx3.1 is one of the earliest markers of the developing prostatic epithelium. Functional studies indicate that Nkx3.1 is a differentiating factor for the prostate gland, and its deletion in mice results in defects in prostate branching morphogenesis, epithelial cell differentiation and growth.[7–9] Although no mutations have been found in the *NKX3.1* gene in human prostate tumors to date, loss of expression of the NKX3.1 protein has been observed in ~40% of human prostate tumors and 20% of PIN lesions.[10]

Mice lacking *Nkx3.1* develop prostatic epithelial hyperplasia that progresses to PIN over time.[7,9] Furthermore, mice with conditional deletion of *Nkx3.1* in the mature prostate also develop hyperplasia and PIN.[9] The latter finding is consistent with the loss of NKX3.1 expression observed in human PIN lesions because the PIN lesions in the conditional knockout mice arise independent of the prostate developmental defects observed in regular *Nkx3.1* knockout animals. PIN lesions in *Nkx3.1* mutant mice do not rapidly progress to invasive carcinoma, implying that while loss of *Nkx3.1* is involved in the development of precursor lesions, additional genetic alterations are required to facilitate tumor progression. Analyses of compound mutant mice support this conclusion. Mice with mutations in both *Nkx3.1* and *Pten* or $p27^{kip1}$ tumor suppressor genes develop more advanced lesions compared to mice with mutations in a single tumor suppressor gene.[11,12] Additional evidence for the role of *Nkx3.1* in prostate tumor initiation comes from gene expression analyses performed on the prostates of genetically engineered mice with a propensity for the development of prostate cancer. Loss of Nkx3.1 expression was observed in a Myc-driven model of the prostate,[13] in TRAMP mice that overexpress the SV40 T antigen in the prostate (S. Abdulkadir, unpublished observations), as well as in mice with prostate-specific deletion of the *Pten* tumor suppressor gene.[14] Interestingly, in Myc transgenic mice, loss of Nkx3.1 was gradual and correlated with tumor stage, suggesting that there is selective pressure for the loss of Nkx3.1 during tumor progression.[13] On the other hand, conditional deletion of *Pten* resulted in sudden loss of Nkx3.1, perhaps implying direct regulation of Nkx3.1 by the Pten pathway.[14]

There are several outstanding questions regarding the mechanism by which loss of Nkx3.1 contributes to prostate tumor initiation. These include, How does Nkx3.1 engage the cell cycle machinery to regulate prostate epithelial cell growth? What is the relationship between Nkx3.1, an androgen-induced transcription factor, and androgen-regulated gene programs in normal and malignant prostate cells? And finally, what is the molecular mechanism for haploinsufficient tumor suppression by Nkx3.1? Recently, Magee *et al.* have used a combination of a castration/testosterone replacement regimen and oligonucleotide microarray analyses in *Nkx3.1* mutant mice to begin to investigate some of these issues.[15] Following castration, the rodent prostate undergoes involution by a program of apoptosis. After testosterone replacement, an androgen-responsive population of transiently proliferating cells repopulates the luminal compartment. The luminal cells will eventually terminally differentiate and exit the cell cycle. In this castration/testosterone replacement scheme, *Nkx3.1*$^{-/-}$ and *Nkx3.1*$^{+/-}$ luminal epithelial cells exhibited a significant delay in exiting from the cell cycle.[15] These results suggest that an extended proliferative phase during the course of normal epithelial cell turnover underlies the epithelial hyperplasia seen in *Nkx3.1*$^{-/-}$ and *Nkx3.1*$^{+/-}$ mutant mice.

Gene expression profiling also identified several genes that are coregulated by Nkx3.1 and androgen in the mouse prostate.[15] Several androgen-regulated genes, such as probasin, beta-microseminoprotein (PSP94), and renin1 are not induced by testosterone treatment in *Nkx3.1*-deficient prostates, consistent with the fact that Nkx3.1 itself is rapidly induced by testosterone. An unexpected finding, however, was the identification of a group of genes that is induced by testosterone selectively in *Nkx3.1*-null prostates. These genes, which are unmasked as androgen target genes by *Nkx3.1* deficiency include angiopoietin 2, elafin-like II, and Fam3c. This observation illustrates how mutant cells (with loss of a tumor suppressor gene [TSG] or gain of an oncogene) may express a distinct androgen-regulated gene program compared to wild-type cells. If this translates to different functional outcomes, it will have important implications for interpretation of studies that catalog androgen target genes in prostate cells.

## NKx3.1 AS A PARADIGM FOR STOCHASTIC, DOSAGE-SENSITIVE GENE REGULATION IN TUMOR INITIATION

Heterozygous *Nkx3.1* mutant mice develop hyperplastic lesions that retain expression from the remaining wild-type allele.[9,15] The phenomenon of haploinsufficiency is being increasingly recognized as a common occurrence in somatic tumorigenesis. Haploinsufficiency of TSGs has been invoked as a possible mechanism to explain the observed high incidence of cancer in the human population. Since loss of one allele of a haploinsufficient TSG could lead to the clonal expansion

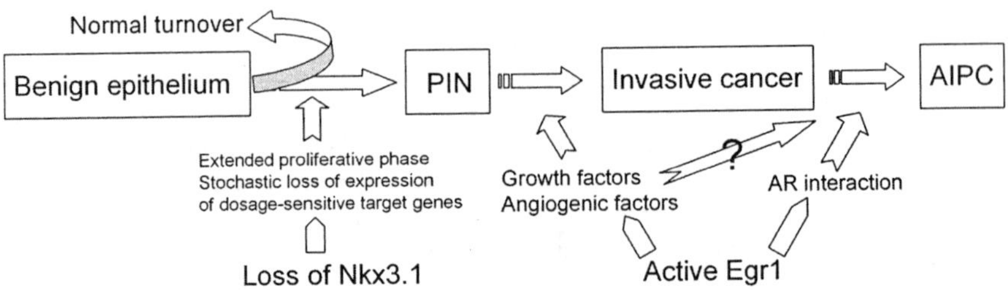


**FIGURE 1.** Model depicting the roles of Nkx3.1 and Egr1 in prostate tumorigenesis. Reduction in Nkx3.1 dosage leads to stochastic loss of target gene expression and an extended proliferative phase during normal epithelial turnover leading to hyperplasia and PIN. Increased Egr1 activity due to overexpression of Egr1 and/or loss of the Egr1 corepressor Nab2 promotes the PIN-to-carcinoma transition via activation of growth and angiogenic factors. Functional interaction between Egr1 and the androgen receptor (AR) promotes androgen independent prostate cancer (AIPC). Egr1-induced growth/angiogenic factors may contribute to the development of AIPC as well.

of the mutant cells, this could lead to an increase in the size of the target cell population susceptible to a second genetic hit.[16] At the gene expression level, a reduction in Nkx3.1 dosage results in a spectrum of responses among Nkx3.1-activated genes.[15] Some genes, such as intelectin, were exquisitely sensitive to a reduction in Nkx3.1 dosage, while others such as probasin were only slightly affected. Interestingly, dosage-sensitive gene regulation was not observed for any of the Nkx3.1-repressed genes examined, indicating perhaps distinct regulatory mechanisms for activation versus repression by Nkx3.1. The expression of dosage-sensitive Nkx3.1 target genes followed a stochastic, on/off pattern in which reduction in Nkx3.1 dosage reduced the proportion of cells expressing the target gene. These results are consistent with a model of haploinsufficient tumor suppression in which reduction in Nkx3.1 dosage increases the probability of complete loss of expression of select target genes in luminal epithelial cells (FIG. 1). This will result in a null phenotype for the particular target gene in the affected cell. This model may be a widely utilized mechanism for haploinsufficiency by transcription factors.

## EGR1 AND THE PIN-TO-CARCINOMA TRANSITION

The transition from PIN to invasive carcinoma is a key step in the progression sequence to prostate cancer. This complex process involves the disruption of the basement membrane and extracellular matrix by proteolytic enzymes, changes in cellular motility and adhesion properties, as well as the initiation of angiogenesis.[17] A better understanding of this transition will facilitate the development of efficient strategies for the prevention of prostate cancer. Recent studies using transgenic mice indicate that the transcription factor Egr1 is involved in regulating the PIN-to-carcinoma transition.

*Egr1* (early growth response gene 1; also known as *NGFI-A*, *Zif268*, *Krox24*, and *Tis8*) encodes a zinc finger transcription factor that is rapidly induced by a variety of stimuli, including growth factors, hypoxia, and free radicals without the need for prior protein synthesis.[18–21] *Egr1*, together with the related proteins *Egr2, Egr3,* and *Egr4* form a conserved gene family whose products regulate target gene transcription by binding to a GC-rich DNA motif that is also shared by the Wilm's tumor suppressor gene product, WT1. As a result of this shared DNA binding site, Egr1 and WT1 can antagonize each other's function by competing for binding to the same site.[22] For example, in baby rat kidney cells, Egr1 overexpression enhances growth and WT1 expression antagonizes this effect.[23]

Several groups have reported EGR1 overexpression in prostate cancer. In the study by Eid *et al.*, EGR1 mRNA was quantified in 96 prostate specimens representing different Gleason scores, as well as in 10 benign tissues.[24] EGR1 was found to be expressed at significantly higher levels in the cancers than in normal prostates ($P < 0.001$). Furthermore, EGR1 expression correlated with the Gleason score ($P < 0.005$). In addition, immunohistochemical analysis confirmed EGR1 protein overexpression in the prostate carcinoma specimens.[24] These findings are substantiated by studies from several other groups, including our own.[25–28] The mechanisms underlying EGR1 overexpression in prostate cancers remain unexplored, although several stimuli that may be present in tumors *in vivo*, such as hypoxia or growth factors, are potent inducers of EGR1. Among Egr1-binding proteins, two molecules, Nab1 and Nab2, [29,30] bind to and repress the transcriptional activation function of Egr1. Nab2, which itself is an Egr1 target gene, may be part of a negative feedback loop that physiologically serves to restrain Egr1 function.[29,30] Interestingly, NAB2 expression is downregulated in human and mouse prostate tumors and PIN lesions.[26] Thus, upregulation of EGR1 and downregulation of NAB2 may lead to an increased EGR1 activity in prostate cancer.

To explore the roles played by Egr1 overexpression in prostate tumorigenesis *in vivo*, we crossed two different prostate cancer-prone mice that express the SV40T antigen in the prostatic epithelium (TRAMP[31] and CR2-TAg mice[32]) with mice that lack *Egr1*. The results indicate that *Egr1* deficiency results in a significant delay in tumor incidence and mortality.[27] Lack of Egr1 specifically delayed progression from PIN to invasive carcinoma without a discernible effect on tumor initiation (i.e., incidence of PIN). $Egr1^{-/-}$ mice demonstrated defects in angiogenesis as well as in the expression of Egr1 target genes such as Pdgf-$\alpha$ and TGF$\beta$1. Subsequently, several studies were published showing that Egr1 is able to transform prostate epithelial cells and that inhibition of Egr1 expression could reverse the transformation of prostate carcinoma cells.[33,34]

In contrast to its pro-tumorigenic role in prostate cancer, Egr1 expression is reduced in other tumor types, such as glioblastomas and astrocytomas, and when overexpressed in cell lines it can lead to growth suppression.[35,36] These observations have led to the notion that Egr1 functions as a negative regulator of growth in some tissues. In fibrosarcoma cell lines, growth suppression by Egr1 has been attributed to induction of TGF$\beta$1.[35] Nevertheless, no inactivating mutations have been found to date in the *Egr1* gene in any human or animal tumors, nor have there been any studies to our knowledge showing the mechanism (such as promoter methylation) by which Egr1 expression may be silenced in tumors. The accumulated evidence therefore indicates a specific role for Egr1 in promoting prostate tumor progression, which does not appear to extend to other tumor types, such as gliomas or fibrosarcomas, thus underlining the importance of a cellular context in determining the functional outcome of Egr1 expression. A possible explanation for this dichotomy may relate to the recent finding that Egr1 functionally interacts with the androgen receptor (AR) and appears to promote AR nuclear translocation[37] (FIG. 1). Another finding that highlights the importance of the cellular context for Egr1 function is the recent report that acetylation of Egr1 by p300/CBP influences the divergent outcomes mediated by Egr1 (proliferation versus apoptosis) on the responses of cells to various stimuli.[38]

## CONCLUSION

Prostatic intraepithelial neoplasia is widely regarded as a precursor for human prostate cancer. The homeodomain transcription factor Nkx3.1 is an important regulator of prostate growth and differentiation, the loss of which leads to the development of PIN lesions. A reduction in Nkx3.1 dosage can lead to the selective inactivation of a dosage-sensitive gene program that could be the basis for haploinsufficiency. Progression from PIN to invasive carcinoma, on the other hand, is facilitated by the zinc finger transcription factor Egr1. A better understanding of the molecular mechanisms through which PIN lesions arise and through which they progress to invasive carcinoma will have enormous implications for developing new strategies for the prevention of prostate cancer.

## ACKNOWLEDGMENTS

This work was supported by Grants CA94858 and CA10491 from the National Cancer Institute.

### REFERENCES

1. BOVA, G.S. *et al.* 1993. Homozygous deletion and frequent allelic loss of chromosome 8p22 loci in human prostate cancer. Cancer Res. **53:** 3869–3873.
2. MACOSKA, J.A. *et al.* 1995. Evidence for three tumor suppressor gene loci on chromosome 8p in human prostate cancer. Cancer Res. **55:** 5390–5395.
3. VOCKE, C.D. *et al.* 1996. Analysis of 99 microdissected prostate carcinomas reveals a high frequency of allelic loss on chromosome 8p12-21. Cancer Res. **56:** 2411–2416.
4. EMMERT-BUCK, M.R. *et al.* 1995. Allelic loss on chromosome 8p12-21 in microdissected prostatic intraepithelial neoplasia. Cancer Res. **55:** 2959–2962.
5. HE, W.W. *et al.* 1997. A novel human prostate-specific, androgen-regulated homeobox gene (NKX3.1) that maps to 8p21, a region frequently deleted in prostate cancer. Genomics **43:** 69–77.
6. BIEBERICH, C.J. *et al.* 1996. Prostate-specific and androgen-dependent expression of a novel homeobox gene. J. Biol. Chem. **271:** 31779–31782.
7. BHATIA-GAUR, R. *et al.* 1999. Roles for Nkx3.1 in prostate development and cancer. Genes Dev. **13:** 966–977.
8. TANAKA, M. *et al.* 2000. Nkx3.1, a murine homolog of drosophila bagpipe, regulates epithelial ductal branching and proliferation of the prostate and palatine glands. Dev. Dyn. **219:** 248–260.
9. ABDULKADIR, S.A. *et al.* 2002. Conditional loss of nkx3.1 in adult mice induces prostatic intraepithelial neoplasia. Mol. Cell. Biol. **22:** 1495–1503.

10. BOWEN, C. *et al.* 2000. Loss of NKX3.1 expression in human prostate cancers correlates with tumor progression. Cancer Res. **60:** 6111–6115.
11. KIM, M.J. *et al.* 2002. Cooperativity of Nkx3.1 and Pten loss of function in a mouse model of prostate carcinogenesis. Proc. Natl. Acad. Sci. USA **99:** 2884–2889.
12. GARY, B. *et al.* 2004. Interaction of Nkx3.1 and p27kip1 in prostate tumor initiation. Am. J. Pathol. **164:** 1607–1614.
13. ELLWOOD-YEN, K. *et al.* 2003. Myc-driven murine prostate cancer shares molecular features with human prostate tumors. Cancer Cell **4:** 223–238.
14. WANG, S. *et al.* 2003. Prostate-specific deletion of the murine Pten tumor suppressor gene leads to metastatic prostate cancer. Cancer Cell **4:** 209–221.
15. MAGEE, J.A., S.A. ABDULKADIR & J. MILBRANDT. 2003. Haploinsufficiency at the Nkx3.1 locus. A paradigm for stochastic, dosage-sensitive gene regulation during tumor initiation. Cancer Cell **3:** 273–283.
16. QUON, K.C. & A. BERNS. 2001. Haplo-insufficiency? Let me count the ways. Genes Dev. **15:** 2917–2921.
17. NAGLE, R.B. *et al.* 1992. New relationships between prostatic intraepithelial neoplasia and prostatic carcinoma. J. Cell. Biochem. Suppl. **16H:** 26–29.
18. SUKHATME, V.P. *et al.* 1988. A zinc finger-encoding gene coregulated with c-fos during growth and differentiation, and after cellular depolarization. Cell **53:** 37–43.
19. MILBRANDT, J. 1987. A nerve growth factor-induced gene encodes a possible transcriptional regulatory factor. Science **238:** 797–799.
20. CHRISTY, B.A., L.F. LAU & D. NATHANS. 1988. A gene activated in mouse 3T3 cells by serum growth factors encodes a protein with "zinc finger" sequences. Proc. Natl. Acad. Sci. USA **85:** 7857–7861.
21. CHAVRIER, P. *et al.* 1988. Characterization of a mouse multigene family that encodes zinc finger structures. Mol. Cell. Biol. **8:** 1319–1326.
22. HAMILTON, T.B., F. BOREL & P.J. ROMANIUK. 1998. Comparison of the DNA binding characteristics of the related zinc finger proteins WT1 and EGR1. Biochemistry **37:** 2051–2058.
23. SCHARNHORST, V. *et al.* 2000. EGR-1 enhances tumor growth and modulates the effect of the Wilms' tumor 1 gene products on tumorigenicity. Oncogene **19:** 791–800.
24. EID, M.A. *et al.* 1998. Expression of early growth response genes in human prostate cancer. Cancer Res. **58:** 2461–2468.
25. THIGPEN, A.E. *et al.* 1996. Increased expression of early growth response-1 messenger ribonucleic acid in prostatic adenocarcinoma. J. Urol. **155:** 975–981.
26. ABDULKADIR, S.A. *et al.* 2001. Frequent and early loss of the EGR1 corepressor NAB2 in human prostate carcinoma. Hum. Pathol. **32:** 935–939.
27. ABDULKADIR, S.A. *et al.* 2001. Impaired prostate tumorigenesis in Egr1-deficient mice. Nat. Med. **7:** 101–107.
28. SVAREN, J. *et al.* 2000. EGR1 target genes in prostate carcinoma cells identified by microarray analysis. J. Biol. Chem. **275:** 38524–38531.
29. RUSSO, M.W., B.R. SEVETSON & J. MILBRANDT. 1995. Identification of NAB1, a repressor of NGFI-A- and Krox20-mediated transcription. Proc. Natl. Acad. Sci. USA **92:** 6873–6877
30. SVAREN, J. *et al.* 1996. NAB2, a corepressor of NGFI-A (Egr-1) and Krox20, is induced by proliferative and differentiative stimuli. Mol. Cell. Biol. **16:** 3545–3553.
31. GREENBERG, N.M. *et al.* 1995. Prostate cancer in a transgenic mouse. Proc. Natl. Acad. Sci. USA **92:** 3439–3443.
32. GARABEDIAN, E.M., P.A. HUMPHREY & J.I. GORDON. 1998. A transgenic mouse model of metastatic prostate cancer originating from neuroendocrine cells. Proc. Natl. Acad. Sci. USA **95:** 15382–15387.
33. BARON, V. *et al.* 2003. Inhibition of Egr-1 expression reverses transformation of prostate cancer cells in vitro and in vivo. Oncogene **22:** 4194–4204.
34. VIROLLE, T. *et al.* 2003. Egr1 promotes growth and survival of prostate cancer cells. Identification of novel Egr1 target genes. J. Biol. Chem. **278:** 11802–11810.
35. LIU, C. *et al.* 1999. The transcription factor EGR-1 suppresses transformation of human fibrosarcoma HT1080 cells by coordinated induction of transforming growth

factor-beta1, fibronectin, and plasminogen activator inhibitor-1. J. Biol. Chem. **274:** 4400–4411.

36. LIU, C. *et al.* 1996. EGR-1, the reluctant suppression factor: EGR-1 is known to function in the regulation of growth, differentiation, and also has significant tumor suppressor activity and a mechanism involving the induction of TGF-beta1 is postulated to account for this suppressor activity. Crit. Rev. Oncog. **7:** 101–25.
37. YANG, S.-Z. & S.A. ABDULKADIR. 2003. Early growth response gene 1 modulates androgen receptor signaling in prostate carcinoma cells. J. Biol. Chem. **278:** 39906–39911.
38. YU, J. *et al.* 2004. Coactivating factors p300 and CBP are transcriptionally crossregulated by Egr1 in prostate cells, leading to divergent responses. Mol. Cell **15:** 83–94.

# Sulindac Sulfone Is Most Effective in Modulating β-Catenin-Mediated Transcription in Cells with Mutant APC

WEN-CHI L. CHANG,[a] LYNETTE C. EVERLEY,[a] GORDON R. PFEIFFER II,[a] HARRY S. COOPER,[b] ALAN BARUSEVICIUS,[b,c] AND MARGIE L. CLAPPER[a]

*Divisions of Population Science[a] and Medical Science,[b] Fox Chase Cancer Center, Philadelphia, Pennsylvania 19111, USA*

**ABSTRACT: Sulindac sulfone (FGN-1, Aptosyn), a metabolite of the nonsteroidal anti-inflammatory drug sulindac, lacks cyclooxygenase inhibitory activity. Although its ability to inhibit tumorigenesis in both carcinogen-treated animals and patients with familial adenomatous polyposis has been attributed to the induction of apoptosis, its complete mechanism of action remains unclear. The purpose of the present study was to determine the ability of sulindac metabolites to regulate cellular levels of β-catenin and downstream targets of the adenomatous polyposis coli (APC)/β-catenin pathway *in vitro*. Sulindac sulfone was consistently more potent than the sulfide metabolite in all analyses, significantly decreasing the expression of total cellular β-catenin (50% of control), pro-caspase 3 (49%), cyclin D1 (51%), and PPARδ (65%) in SW480 cells. No significant alteration in pro-caspase 3 or β-catenin expression was found in HCA7, LS174, or Caco-2 cells treated with sulindac sulfone. A dose-dependent reduction in TCF-mediated transcriptional activity was also observed in SW480 cells. These data demonstrate that sulindac sulfone can modulate the APC/β-catenin pathway *in vitro* and that its efficacy is dependent upon the mutational status of *APC* and β-catenin.**

**KEYWORDS: sulindac sulfone; APC; β-catenin; colon**

## INTRODUCTION

Mutations in the adenomatous polyposis coli (*APC*) tumor suppressor gene occur in most sporadic colorectal cancers. A germline mutation in this gene results in familial adenomatous polyposis (FAP), an autosomal dominant condition characterized by the development of hundreds to thousands of colonic adenomas and the early onset of colorectal cancer.[1] Although hundreds of distinct mutations have been identified, the majority of these are localized to the 5′ region of the β-catenin binding domain.[2] The *APC* gene encodes a large multidomain protein that interacts with at

Address for correspondence: Wen-Chi L. Chang, Ph.D., Division of Population Science, Fox Chase Cancer Center, 333 Cottman Avenue, Philadelphia, PA 19111. Voice: 215-728-5368; fax: 215-214-1622.

wen-chi.chang@fccc.edu

[c]Present address: MDR Global Systems, LLC, 425 Park Place, Windber, PA 15963.

**Ann. N.Y. Acad. Sci. 1059: 41–55 (2005). © 2005 New York Academy of Sciences.**
**doi: 10.1196/annals.1339.020**

least six other proteins, including β-catenin and glycogen synthase kinase-3β (GSK3β).[3,4] Interactions of wild-type *APC* with β-catenin result in the maintenance of low levels of β-catenin. In contrast, loss of APC function or mutation of β-catenin leads to the accumulation of β-catenin in the cytoplasm, its translocation to the nucleus, and T cell factor (TCF)-4–mediated transcriptional activation.[5] Numerous downstream targets of the APC/β-catenin pathway have been identified, including cyclin D1,[6] *c-myc*,[7] and peroxisome proliferator-activated receptor δ (PPARδ).[8]

Immunohistochemical characterization of the cellular distribution of β-catenin in colon tumors and normal colonic mucosa from FAP patients has provided additional support for the proposed cascade of events leading to the induction of gene transcription. Staining of β-catenin was confined to cell–cell contacts in the normal tissue and localized primarily in the nucleus and cytoplasm of adenomas and carcinomas.[9] Approximately 45% of colorectal tumors without mutant *APC* possess mutations in the $NH_2$-regulatory domain of β-catenin.[10] Corresponding intracellular accumulation of β-catenin has been observed and attributed to the alteration of potential GSK3β phosphorylation sites of β-catenin.[5] These findings suggest that APC and β-catenin mediate similar cellular effects and that mutational activation of β-catenin may be a critical event in some colorectal cancers.

The protective effects of the nonsteroidal anti-inflammatory drug (NSAID) sulindac against both carcinogen-induced colonic tumors in animals[11,12] and premalignant polyps in FAP patients[13,14] have been demonstrated and attributed to cyclooxygenase (COX) inhibition. However, the renal and gastrointestinal toxicities of sulindac and its sulfide metabolite have precluded their long-term use. In contrast to sulindac, its irreversibly oxidized metabolite, sulindac sulfone, lacks COX inhibitory activity.[15] Chronic administration of sulindac sulfone to azoxymethane (AOM)-treated rats led to a dose-dependent reduction in the incidence and multiplicity of both colon adenomas and carcinomas, as compared to controls.[16] Recent data indicated that sulindac sulfone is most effective when administered early during colon carcinogenesis.[17] However, it should be noted that polyp number was unaffected by phase I administration of sulindac sulfone to patients with FAP.[18]

The ability of sulindac sulfone to inhibit AOM-induced tumorigenesis in the absence of COX-1/2 inhibition suggests that its mechanism of action may involve COX-independent pathway(s). Treatment of colon carcinoma cells with sulindac sulfone increases *APC* mRNA expression fivefold, implicating a role for the APC/β-catenin pathway in the action of sulindac sulfone.[19] In addition, sulindac sulfone regulates the DNA binding activity of PPARδ, a downstream target of the APC/β-catenin pathway.[8] These data, when combined with the ability of sulindac sulfone to induce apoptosis[15] and the putative role of the APC pathway in apoptosis,[20] provide strong support for the involvement of the APC/β-catenin pathway in the mechanism of action of sulindac sulfone.

The hypothesis of the present study is that sulindac sulfone can effectively modulate cellular β-catenin levels only in cells with mutant *APC*. This hypothesis has been addressed by examining both the expression and cellular localization of β-catenin in human colon carcinoma cells with defined mutations of *APC* and β-catenin, with and without exposure to sulindac metabolites. The effect of the drug on the expression of pro-caspase 3 (an apoptotic marker), cyclin D1, PPARδ, and TCF-dependent transcriptional activity has been evaluated. The resulting data suggest that, in addition to inducing apoptosis, sulindac sulfone can specifically ameliorate the deleterious effects of mutant *APC*, but not β-catenin, by decreasing both nuclear levels of β-catenin and the expression of downstream targets of the APC/β-catenin pathway.

## MATERIALS AND METHODS

### *Cell Lines and Culture*

Four human colon carcinoma cell lines bearing either wild-type *APC* and wild-type β-catenin (HCA7), mutant *APC* and wild-type β-catenin (SW480), wild-type *APC* and mutant β-catenin (LS174), or mutant *APC* and mutant β-catenin (Caco-2)[21] were maintained *in vitro* under recommended culture conditions. HCA7 cells were provided by Dr. Susan Kirkland (Imperial College of Science, Technology and Medicine, London, UK). SW480, LS174, and Caco-2 cells were obtained from the American Type Culture Collection (Rockville, MD).

### *Sulindac Metabolites Treatment*

Sulindac sulfide and sulindac sulfone were obtained from BIOMOL Research Laboratories, Inc. (Plymouth Meeting, PA). Four human colon carcinoma cell lines were treated at 50–70% confluency for 48 h with either 0.1% dimethylsulfoxide (DMSO; vehicle), sulindac sulfone (240 or 360 μM), or sulindac sulfide (40 or 60 μM). The dose of sulindac sulfone employed was selected from a dose–response curve where the optimal dose was that which caused a 50% reduction in the number of attached viable cells: 360 μM sulindac sulfone for HCA7, SW480, and Caco-2 cells; and 240 μM sulindac sulfone for LS174 cells. The dose of sulindac sulfide was selected based on previous data that indicate that sulindac sulfone is sixfold less potent than sulindac sulfide in its ability to induce apoptosis.[15] Attached cells were harvested at 12, 24, and 48 h post-treatment, trypsinized, pelleted by centrifugation, washed twice with phosphate buffered saline (PBS), and processed for either immunohistochemical staining or Western blot analyses.

### *Treatment of Proteasome Inhibitor*

The proteasome inhibitor Z-Leu-Leu-Leu-B$(OH)_2$ was obtained from Boston Biochem (Cambridge, MA). SW480 cells were treated with 0.1 nM Z-Leu-Leu-Leu-B$(OH)_2$ for 15 min prior to treatment with either 0.1% DMSO, 360 μM sulindac sulfone, or 60 μM sulindac sulfide. SW480 cells were harvested at 48 h post-treatment and processed for Western blot analysis of β-catenin.

### *Plasmids, Transient Transfection, and Luciferase Assays*

pGL3-OT and pGL3-OF (gifts from Dr. Bert Vogelstein) are luciferase reporter constructs containing three wild-type or mutated *TCF* binding sites, respectively.[5] The pGL3-basic vector was obtained from Promega (Madison, WI). Transfection experiments were performed in duplicate on independent days, while triplicate replicates were included in each experiment. All cells were co-transfected with a pCMV-β-galactosidase control plasmid (gift from Dr. Maureen Murphy, Fox Chase Cancer Center [FCCC]) to monitor transfection efficiency.

Twenty-four hours before transfection, SW480 cells were seeded on 6-well plates with $4 \times 10^5$ cells/well. Cells were transfected with 0.5 μg of luciferase reporter plasmid, 0.5 μg of pCMV-β-galactosidase control plasmid, and empty pGL3–basic vector (a total of 2.5 μg of plasmid DNA) using SuperFect Transfection Reagent (QIAGEN, Valencia, CA). Three hours post-transfection, cells were washed with PBS and placed in new media. After 3 h of recovery, cells were treated with DMSO (vehicle, negative control) or 120 μM, 240 μM, or 360 μM of sulindac sulfone for 48 h and lysed. Luciferase and β-galactosidase activities were determined using enzyme assay kits (Promega) and standardized per microgram of protein. Luciferase activity was normalized to β-galactosidase activity (ratio) and expressed as arbitrary units.

### *Immunohistochemical Detection of* β*-Catenin*

Cells for immunohistochemical analysis were fixed in 10% neutral buffered formalin and embedded in paraffin. Heat-induced epitope retrieval was performed. Sections were stained with polyclonal antibodies against β-catenin (amino acids 768-781) (Sigma, St. Louis, MO) at a dilution of 1:4000 using an automated Techmate 1000. Biotinylated sheep anti-rabbit (Vector Laboratories, Burlingame, CA) was used as secondary antibody. Controls for β-catenin expression were normal and neoplastic colonic lesions from mice possessing a germline mutation in the *APC* gene. Nonimmune rabbit IgG of a similar protein concentration was substituted for β-catenin antibodies as a negative control.

### *Immunoblotting*

Cells were lysed with RIPA buffer (10 mM Tris, pH 7.2; 150 mM NaCl, 1% sodium deoxycholate, 1% triton X-100, 0.1% SDS, 0.1 mM $Na_3VO_4$; 50 mM NaF), containing a protease inhibitor cocktail (Boehringer Mannheim, GmbH, Germany). Cells were homogenized on ice, passed through a 25-gauge needle and left on ice for 30 min to ensure total cell lysis. Supernatants were collected for analysis after centrifugation at $12{,}000 \times g$ for 15 min at 4°C.

The expression of select proteins was examined by Western blot. β-Actin expression served as an internal loading control. The protein concentration of each cell lysate was determined using the Bradford assay (Bio-Rad, Hercules, CA). Equivalent amounts of protein were electrophoretically separated on polyacrylamide gels and transferred to PVDF membranes by electroblotting (Millipore, Bedford, MA). Immunoreactive proteins were detected using polyclonal antibodies against β-catenin (1:4000 dilution, Sigma), pro-caspase 3 (1:2000 dilution, PharMingen, San Diego, CA), cyclin D1 (1:200 dilution, NeoMarkers, Inc., Fremont, CA), PPARδ (1:500 dilution, Affinity Bioreagents, Inc., Golden, CO), axin (1:200 dilution, Invitrogen Corp., Carlsbad, CA), GSK3β (1:1500 dilution, Transduction Laboratories, Lexington, KY), and β-actin (1:5000 dilution, Sigma), and developed using enhanced chemiluminescence detection (Amersham Pharmacia, Arlington Heights, IL). The resulting images were scanned using an Alpha Imager (Alpha Innotech Corp., San Leandro, CA) and quantitatively analyzed using Alpha Ease™ Stand Alone Software.

### *Statistical Analysis*

The $t$ test was used to compare the expression of proteins with and without drug treatment. A $P < 0.05$ was considered significant.

## RESULTS

### *Induction of Apoptosis*

Initial experiments were performed to confirm the ability of the sulfone and sulfide metabolites of sulindac to induce apoptosis in the selected human colon carcinoma cell lines. Apoptosis was measured in control and drug-treated cells by quantifying the level of pro-caspase 3, an early marker of apoptosis, by Western blot. Pro-caspase 3 levels were reduced in cells undergoing apoptosis due to self-proteolysis and/or cleavage of this 32 kDa protein to its active subunit. Exposure of SW480 cells, bearing mutant *APC* and wild-type β-catenin, to sulindac sulfone for 48 h significantly decreased levels of pro-caspase 3 by 49% as compared to DMSO-treated controls ($P = 0.02$) (FIG. 1). Sulindac sulfone was less efficient in reducing pro-caspase 3 levels in the presence of wild-type *APC* (8% and 12% reduction for HCA7 and LS174 cells, respectively), regardless of the mutational status of β-catenin. However, sulindac sulfone did not alter the expression of pro-caspase 3 significantly in Caco-2 cells bearing both mutant *APC* and β-catenin.

Although a reduction of pro-caspase 3 was observed in SW480 cells following sulindac sulfide treatment (22%, $P = 0.09$), sulindac sulfide did not alter the expression of pro-caspase 3 significantly in the other three cell lines.

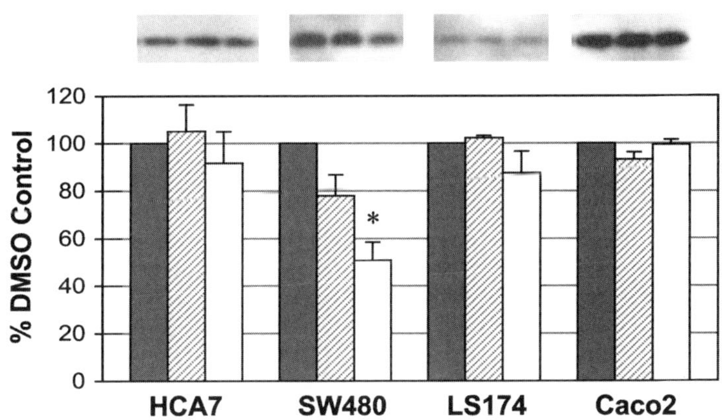


**FIGURE 1.** Analysis of pro-caspase 3 expression in extracts of human colon carcinoma cells treated with sulindac metabolites. Cells were treated for 48 h with DMSO (*dark gray bars*), sulindac sulfide (*hatched bars*), or sulindac sulfone (*open bars*). Immunoreactive proteins were detected by Western blot and quantified. Data are expressed as percent control (mean ± standard error) ($n = 3$). $*P < 0.05$ by Student's $t$ test.

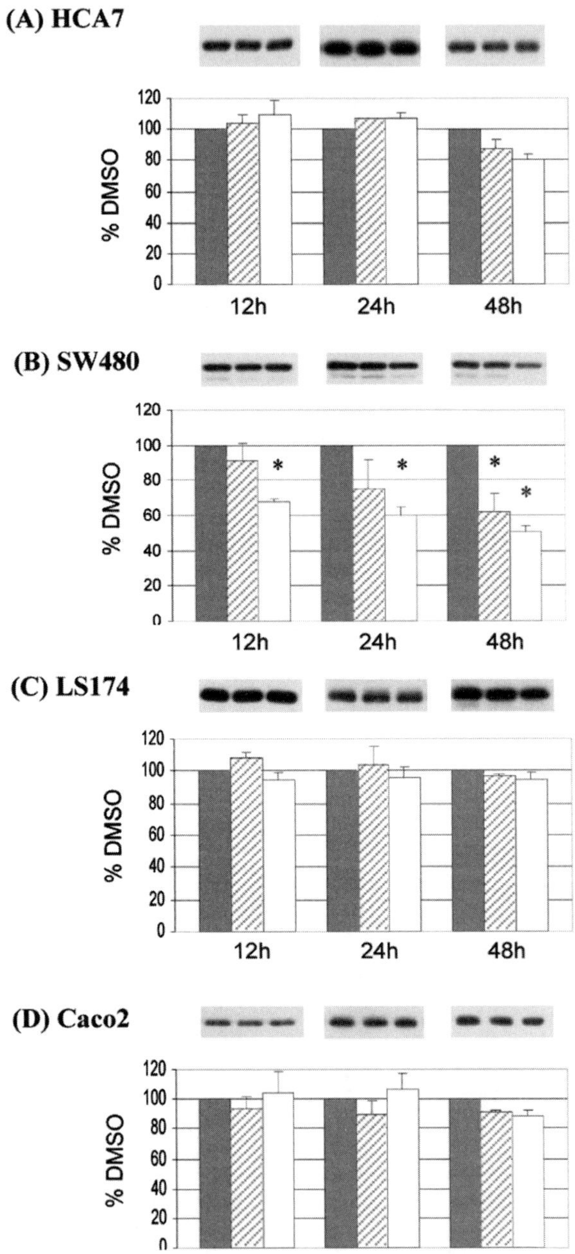


**FIGURE 2.** Analysis of β-catenin expression in cell extracts of human colon carcinoma cells treated with sulindac metabolites. Cells were treated with DMSO (*dark gray bars*), sulindac sulfide (*hatched bars*), or sulindac sulfone (*open bars*). Immunoreactive proteins were detected by Western blot and quantified. Data are expressed as percent control (mean ± standard error) ($n = 3$). $*P < 0.05$ by Student's $t$ test.

### *Expression of Total Cellular β-Catenin*

In order to evaluate the ability of sulindac metabolites to downregulate β-catenin in colon carcinoma cells bearing defined mutations in *APC* and β-catenin, Western blot analyses were employed, and the expression of total cellular β-catenin in vehicle and drug-treated cells was compared. The effect of sulindac sulfide and sulfone on the expression of total cellular β-catenin varied with the mutational status of *APC* and β-catenin and was time dependent. Expression of β-catenin in SW480 cells was decreased by 32% (12 h), 40% (24 h), and 50% (48 h) as compared to vehicle-treated control (DMSO) following sulindac sulfone exposure (FIG. 2). However, no significant reductions in total cellular β-catenin expression were observed in HCA7, LS174, and Caco-2 cells following 12 and 24 h of drug exposure; the expression of β-catenin was reduced by less than 20% in each of these three cell lines following exposure to sulindac sulfone for 48 h.

Sulindac sulfide also had a similar effect on the expression of total cellular β-catenin in SW480 cells. SW480 cells treated with 60 μM sulindac sulfide for 12, 24, or 48 h had 91%, 75%, and 62%, respectively, of the level of β-catenin present in vehicle-treated cells examined at the same time points. Sulindac sulfide did not significantly alter β-catenin levels in HCA7, LS174, and Caco-2 cells at any of the time points tested.

### *Nuclear Staining of β-Catenin*

The established nuclear localization of β-catenin in cells with mutant *APC* provided a visual biomarker by which to assess the ability of sulindac metabolites to modulate β-catenin levels within the nucleus. Cells were evaluated 48 h following drug treatment when maximum reductions in β-catenin by sulindac sulfone were observed (FIG. 2). Sections from control and drug-treated cell blocks were stained with polyclonal antibodies against β-catenin.

The ability of sulindac sulfone to alter the cellular localization of β-catenin was dependent on the mutational status of *APC* and β-catenin. β-Catenin was primarily detected on the cell membrane and in the cytosol of untreated LS174 (FIG. 3), HCA7, and Caco-2 cells. After treatment with either sulindac sulfone or sulfide, no alterations in either β-catenin distribution or staining intensity were found in any of these cell lines. In contrast, vehicle-treated SW480 cells bearing mutant *APC* and wild-type β-catenin exhibited intense staining of β-catenin in both the cytoplasm and nucleus (FIG. 3). After treatment with sulindac sulfone, the intensity of both nuclear and total cellular β-catenin staining was decreased as compared to that of SW480 cells treated with DMSO.

### *Cyclin D1 and PPARδ Expression*

The effect of sulindac sulfide and sulfone on the β-catenin signaling cascade was further evaluated by quantifying the expression of cyclin D1 and PPARδ, downstream targets of the APC/β-catenin pathway, in cells with and without mutant *APC* and/or β-catenin, before and after drug treatment.

Western blot analyses revealed that sulindac sulfone significantly reduced the levels of cyclin D1 in SW480 cells to 49% of DMSO-treated controls ($P = 0.005$) (FIG. 4). In contrast, sulindac sulfone did not significantly change the level of

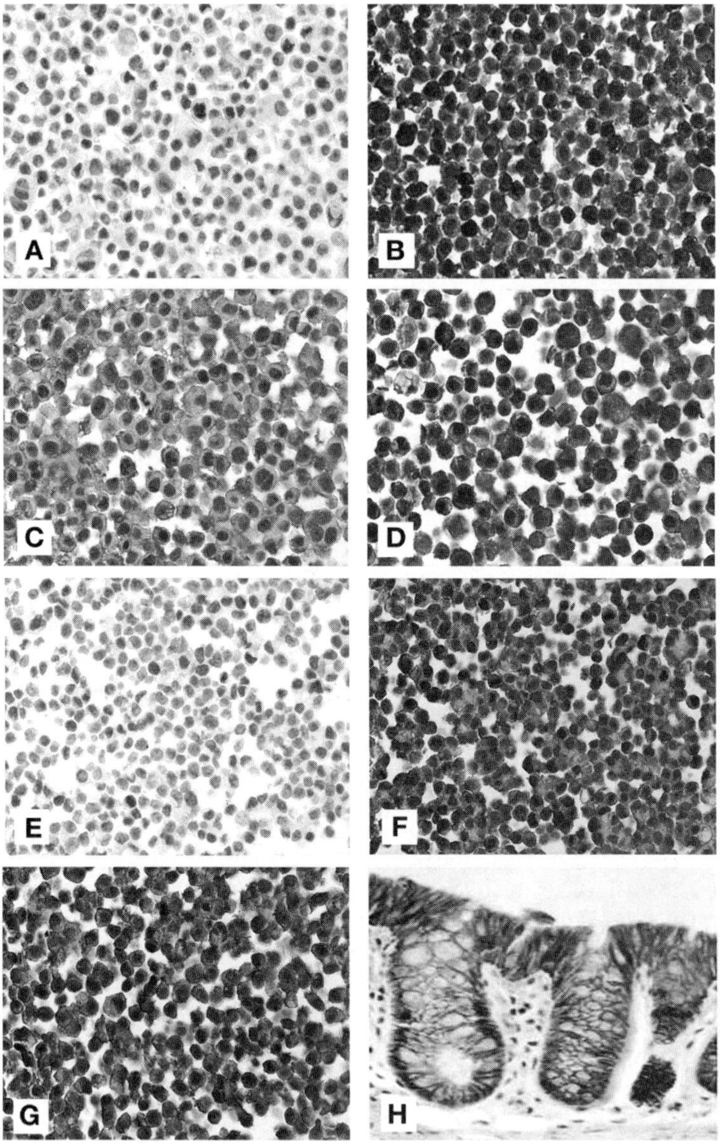


**FIGURE 3.** Immunohistochemical staining of β-catenin in SW480 (**panels A–D**) and LS174 (**panels E–G**) cells. Formalin-fixed sections were incubated with β-catenin antibodies and stained according to the ABC peroxidase method. Sections in **A** and **E** represent negative controls stained with normal rabbit serum. **B** and **F** contain cells treated with vehicle (DMSO), while cells in **C** and **G** have been exposed to sulindac sulfone. In **D**, SW480 cells were treated with an irreversible proteasome inhibitor prior to sulindac sulfone exposure. **H** is a section of normal mouse colon, which serves as a positive control for β-catenin staining.

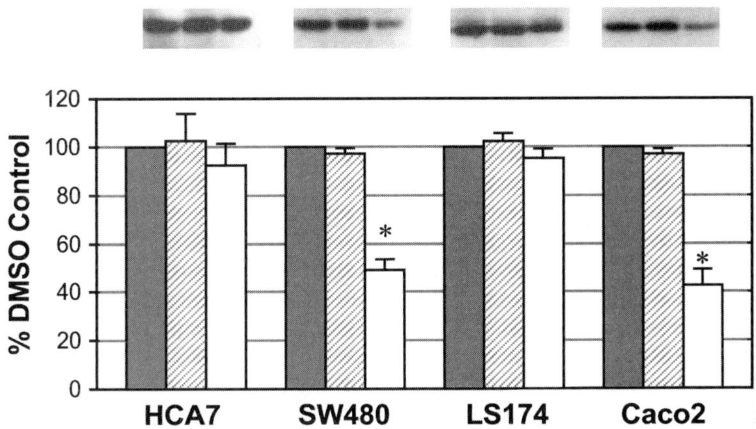


**FIGURE 4.** Analysis of cyclin D1 expression in extracts of human colon carcinoma cells treated with sulindac metabolites. Cells were treated for 48 h with DMSO (*dark gray bars*), sulindac sulfide (*hatched bars*), or sulindac sulfone (*open bars*). Immunoreactive proteins were detected by Western blot. Data are expressed as percent control (mean ± standard error) ($n = 3$). *$P < 0.05$ by Student's $t$ test.

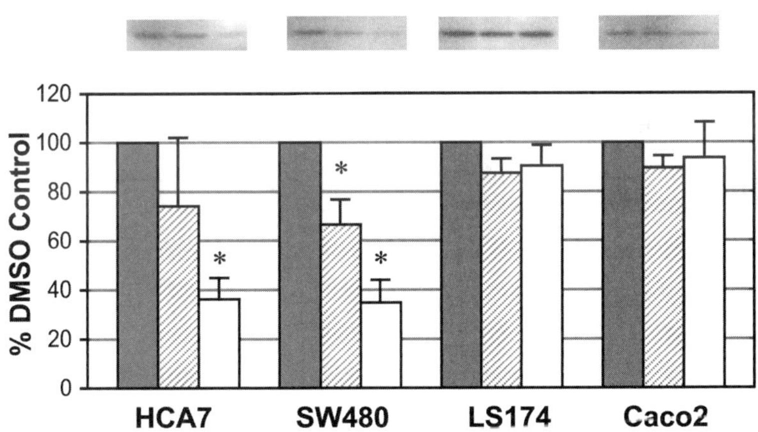


**FIGURE 5.** Analysis of PPARδ expression in extracts of human colon carcinoma cells treated with sulindac metabolites. Cells were treated for 48 h with DMSO (*dark gray bars*), sulindac sulfide (*hatched bars*), or sulindac sulfone (*open bars*). Immunoreactive proteins were detected by Western blot. Data are expressed as percent control (mean ± standard error) ($n = 3$). *$P < 0.05$ by Student's $t$ test.

cyclin D1 in either HCA7 cells (wild-type *APC* and wild-type β-catenin) or LS174 cells (wild-type *APC* and mutant β-catenin). However, sulindac sulfone decreased the level of cyclin D1 in Caco-2 cells to 43% of that of controls ($P = 0.009$). The level of cyclin D1 in HCA7, SW480, LS174, and Caco-2 cells following exposure to sulindac sulfide was similar to that of DMSO-treated controls.

Expression of PPARδ was also determined in cells treated with sulindac sulfone or sulfide (FIG. 5). A reduction in PPARδ was observed in SW480 cells treated for

48 h with sulindac sulfone (35% of that of DMSO-treated control, $P = 0.004$). No alteration in PPARδ expression was found in either LS174 or Caco-2 cells following sulindac sulfone exposure. However, sulindac sulfone decreased the level of PPARδ in HCA7 cells to 39% of that of control ($P = 0.03$). Sulindac sulfide reduced the level of PPARδ in SW480 cells (67% of control, $P = 0.03$), but did not significantly change the level of PPARδ in HCA7, LS174, and Caco-2 cells.

### *Proteasomal Degradation of β-Catenin*

The potential ability of sulindac sulfone to induce the degradation of β-catenin via the ubiquitin-proteasome pathway was examined in SW480 cells. Cells were pretreated with either Z-Leu-Leu-Leu-B$(OH)_2$ (proteasome inhibitor) or vehicle and subsequently exposed to either DMSO, sulindac sulfone, or sulindac sulfide (FIG. 6). A dose-dependent reduction in β-catenin expression was observed in SW480 cells pretreated with 0.1% DMSO, the vehicle for the proteasome inhibitor; subsequently, the cells were exposed to sulindac sulfone for 48 h. However, no decrease in cellular β-catenin levels was observed when cells were incubated with Z-Leu-Leu-Leu-B$(OH)_2$ prior to drug exposure. A similar cellular response to the proteasome inhibitor was observed in cells treated with sulindac sulfide.

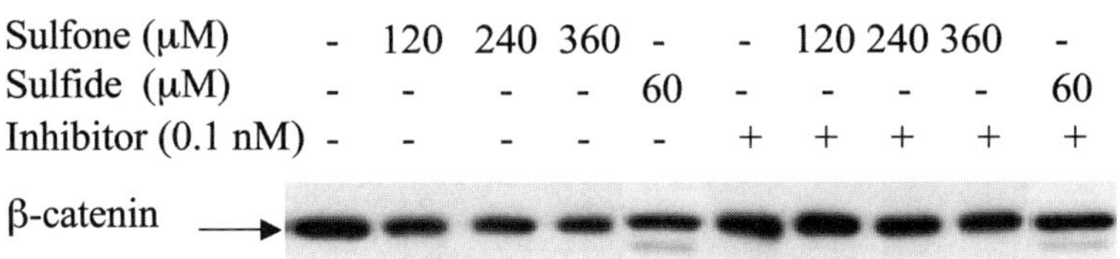


**FIGURE 6.** Analysis of β-catenin expression in extracts of human colon carcinoma cells treated with an irreversible proteasome inhibitor prior to exposure to sulindac metabolites. Cells were pretreated with Z-Leu-Leu-Leu-B$(OH)_2$, followed by exposure to vehicle (DMSO), sulindac sulfide, or sulindac sulfone. Immunoreactive proteins were detected by Western blot.

### *Sulindac Sulfone Decreased Tcf-dependent Transcriptional Activity*

In order to confirm that sulindac sulfone could downregulate downstream targets of the APC/β-catenin pathway in SW480 cells, the ability of sulindac sulfone to modulate TCF-dependent transcriptional activity was evaluated (FIG. 7). Sulindac sulfone altered the luciferase activity of SW480 cells transfected with pGL3-OT, a luciferase reporter construct containing three copies of the wild-type *TCF* binding element, in a dose-dependent manner (luciferase activity was 53%, 19% and 3.5% of that of DMSO-treated cells after exposure (48 h) to 120, 240, and 360 μM sulindac sulfone, respectively). The luciferase activity of cells transfected with pGL3-OF, containing three copies of the mutant *TCF* binding element, was similar to that of both cells transfected with empty pGL3-basic construct and untransfected cells, irrespective of sulindac sulfone treatment.

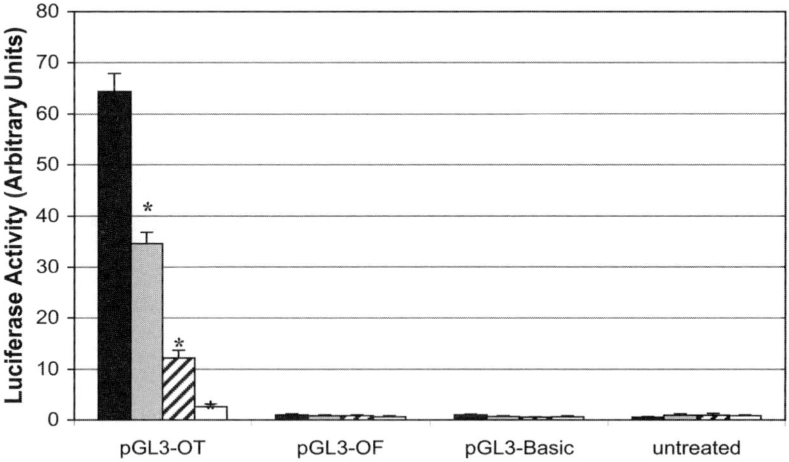


**FIGURE 7.** Sulindac sulfone reduces Tcf-dependent transcriptional activity in a dose-response manner. SW480 cells were transfected with pGL3-OT or pGL3-OF, luciferase reporter constructs containing three copies of either the wild-type or mutated *TCF* binding element, respectively. All cells were co-transfected with a β-galactosidase construct to monitor transfection efficiency. Cells were treated with DMSO (vehicle, *black bars*) or 120 μM (*light gray bars*), 240 μM (*hatched bars*), or 360 μM (*open bars*) sulindac sulfone. After 48 h, cells were lysed and luciferase and β-galactosidase activities were determined. *$P < 0.05$ by Student's *t* test.

### *Axin and GSK3β Expression*

The ability of sulindac sulfone to modulate the APC/β-catenin pathway was also investigated by quantifying the expression of axin and GSK3β by Western blot. Sulindac sulfone did not alter the expression of axin in SW480, LS174, and Caco-2 cells significantly, even though axin expression tended to be higher after drug treatment. The only statistically significant response was observed in HCA7 cells where sulindac sulfone increased the expression of axin above that of control DMSO-treated cells ($P = 0.02$). Although sulindac sulfone did not alter the expression of GSK3β in HCA7, LS174, and Caco-2 cells, it marginally decreased expression of GSK3β in SW480 cells ($P = 0.055$). Sulindac sulfide did not alter the expression of either axin or GSK3β in any of the cell lines.

## DISCUSSION

The present study suggests for the first time that sulindac metabolites are most effective in inducing apoptosis in cells with mutant *APC* and wild-type β-catenin. Pro-caspase 3 levels in SW480 cells treated with sulindac sulfone were two- to five-fold less than those of HCA7, LS174, or Caco-2 cells treated in an identical manner. In order to confirm that this drug response was not specific to SW480 cells, the experiment was repeated with DLD1 colon carcinoma cells, also bearing mutant *APC*, and similar results were obtained. Expression of β-catenin in DLD1 cells was decreased by 35% as compared to vehicle-treated controls (DMSO) following 48 h of sulindac sulfone exposure.

Although previous studies have established that sulindac sulfone induces apoptosis, the molecular basis for this activity remains to be elucidated. The contribution of either inhibition of prostaglandin synthesis,[16,22,23] p53, or bcl-2 to this response appears unlikely.[15,24,25] Our data suggest that this sulindac metabolite induces apoptosis by restoring the function of a mutated APC/β-catenin pathway. Support for this mechanism is provided by the following post-treatment observations in cells with mutant *APC*: (1) cytoplasmic and nuclear levels of β-catenin are decreased significantly *in vitro*; (2) β-catenin staining becomes more apparent at the cell membrane *in vitro*; and (3) reductions in pro-caspase 3 are accompanied by downregulation of TCF-dependent transcription activity, cyclin D1, and PPARδ; established downstream targets of the APC/β-catenin pathway. Although our *in vitro* observations in SW480 cells are in agreement with the findings of Li *et al.*,[26] neither the response of other cell lines (control nonmutated, mutant β-catenin) nor the ability of this sulindac metabolite to directly modulate β-catenin–mediated transcription was investigated.

Although specific apoptotic genes have not been identified to date as downstream targets of the APC/β-catenin pathway, the role of *APC* in the induction of apoptosis has been demonstrated. Expression of wild-type *APC* in HT29 human colon carcinoma cells with inactive *APC* alleles leads to the induction of apoptosis.[20] These data, when combined with the putative function of *APC* as the "gatekeeper of colorectal carcinogenesis," suggest the importance of aberrant apoptosis in the early development of colorectal tumors, the period when sulindac sulfone was most effective in inhibiting tumor formation *in vivo*.[17]

The anti-neoplastic activity of sulindac sulfone appears to be due at least in part to its ability to enhance the degradation of β-catenin. Treatment of SW480 cells with a potent irreversible proteasome inhibitor prior to sulindac sulfone exposure blocked both the downregulation of β-catenin and its drug-induced redistribution within the cell. Indirect support for this finding has been provided by Northern blot analyses, which indicate no significant difference in the levels of β-catenin transcripts in cells treated with vehicle vs. those exposed to sulindac sulfone (data not shown). Because targeted phosphorylation of the highly conserved serine and threonine residues of β-catenin is required for proteasomal degradation, protein kinases may serve as mediators of the sulindac sulfone-induced response. Recent studies have demonstrated that β-catenin is a substrate for cGMP-dependent protein kinase, a kinase that is induced following sulindac sulfone exposure.[27] However, it should be noted that at least six kinases, including GSK3β,[28] epidermal growth factor receptor,[29] and *c-erb*B-2,[30] are known to phosphorylate β-catenin. The effect of sulindac sulfone on the activity of other kinases remains to be established.

These data confirm the importance of genetic background in predicting cellular response to NSAIDs. First, the ineffectiveness of sulindac sulfone in reducing β-catenin levels in LS174 and Caco-2 cells suggests that nonmutated β-catenin may be required to achieve drug-induced depletion of cellular β-catenin levels. This observation is consistent with the ability of mutations in β-catenin to inhibit its ubiquitination and proteasomal degradation, thus increasing its activity as a transcriptional activator.[31] Second, sulindac sulfone was effective in reducing cyclin D1 expression only in cells with mutant *APC*, irrespective of the mutational status of β-catenin. Alternatively, because GSK3β can phosphorylate cyclin D1 directly and target it for degradation,[32] it is possible that sulindac sulfone also enhanced the proteasomal degradation of cyclin D1 in Caco-2 cells. The relevance of *in vitro* data from Caco-2 cells to human colon cancers remains questionable because no human colon tumors have been identified to date that harbor mutations in both *APC* and β-catenin.[10] Third, in contrast to the cyclin D1 data, reductions in PPARδ were observed following exposure to sulindac metabolites only in cells bearing wild-type β-catenin. These data are in agreement with those of He and colleagues,[8] which demonstrated that expression of oncogenic mutations in β-catenin can activate the PPARδ reporter. Although the contribution of prostaglandins to the observed response is unknown, it should be noted that HCA7 cells have high levels of COX-2[33] and that both the sulfide and sulfone metabolites of sulindac can inhibit prostaglandin $E_2$ production in this cell line.[34] Further interpretation of the present data is compromised by our limited understanding of both the mechanism of action of sulindac sulfone and the identity of proapoptotic downstream targets of the APC/β-catenin pathway.

Since mutations in *APC* represent a common genetic event in humans, it can be inferred that a large population of high-risk individuals could benefit from early intervention with agents targeting the malfunctioned APC/β-catenin pathway. Potential candidates for chemopreventive therapy include individuals with heritable colorectal syndromes as well as those at risk for sporadic colon carcinomas. The role of a defective APC/β-catenin pathway in the development of neoplasias of the prostate[35,36] and breast[37] has also been suggested. Thus, drug-induced restoration of a mutant APC/β-catenin pathway represents a promising strategy for the clinical chemoprevention of a broad range of tumor types.

## ACKNOWLEDGMENTS

This work was supported by USPHS grants CA-06927, a supplement to CA-06927, CA-82624, and CA-87817. Its contents are solely the responsibility of the authors and do not necessarily represent the official views of the National Cancer Institute. This work was also supported by an appropriation from the Commonwealth of Pennsylvania.

We wish to gratefully acknowledge Gerard Caprio for technical assistance, the Cell Culture Facility for media preparation, Dr. Alfonso Bellacosa for reviewing this manuscript, and Maureen Climaldi for her excellent assistance in preparing this manuscript for publication.

## REFERENCES

1. Cottrell, S., D. Bicknell, L. Kaklamanis, *et al.* 1992. Molecular analysis of APC mutations in familial adenomatous polyposis and sporadic colon carcinomas. Lancet **340:** 626–630.
2. Polakis, P. 1997. The adenomatous polyposis coli (APC) tumor suppressor. Biochim. Biophys. Acta **1332:** F127–F147.
3. Rubinfeld, B., B. Souza, I. Albert, *et al.* 1993. Association of the *APC* gene product with β-catenin. Science **262:** 1731–1734.

4. Su, L.K., B. Vogelstein & K.W. Kinzler. 1993. Association of the APC tumor suppressor protein with catenins. Science **262:** 1734–1737.
5. Korinek, V., N. Barker, P.J. Morin, *et al.* 1997. Constitutive transcriptional activation by a β-catenin-Tcf complex in APC–/– colon carcinoma. Science **275:** 1784–1787.
6. Shtutman, M., J. Zhurinsky, I. Simcha, *et al.* 1999. The cyclin D1 gene is a target of the β-catenin/LEF-1 pathway. Proc. Natl. Acad. Sci. USA **96:** 5522–5527.
7. He, T.-C., A.B. Sparks, C. Rago, *et al.* 1998. Identification of c-*MYC* as a target of the APC pathway. Science **281:** 1509–1512.
8. He, T.C., T.A. Chan, B. Vogelstein, *et al.* 1999. PPARδ is an APC-regulated target of nonsteroidal anti-inflammatory drugs. Cell **99:** 335–345.
9. Inomata, M., A. Ochiai, S. Akimoto, *et al.* 1996. Alteration of β-catenin expression in colonic epithelial cells of familial adenomatous polyposis patients. Cancer Res. **56:** 2213–2217.
10. Sparks, A.B., P.J. Morin, B. Vogelstein, *et al.* 1998. Mutational analysis of the APC/β-catenin/Tcf pathway in colorectal cancer. Cancer Res. **58:** 1130–1134.
11. Moorghen, M., P. Ince, K.J. Finney, *et al.* 1988. A protective effect of sulindac against chemically-induced primary colonic tumors in mice. J. Pathol. **156:** 341–347.
12. Skinner, S.A., A.G. Penney & P.E. O'Brien. 1991. Sulindac inhibits the rate of growth and appearance of colon tumors in the rat. Arch. Surg. **126:** 1094–1096.
13. Labayle, D., D. Fischer, P. Vielh, *et al.* 1991. Sulindac causes regression of rectal polyps in familial adenomatous polyposis. Gastroenterology **101:** 635–639.
14. Giardiello, F.M., S.R. Hamilton, A.J. Krush, *et al.* 1993. Treatment of colonic and rectal adenomas with sulindac in familial adenomatous polyposis. N. Engl. J. Med. **328:** 1313–1316.
15. Piazza, G.A., A.K. Rahm, T.S. Finn, *et al.* 1997. Apoptosis primarily accounts for the growth-inhibitory properties of sulindac metabolites and involves a mechanism that is independent of cyclooxygenase inhibition, cell cycle arrest, and p53 induction. Cancer Res. **57:** 2452–2459.
16. Piazza, G.A., D.S. Alberts, L.J. Hixson, *et al.* 1997. Sulindac sulfone inhibits azoxymethane-induced colon carcinogenesis in rats without reducing prostaglandin levels. Cancer Res. **57:** 2909–2915.
17. Reddy, B.S., T. Kawamori, R.A. Lubet, *et al.* 1999. Chemopreventive efficacy of sulindac sulfone against colon cancer depends on time of administration during carcinogenic process. Cancer Res. **59:** 3387–3391.
18. van Stolk, R., G. Stoner, W.L. Hayton, *et al.* 2000. Phase I trial of exisulind (sulindac sulfone, FGN-1) as a chemopreventive agent in patients with familial adenomatous polyposis. Clin. Cancer Res. **6:** 78–89.
19. Schnitzler, M., T. Dwight & B.G. Robinson. 1996. Sulindac increases the expression of APC mRNA in malignant colonic epithelial cells: an *in vitro* study. Gut **38:** 707–713.
20. Morin, P.J., B. Vogelstein & K.W. Kinzler. 1996. Apoptosis and *APC* in colorectal tumorigenesis. Proc. Natl. Acad. Sci. USA **93:** 7950–7954.
21. Ilyas, M., I.P.M. Tomlinson, A. Rowan, *et al.* 1997. β-catenin mutations in cell lines established from human colorectal cancers. Proc. Natl. Acad. Sci. USA **94:** 10330–10334.
22. Hixson, L., D.S. Alberts, M. Krutzsch, *et al.* 1994. Antiproliferative effect of nonsteroidal antiinflammatory drugs against human colon cancer cells. Cancer Epidemiol. Biomarkers Prev. **3:** 433–437.
23. Alberts, D.S., L. Hixson, D. Ahnen, *et al.* 1995. Do non-steroidal anti-inflammatory drugs (NSAIDs) exert their colon cancer chemoprevention activities through inhibition of colonic mucosal prostaglandin synthetase? J. Cell. Biochem. Suppl. **22:** 18–23.
24. Lim, J.T., G.A. Piazza, E.K. Han, *et al.* 1999. Sulindac derivatives inhibit growth and induce apoptosis in human prostate cancer cell lines. Biochem. Pharmacol. **58:** 1097–1107.
25. Piazza, G., A. Rahm, R. Pamukcu, *et al.* 1996. Induction of apoptosis by sulindac metabolites involves a p53 and bcl-2 independent mechanism and does not require cell cycle arrest. Gastroenterology **110:** A577.

26. Li, H., L. Liu, M.L. David, *et al.* 2002. Pro-apoptotic actions of exisulind and CP461 in SW480 colon tumor cells involve beta-catenin and cyclin D1 down-regulation. Biochem. Pharmacol. **64:** 1325–1336.
27. Thompson, W.J., G.A. Piazza, H. Li, *et al.* 2000. Exisulind induction of apoptosis involves guanosine 3′,5′-cyclic monophosphate phosphodiesterase inhibition, protein kinase G activation, and attenuated beta-catenin. Cancer Res. **60:** 3338–3342.
28. Rubinfeld, B., I. Albert, E. Porfiri, *et al.* 1996. Binding of GSK3β to the APC-β-catenin complex and regulation of complex assembly. Science **272:** 1023–1026.
29. Shiozaki, H., T. Kadowaki, Y. Doki, *et al.* 1995. Effect of epidermal growth factor on cadherin-mediated adhesion in a human oesophageal cancer cell line. Br. J. Cancer. **71:** 250–258.
30. Ochiai, A., S. Akimoto, Y. Kanai, *et al.* 1994. c-erbB-2 gene product associates with catenins in human cancer cells. Biochem. Biophys. Res. Commun. **205:** 73–78.
31. Morin, P.J., A.B. Sparks, V. Korinek, *et al.* 1997. Activation of β-catenin-Tcf signaling in colon cancer by mutations in β-catenin or APC. Science **275:** 1787–1790.
32. Diehl, J.A., M. Cheng, M.F. Roussel, *et al.* 1998. Glycogen synthase kinase-3β regulates cyclin D1 proteolysis and subcellular localization. Genes Dev. **12:** 3499–3511.
33. Shao, J., H. Sheng, H. Inoue, *et al.* 2000. Regulation of constitutive cyclooxygenase-2 expression in colon carcinoma cells. J. Biol. Chem. **275:** 33951–33956.
34. Williams, C.S., A.P. Goldman, H. Sheng, *et al.* 1999. Sulindac sulfide, but not sulindac sulfone, inhibits colorectal cancer growth. Neoplasia **1:** 170–176.
35. Watanabe, M., H. Kakiuchi, H. Kato, *et al.* 1996. *APC* gene mutations in human prostate cancer. Jpn. J. Clin. Oncol. **26:** 77–81.
36. Voeller, H.J., C.I. Truica & E.P. Gelmann. 1998. β-Catenin mutations in human prostate cancer. Cancer Res. **58:** 2520–2523.
37. Redston, M., K.L. Nathanson, Z.Q. Yuan, *et al.* 1998. The APCI1307K allele and breast cancer risk. Nat. Genet. **20:** 13–14.

# Targeting Ligand Cleavage to Inhibit the ErbB Pathway in Cancer

BIN-BING S. ZHOU

*Drug Discovery Biology, Incyte Corporation, Wilmington, Delaware 19880, USA*

**ABSTRACT: ADAMs (a disintegrin and metalloproteases) are zinc-dependent transmembrane metalloproteases that shed the extracellular domains of membrane-bound growth factors, cytokines, and receptors. Recently, ADAMs have emerged in ErbB signaling pathways as sheddases or multiple ErbB ligands. As the ErbB pathway is a validated target for anticancer drugs, upstream activators of ErbB ligands, their sheddases, become new drug targets in the ErbB pathway. We have identified selective small molecule inhibitors of ADAM proteases that block shedding and activation of multiple ErbB ligands, and we are planning to test the compounds in the clinic.**

**KEYWORDS: ADAM protease; ErbB pathway; ligand; shedding; cancer**

Cancer cells can synthesize and secrete various growth factors and express their cognate receptors, allowing their secreted growth factors to stimulate tumor growth through autocrine and/or paracrine mechanisms.[1–4] Based on these early observations, the idea has been developed that preventing the binding of a growth factor to its receptor could inhibit the proliferation of tumor cells.[5] This can be achieved by antibodies that can block the physical binding of growth factors to their receptors or small molecules that inhibit the activation and/or maturation of growth factors.

The ErbB family of receptor tyrosine kinases and their ligands are important regulators of cell proliferation, differentiation, and survival, and have been the targets of intensive cancer drug discovery efforts.[6] There are four receptors in the ErbB family, including EGFR (Her-1 or ErbB1), Her-2 (neu or ErbB2), Her-3 (ErbB3), and Her-4 (ErbB4).[7] Among them, EGFR, Her-2, and Her-4 have tyrosine kinase activities, which can be inhibited by small molecule kinase inhibitors. On the other hand, Her-3 has a truncated kinase domain that is not functional.[8] Eleven ligands have been reported to bind to the ErbB receptor family, including epidermal growth factor (EGF), transforming growth factor α (TGF-α), heparin-binding EGF-like ligand (HB-EGF), amphiregulin (AR), betacellulin (BTC), epiregulin (EPR), epigen (EPG), and heregulin (HRG)/neuregulin (NRG) family members.[9] These ligands bind directly to EGFR, Her-3 or Her-4, resulting in the formation of hetero- or homodimers, activation of the tyrosine kinase domain(s), and receptor autophosphorylation. ErbB ligand binding has been the target of several anti-ErbB antibodies.

Address for correspondence: Bin-Bing S. Zhou, Drug Discovery Biology, Incyte Corporation, Experimental Station, Rt. 141 and Henry Clay Road, Bldg. 400, Wilmington, DE 19880. Voice: 302-498-6813; fax: 302-425-2760.

bzhou@incyte.com

**Ann. N.Y. Acad. Sci. 1059: 56–60 (2005). © 2005 New York Academy of Sciences.**
**doi: 10.1196/annals.1339.022**

After ligand binding, the activated ErbB receptors can trigger multiple downstream signaling cascades, including MEK-MAPK, PI3K-Akt, and STATs, which each have pleiotropic oncogenic effects when dysregulated.[7] Different from prototypical receptor tyrosine kinases, Her-2 has no validated extracellular ligand. Rather, it is the preferred partner for heterodimerization with other ErbB family receptors upon ligand activation.[10,11] In addition to kinase and ligand binding, recent understanding of ErbB ligand processing and activation offered new opportunity for the therapeutic intervention in ErbB pathway.[12]

ErbB ligands are structurally and functionally related membrane proteins that can be proteolytically cleaved and released from cells for signaling through autocrine and paracrine mechanisms.[13–15] This cleavage event is critical for the activation of the ligands under a variety of circumstances and is thought to be mediated by ADAMs (a disintegrin and metalloproteases),[14,16,17] which are zinc-dependent transmembrane metalloproteases that cleave the extracellular domains of membrane-bound growth factors, cytokines, and receptors. One of the first connections between ADAMs and the ErbB pathway came from the observation that ADAM17 is crucial for activating EGFR during mouse development.[18] ADAM17-deficient cells have been shown to be defective in the shedding of TGF-α, HB-EGF, EPR, and AR.[14,18–20] Several defects in ADAM17–/– mice may result from a lack of ErbB ligand processing, including the defects in the maturation and morphogenesis of epithelial structures that resemble those of TGF-α–/– or EGFR–/– mice,[18] defects in branching morphogenesis of the lung,[21] thickened and misshapen heart valves that resemble those of HBEGF–/– mice,[22–24] and defects in branching morphogenesis during development of the mammary gland that are similar to those seen in mice lacking AR.[16,25] To date, the ADAM family members that have also been suggested to affect ErbB ligand shedding include ADAM10, ADAM12, and ADAM9.[14] ADAM10 is potentially the main sheddase of EGF and BTC in mouse embryonic fibroblasts.[14] It should also be mentioned that, although ligand processing does appear to be a necessary activating event for signaling in most cases, others have shown that membrane-bound ErbB ligands can also engage in juxtacrine signaling in some model systems.[26,27] Importantly, a recent report suggests that even juxtacrine activation of the EGFR by TGF-α requires ADAM activity, perhaps because ligands that remain tethered to the plasma membrane do not have the conformational freedom to assume a functional orientation.[15,16] It is apparent that ADAMs regulate the availability of these ligands by liberating active forms and, as a result, ErbB signaling.

Dysregulation of the ErbB signaling pathways through the autocrine mechanism has been observed in numerous cancers, including breast, lung, and colon.[11,13] Overexpression of EGFR is frequent in human cancer; however, *in vitro* studies suggest that overexpression of the wild-type receptor leads to transformation only in the presence of ligand.[7,28] Accordingly, increased expression of ErbB ligands often accompanies expression of their cognate receptors in tumor cells, and autocrine activation of the EGFR pathway has been linked to resistance to therapeutic intervention and tumor metastasis resulting in a poor prognosis.[29] Of all the ErbB ligands implicated in cancer, TGF-α is the best characterized. TGF-α and EGFR are co-expressed in several types of carcinomas,[7] and expression of TGF-α, particularly in lung, ovary, and colon tumors co-expressing EGFR, correlates with a poor prognosis.[30] Autocrine expression of ErbB ligands and receptors clearly play an important role during tumor progression and in response to therapy.

It is now clear that inhibition of the ErbB pathway has considerable potential to uncouple diverse mitogenic and prosurvival inputs. Several anti-ErbB agents, including antibodies and small molecule kinase inhibitors, have been developed and recently approved to treat various human cancers.[31,32] The humanized monoclonal antibody cetuximab (Erbitux®), which can block EGFR ligand binding, has been shown to improve the survival of patients with metastatic colon cancer,[5,33] validating clinically the approach of targeting ErbB ligands in treating cancer patients. The EGFR tyrosine kinase inhibitors, gefitinib (Iressa®) and erlotinib (Tarceva®), have also shown efficacy in patients with non–small cell lung carcinomas,[32] especially in a subgroup of patients who have mutations in the EGFR kinase domain which make the kinase activity more susceptible to inhibition by these molecules.[34–36] Different from many other growth factor receptors, these mutant EGFR proteins are not constitutively active, and require ligand for their activities.[35] In addition, pulmonary adenocarcinoma specimens containing these mutant receptors showed strong expression of both TGF-α and EGF in the tumor cells, but not in the surrounding stromal cells.[37] Therefore, pulmonary adenocarcinomas with EGFR mutations are similar to more common forms of lung cancer, in which autocrine secretion of EGFR ligands by tumor cells stimulates the receptors.

Despite the efficacy of the antibodies and kinase inhibitors targeting the ErbB pathway, the majority of patients do not show long-term benefit from these therapies, and drug resistance is fairly common in the patients who have received the treatments. Data from preclinical models suggest that combining these therapies may be more effective than any single agent alone,[38–40] and it may be advantageous to simultaneously block the ErbB pathways at multiple levels. The intervention of ErbB pathways by selectively inhibiting ADAM family metalloproteases may represent a novel and effective approach for treating human cancers where the activation of ErbB pathways plays a causal role. A potent and selective ADAM inhibitor would fulfill this role by controlling the availability of multiple ErbB ligands.

Through our drug discovery efforts, we have identified selective, orally bioavailable, small molecule inhibitors against ADAM family metalloproteases. Different from other available metalloprotease inhibitors such as marimastat, our inhibitor is selective against the ADAM family but not the MMP (matrix metalloproteinase) family of metalloprotease (unpublished data). Our selective ADAM inhibitor can block shedding of a number of ErbB ligands including TGF-α and heregulin, and shows significant *in vivo* anti-tumor activities in several xenograft models. The ADAM inhibitor showed no toxicities in a four-week rodent study, including no evidence of fibroplasia (unpublished data), the dose-limiting toxicity associated with broad-spectrum matrix metalloprotease inhibitors.[41] These preliminary results suggest that our selective ADAM inhibitor is a desirable candidate to test in the clinic the idea of inhibiting ligand processing to abrogate the ErbB pathway. Clearly, strategies targeting ADAMs might be an important complement to existing anti-ErbB approaches, and potentially could be used in combination with different anti-ErbB agents.

## ACKNOWLEDGMENT

I thank Peggy Scherle for comments on the manuscript.

## REFERENCES


1. Barnes, D. & G. Sato. 1980. Serum-free cell culture: a unifying approach. Cell **22:** 649–655.
2. Sporn, M.B. & G.J. Todaro. 1980. Autocrine secretion and malignant transformation of cells. N. Engl. J. Med. **303:** 878–880.
3. Osborne, C.K. & C.L. Arteaga. 1990. Autocrine and paracrine growth regulation of breast cancer: clinical implications. Breast Cancer Res. Treat. **15:** 3–11.
4. Carpenter, G. & S. Cohen. 1990. Epidermal growth factor. J. Biol. Chem. **265:** 7709–7712.
5. Mendelsohn, J. 1997. Epidermal growth factor receptor inhibition by a monoclonal antibody as anticancer therapy. Clin. Cancer Res. **3:** 2703–2707.
6. Gschwind, A., O.M. Fischer & A. Ullrich. 2004. The discovery of receptor tyrosine kinases: targets for cancer therapy. Nat. Rev. Cancer **4:** 361–370.
7. Yarden, Y. & M.X. Sliwkowski. 2001.Untangling the ErbB signalling network. 2001. Nat. Rev. Mol. Cell. Biol. **2:** 127–137.
8. Guy, P.M., J.V. Platko, L.C. Cantley, *et al.* 1994. Insect cell-expressed p180erbB3 possesses an impaired tyrosine kinase activity. Proc. Natl. Acad. Sci. USA **91:** 8132–8136.
9. Harris, R.C., E. Chung & R.J. Coffey. 2003. EGF receptor ligands. Exp. Cell. Res. **284:** 2–13.
10. Graus-Porta, D., R.R. Beerli, J.M. Daly & N.E. Hynes. 1997. ErbB-2, the preferred heterodimerization partner of all ErbB receptors, is a mediator of lateral signaling. EMBO J. **16:** 1647–1655.
11. Mosesson, Y. & Y. Yarden. 2004. Oncogenic growth factor receptors: implications for signal transduction therapy. Semin. Cancer Biol. **14:** 262–270.
12. Zhou, B.-B. *et al.* 2005. ADAM proteases, ErbB pathways and cancer. Expert Opin. Investig. Drugs **14:** 591–606.
13. Normanno, N., C. Bianco, A. De Luca & D.S. Salomon. 2001. The role of EGF-related peptides in tumor growth. Front. Biosci. **6:** D685–707.
14. Sahin, U. *et al.* 2004. Distinct roles for ADAM10 and ADAM17 in ectodomain shedding of six EGFR ligands. J. Cell Biol. **164:** 769–779.
15. Borrell-Pages, M., F. Rojo, J. Albanell, *et al.* 2003. TACE is required for the activation of the EGFR by TGF-alpha in tumors. EMBO J. **22:** 1114–1124.
16. Blobel, C.P. 2005. ADAMs: key components in EGFR signalling and development. Nat.Rev. Mol. Cell. Biol. **6:** 32–43.
17. Gee, J.M. & J.M. Knowlden. 2003. ADAM metalloproteases and EGFR signalling. Breast Cancer Res. **5:** 223–224.
18. Peschon, J.J. *et al.* 1998. An essential role for ectodomain shedding in mammalian development. Science **282:** 1281–1284.
19. Merlos-Suarez, A., S. Ruiz-Paz, J. Baselga & J. Arribas. 2001. Metalloprotease-dependent protransforming growth factor-alpha ectodomain shedding in the absence of tumor necrosis factor-alpha-converting enzyme. J. Biol. Chem. **276:** 48510–48517.
20. Sunnarborg, S.W. *et al.* 2002. Tumor necrosis factor-alpha converting enzyme (TACE) regulates epidermal growth factor receptor ligand availability. J. Biol. Chem. **277:** 12838–12845.
21. Zhao, J. *et al.* 2001. Pulmonary hypoplasia in mice lacking tumor necrosis factor-alpha converting enzyme indicates an indispensable role for cell surface protein shedding during embryonic lung branching morphogenesis. Dev. Biol. **232:** 204–218.
22. Jackson, L.F. *et al.* 2003. Defective valvulogenesis in HB-EGF and TACE-null mice is associated with aberrant BMP signaling. EMBO J. **22:** 2704–2716.
23. Iwamoto, R. *et al.* 2003. Heparin-binding EGF-like growth factor and ErbB signaling is essential for heart function. Proc. Natl. Acad. Sci. USA **100:** 3221–3226.
24. Shi, W. *et al.* 2003. TACE is required for fetal murine cardiac development and modeling. Dev. Biol. **261:** 371–380.
25. Luetteke, N.C. *et al.* 1999. Targeted inactivation of the EGF and amphiregulin genes reveals distinct roles for EGF receptor ligands in mouse mammary gland development. Development **126:** 2739–2750.

26. BRACHMANN, R. *et al.* 1989. Transmembrane TGF-alpha precursors activate EGF/TGF-alpha receptors. Cell **56:** 691–700.
27. WONG, S.T. *et al.* 1989. The TGF-alpha precursor expressed on the cell surface binds to the EGF receptor on adjacent cells, leading to signal transduction. Cell **56:** 495–506.
28. DI MARCO, E. *et al.* 1989. Autocrine interaction between TGF alpha and the EGF-receptor: quantitative requirements for induction of the malignant phenotype. Oncogene **4:** 831–838.
29. UMEKITA, Y., Y.OHI, Y. SAGARA & H. YOSHIDA. 2000. Co-expression of epidermal growth factor receptor and transforming growth factor-alpha predicts worse prognosis in breast-cancer patients. Int. J. Cancer **89:** 484–487.
30. SALOMON, D.S., R. BRANDT, F. CIARDIELLO & N. NORMANNO. 1995. Epidermal growth factor-related peptides and their receptors in human malignancies. Crit. Rev. Oncol. Hematol. **19:** 183–232.
31. BASELGA, J. 2001. Clinical trials of Herceptin(trastuzumab). Eur. J. Cancer **37:** S18–24.
32. HERBST, R.S., M. FUKUOKA & J. BASELGA. 2004. Gefitinib—a novel targeted approach to treating cancer. Nat. Rev. Cancer **4:** 956–965.
33. GRAHAM, J., M. MUHSIN & P. KIRKPATRICK. 2004. Cetuximab. Nat. Rev. Drug Discov. **3:** 549–550.
34. PAEZ, J.G. *et al.* 2004. EGFR mutations in lung cancer: correlation with clinical response to gefitinib therapy. Science **304:** 1497–1500.
35. LYNCH, T.J. *et al.* 2004. Activating mutations in the epidermal growth factor receptor underlying responsiveness of non-small-cell lung cancer to gefitinib. N. Engl. J. Med. **350:** 2129–2139.
36. PAO, W. *et al.* 2004. EGF receptor gene mutations are common in lung cancers from "never smokers" and are associated with sensitivity of tumors to gefitinib and erlotinib. Proc. Natl. Acad. Sci. USA **101:** 13306–13311.
37. RIEMENSCHNEIDER, M.J., D.W. BELL, D.A. HABER & D.N. LOUIS. 2005. Pulmonary adenocarcinomas with mutant epidermal growth factor receptors. N. Engl. J. Med. **352:** 1724–1725.
38. MATAR, P. *et al.* 2004. Combined epidermal growth factor receptor targeting with the tyrosine kinase inhibitor gefitinib (ZD1839) and the monoclonal antibody cetuximab (IMC-C225): superiority over single-agent receptor targeting. Clin. Cancer Res. **10:** 6487–6501.
39. HUANG, S., E.A. ARMSTRONG, S. BENAVENTE, *et al.* 2004. Dual-agent molecular targeting of the epidermal growth factor receptor (EGFR): combining anti-EGFR antibody with tyrosine kinase inhibitor. Cancer Res. **64:** 5355–5362.
40. NORMANNO, N. *et al.* 2002. Cooperative inhibitory effect of ZD1839 (Iressa) in combination with trastuzumab (Herceptin) on human breast cancer cell growth. Ann. Oncol. **13:** 65–72.
41. COUSSENS, L.M., B. FINGLETON & L.M. MATRISIAN. 2002. Matrix metalloproteinase inhibitors and cancer: trials and tribulations. Science **295:** 2387–2392.

# Preclinical Modeling of Combination Treatments: Fantasy or Requirement?

SHANNON DECKER AND EDWARD A. SAUSVILLE

*University of Maryland Marlene and Stewart Greenebaum Cancer Center, Baltimore, Maryland 21201, USA*

**ABSTRACT: Combination chemotherapy is considered the "norm" in cancer chemotherapy. While the development of classical combination regimens took into account factors such as single-agent activity, different toxicity profiles, and advantageous pharmacology of the component drugs, in the era of targeted therapies there are additional considerations such as new mechanisms of resistance due to modulation of pathway dependence. Since it is not feasible to test all of the possible combinations clinically, some method for preclinically identifying and prioritizing promising combinations is necessary. While *in vivo* animal models can be used for safety testing and some pharmacokinetics, even they can quickly become prohibitively resource intensive for the purpose of efficacy determinations. Therefore, factors such as biologic rationale, reliable *in vitro* results in more than one tumor type, achievable *in vivo* pharmacology, and selectivity of primary tumor cell activity become important in the evaluation of potential combination regimens.**

**KEYWORDS: combination chemotherapy; cancer; synergy; preclinical models**

## COMBINATIONS ARE THE "NORM" IN CANCER CHEMOTHERAPY

In cancer treatment, combination chemotherapy has been found more effective than single-drug regimens and, in fact, is accepted as the "norm." Combination therapies have been the basis of the major success stories in the treatment of various cancers. Initial treatment for acute lymphoblastic leukemia (ALL) usually consists of a regimen such as vincristine, prednisone, and anthracycline with or without asparaginase, resulting in complete remissions in a large majority of cases. More than 75% of all newly diagnosed patients with adult Hodgkin's lymphoma can be cured with combination chemotherapy and/or radiation therapy. One of the most effective and least toxic chemotherapy regimens for this disease is known as ABVD and consists of a combination of adriamycin, bleomycin, vinblastine, and dacarbazine. In lung cancer, the combination of carboplatin and paclitaxel is clinically useful. Even in epithelial cancers, such as testis or adjuvant therapies for breast or colon cancers, combination therapies are standard.

Address for correspondence: Edward A. Sausville, University of Maryland Marlene and Stewart Greenebaum Cancer Center, 22 S. Greene Street, Baltimore, MD 21201. Voice: 410-328-7394; fax: 410-328-6896.
esausville@umm.edu

**Ann. N.Y. Acad. Sci. 1059: 61–69 (2005). © 2005 New York Academy of Sciences.**
**doi: 10.1196/annals.1339.024**

One empirical basis for understanding the success of certain combination therapies is that they represent pharmacologically tolerable combinations of drugs that affect the same target but that have often been selected due to different "large" organ toxicities.[1] Three of the four drugs in the ABVD regimen target DNA. While three of the four in the regimen cause decreases in white blood cells and platelets, the nonhematologic toxicities vary. Adriamycin produces cardiac toxicity, vinblastine causes neurotoxicity, and bleomycin has pulmonary side effects.

A different view of how to produce useful combination regimens suggests that in addition to having different spectra of toxicity, preferably with minimal cross resistance, other important criteria are that each of the drugs have proven efficacy as single agents, and they actually have different mechanisms of action in eliciting an antiproliferative effect.[2] Ideally, the drugs should be administered at the maximum tolerated dose for the shortest time compatible with normal cell compartment recovery. In the lung cancer regimen mentioned above, both carboplatin and paclitaxel have some single-agent activity, with carboplatin targeting DNA and paclitaxel acting on tubulin. Both drugs lower white blood cell counts and platelets, with paclitaxel having neurotoxicity as an additional side effect.

## TARGETED THERAPY AND COMBINATION DESIGN

In addition to empirical approaches to combination design, the development of targeted therapies has created the possibility for a "rational" basis for constructing combinations where the drugs are selected to affect different targets and/or circumvent resistance. For example, the use of combinations of reverse transcriptase inhibitors and protease inhibitors is the standard of care in the treatment of AIDS and seems to prevent the facile development of mutant resistant strains of the HIV virus. In this case, two distinct targets—each crucial to creating a successful viral replication cycle—convey a profound antiviral effect when coincidentally inhibited. An analogous strategy is used in the treatment of tuberculosis, which rapidly becomes resistant to monotherapy.

This rational approach to combination design requires consideration of the targets and pathways involved. For instance, one can take into account whether a linear or concentric model of target action applies (FIG. 1). In the classic linear model with a single pathway affected, a series of drugs each acting on its own component of that linear pathway could be imagined as conveying benefit when used in combination. Alternatively and somewhat more likely, the tumor could exist in a "super state" where there are multiple pathways that all contribute to tumor survival and growth. One could then design a combination drug strategy that affects each of the targets contributing to the super state.

Another method for approaching targets and pathways in the context of combination design is to consider what has been described as the six essential alterations in cell physiology in malignancy: evasion of apoptosis; self-sufficiency in growth signals; insensitivity to anti-growth signals; sustained angiogenesis; limitless replicative potential; and capacity for tissue invasion and metastasis.[3] The first three of these alterations can be thought of as the targets of more classical cancer chemotherapy agents, while the latter three are the focus of intense interest for the development of many new targeted therapies. Acting on the more "classical" targets, such as DNA

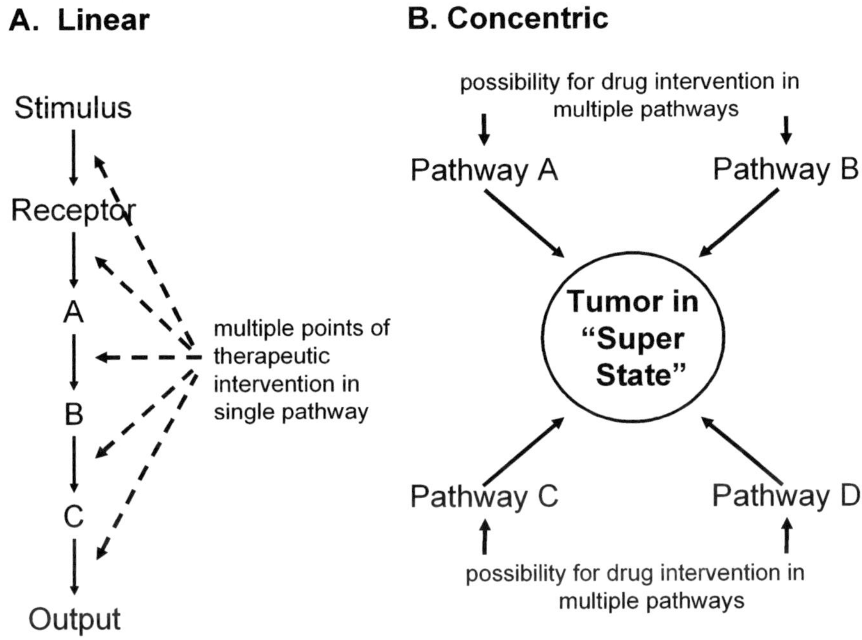


**FIGURE 1.** Models of target action. (**A**) In a classic linear model, a single pathway needs to be affected by candidate agents. (**B**) In a concentric model, multiple pathways contribute to tumor survival and growth.

or tubulin, is in essence a means of evoking a "stress response" leading to the induction of apoptosis. For DNA-interactive agents, this could mean affecting the p53 checkpoint response or p53-induced genes, while for a tubulin-targeted drug the stress evokes a mitotic checkpoint response. Useful targeted agents will also evoke a stress response depending on how important the drug's target is in sustaining an anti-apoptotic influence.

While minimal cross resistance was a desired characteristic of a classical combination regimen, inclusion of targeted therapies in combination regimens offers potential additional avenues of resistance. In addition to the classical mechanisms of drug resistance related to the drug itself, such as efflux, metabolism, and target expression, another means of resistance that arises with targeted agents is through the modulation of pathway dependence. In the super state example in FIGURE 1, if a drug affecting only pathway A were used, the tumor could alter its growth and survival so as to exist without pathway A, rendering that drug alone ineffective. This was actually recently illustrated by the development of resistance to A431 squamous cell carcinoma xenografts to anti-epidermal growth factor receptor (EGFR) monoclonal antibodies for two cycles.[4] A431 cell variants were developed from recurring resistant tumors which grew faster and were clearly less responsive to the anti-EGFR antibodies than the parental line. The investigators looked at the relative expression levels of a number of different targets in these variants, including relative VEGF expression. In five of the six resistant cell variants, VEGF expression levels were elevated relative to the parent line. These results suggest that, at least in this example, acquired resistance can develop to a targeted therapy and can proceed, in part, by selecting advantageous tumor subpopulations which upregulate a different, parallel growth-modulating pathway, in this case modifying the tumor stroma. Resistance does not appear therefore to have arisen in relation to the drug-affected pathway, but with another pathway having been called into play.

Taking into account target, pathway, and resistance issues, one could imagine designing a combination of targeted agents for the treatment of bulk tumor that consisted of an anti-proliferative, a pro-apoptotic, and an anti-vascular therapy. A recent clinical trial of an anti-vascular agent with an anti-proliferative regimen demonstrated that this sort of combination could be beneficial in a patient population.[5] The trial placed patients with previously untreated metastatic colorectal carcinoma into one of three groups: bolus IFL (5-fluorouracil, leucovorin, and irinotecan) + placebo; bolus IFL + the anti-vascular antibody bevacizumab; or 5-fluorouracil, leucovorin, and bevacizumab. The overall response rate for IFL + placebo was 34.7% with a duration of 7.1 months, while IFL + bevacizumab was 44.9% with a duration of 10.4 months (P = 0.029). Improvement was also seen in progression-free survival, 6.2 months for IFL + placebo versus 10.6 months for IFL + bevacizumab ($P < 0.00001$).

Other clinical results from the combination of classical regimens with targeted agents include those with the RAF-kinase and VEGFR inhibitor BAY43-9006. In a phase II randomized discontinuation trial in a variety of advanced solid tumors, there were no complete responses to the single agent, but partial responses in renal (35%), sarcoma (10%), thyroid (40%), and melanoma (2%).[6] A phase II trial in melanoma of BAY-43-9006 with carboplatin and paclitaxel, however, achieved 40% PR and 43% stable disease.[7] Taken together, these data raise the possibility of modulation of sensitivity *in vivo* to platinum by BAY43-9006. One potential mechanism is better delivery of the drug because of the effects of the anti-vascular compound on interstitial fluid pressure.[8]

In contrast to a classical combination regimen where each component of the regimen had some level of activity as a single agent, the possibility exists that the targeted agents may be relatively to completely inactive as single agents. Another design strategy therefore is to combine two or more anti-signaling molecules that alone may not be toxic, but in combination they affect two or more critical pathways or have an augmented effect on one pathway. For preventive therapy, a strategy that combines an anti-mutator, an anti-telomerase, and an anti-invasive could be envisioned.

## PRECLINICAL TESTING OF COMBINATIONS

Clinical trials of combination regimens are extremely expensive and time-consuming. Furthermore, the number of potential combinations is virtually unlimited. So the question is whether it is possible to determine preclinically which combinations will be effective. In April 2003, the U.S. National Cancer Institute Developmental Therapeutics Program (NCI DTP) held a workshop on defining the efficacy of combinations.[9] Some of the goals of the workshop were to attempt to determine what preclinical data would represent convincing evidence that a combination should be tested clinically, and how best to prioritize the possibilities. The outcome of the workshop suggested that one should utilize the *in vitro* data to prioritize for those regimens clearly showing synergy as opposed to mere lack of antagonism. *In vitro* data should represent more than one tumor type. There should be a biologic rationale for the combination. Ideally, evidence should exist for greater activity against tumor cells as opposed to normal cells. *In vivo* tumor efficacy of the combination was not considered necessary, although obviously a plus if present. If possible, clear evidence of likely safety in the *in vivo* models should be demonstrated. Pharmacokinetics, however, should be utilized from early human studies, where available, to model regimens that approximate non-antagonistic interactions *in vitro*. The concentrations studied *in vitro* should clearly be those that are relevant clinically.

## SYNERGY

Given the enormous number of possible combinations of drugs, the idea of prioritizing synergistic combinations and not selecting antagonistic ones is obviously desirable. Synergism in fact is almost critical to define in those situations where the single agents are relatively ineffective on their own. Defining synergy, however, is no simple matter, and a variety of techniques for doing so has been covered in great detail elsewhere.[10]

One of the more straightforward methods for determining synergy is known as fractional effect analysis, where the effect of the drugs alone is multiplied and compared with the effect of the combination at the same drug concentrations. Although simple, it has the significant limitation of assuming a linear concentration–effect relationship for each agent as well as the combination.

The isobologram representation is one of the most commonly used methods for calculating synergy. Concentration– effect curves are calculated for each drug alone and for the effect of a variable concentration of one drug in the presence of a fixed concentration of the other. The "apparent" $IC_{50}$ (50% inhibitory concentration) of the combination is then plotted, representing expected additivity. If the observed effect of the combination falls to the left of the expected curve, there is synergy and to the right, antagonism. In addition to being a very labor-intensive method that does not allow quantitation of synergism, this method also occasionally produces sigmoidal observed curves that lie on both sides of the expected curve. Although there are complicated three-dimensional response surface approaches that overcome some of the limitations of isobolograms, their complexity often dictates against them.

The well-known Chou and Talalay median-drug effect analysis is a somewhat more accessible method to overcome the sigmoidicity problem found with isobolograms.[11] The drug mixture is at constant concentration ratios so that the relative effects of each drug in the mixture are identical. The growth inhibitory effect of each drug, the sigmoidicity of the curves, and an estimated $IC_{50}$ are used to calculate a combination index (CI) that serves as a quantitative measure of synergism. This method has the advantage of allowing evaluation of drug combinations where the drugs interact in the same pathway or in completely separate pathways.

## PROBLEMS IN DESIGNING SIGNALING COMBINATIONS

Definition of synergy is by no means the only issue that remains unresolved in the design of signaling combinations in cancer treatment. We do not know yet how to diagnose the "mixture" of pathways acting in a tumor, and what would be a basis for selecting certain combination regimen drug members. Also unknown is the best time in the natural history of the tumor for intervention with agents affecting combined pathways, whether "up front" or after a certain sequence of standard and investigational therapies. It would also be useful to know whether there are any qualitative differences in the results that are achievable between certain drug types, such as antibodies versus small molecules or between different types of small molecules. If so, why and how can they be exploited?

## COMBINATIONS OF KINASE-DIRECTED AGENTS

A look at any of a number of schematic illustrations of the principal pathways involved for some of the new kinase-directed agents in development reveals the complexity of attempting to select the best possible combinations. Among the combinations of new agents that have been tried preclinically are the cyclin-dependent kinase (CDK) inhibitor flavopiridol with the erbB receptor-directed monoclonal antibody trastuzumab. Flavopiridol has been shown to inhibit CDK4 activity after cyclin D1 expression in MCF7 breast cancer cells.[12] On Western blots, cyclin D1 starts to diminish after 6 h of exposure to flavopiridol and is almost completely gone by 10 h. CDK4 activity follows slightly behind, beginning to diminish at 8 h. Effects on steady-state mRNA levels after treatment with 300 nM flavopiridol show a similar time course. Cyclin D1 is downstream of erbB2, and Nahta *et al.* demonstrated that cyclin D1 functions are essential and rate limiting for erbB2 transformation.[13] These results suggested the combination of drugs active against erbB2 and cyclin D1 (trastuzumab and flavopiridol). They found that these two drugs were synergistically cytotoxic against erbB2-positive breast cancer cell lines and that adding flavopiridol to trastuzumab synergistically lowered erbB2 levels in these cells.

The PDK1-Akt survival pathway (FIG. 2) has also been the focus of numerous drug discovery efforts. The alkylphospholipid perifosine, which is currently in clinical trials, causes almost complete loss of Akt phosphorylation on at least two key sites.[14] Perifosine was further shown to decrease plasma membrane localization of Akt at approximately 5 μM. In patients, a loading dose followed by maintenance dosing produces approximately these levels.[16,17] UCN-01 produced this effect by inhibiting the upstream kinase, PDK1. The combination of perifosine and UCN-01 was tested *in vitro* because these two drugs both produce loss of phosphorylation of Akt, but through different mechanisms.[18] Using the Chou and Talalay method, this combination was shown to be moderately synergistic. Further, cell cycle analysis of the effect of the combination showed an increase in the percentage of cells arresting in G0/G1, 87% for the combination versus 51% for controls, 52% for perifosine-treated, and 69% for UCN-01–treated.

UCN-01 was also tested *in vitro* in combination with the geldanamycin analogue 17-AAG, an antagonist of the molecular chaperone hsp90. Synergistic induction of apoptosis and loss of mitochondrial membrane potential was observed in leukemia

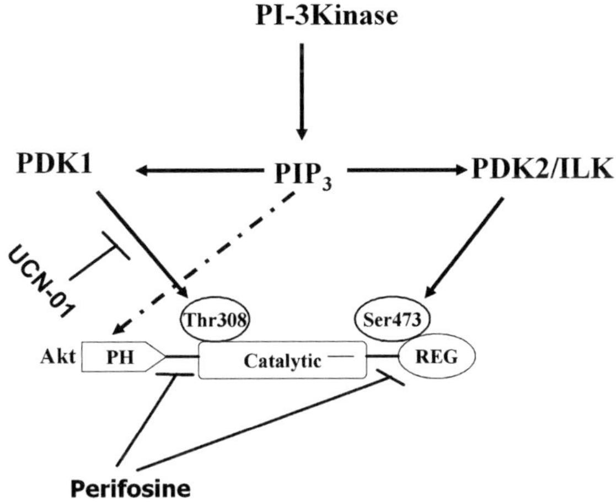


**FIGURE 2.** The PDK1-Akt survival pathway. Points of action of perifosine and UCN-01 are shown. Numerous drug discovery efforts not reviewed here have focused on various other targets in the pathway.

cells.[19] Explication of the basis of this synergy indicated that 17-AAG potentiates UCN-01 cytotoxicity and that interference with both the Akt and Raf-1/MEK/MAP kinase cytoprotective signaling pathways contributes to this effect.

## ANIMAL MODELS AND COMBINATIONS

While the above examples all demonstrate synergy *in vitro*, the question often arises whether *in vitro* combination data are sufficient to justify moving forward to human clinical trials. There are, however, a number of problems with using animal models for the assessment of combinations. An appropriately powered animal experiment with untreated controls, vehicle controls, a Drug A alone group, a Drug B alone group, and a combination group easily exceeds over 100 animals. Logistical and cost issues aside, the pharmacology in mice, or whatever species is desired, must approximate the pharmacology in humans, and even then it will be difficult to predict the pharmacokinetic interactions. One must either control for or actively design pharmacology into the study. Finally, the results can easily show not only additive or synergistic efficacy, but also additive or synergistic toxicity that may or may not be relevant to the human experience.

Animal models have both logistical and technical limitations; therefore, in attempting to define a "roadmap" to the clinic for new combination therapies, the guidelines emerging from the NCI DTP workshop on prioritizing on synergy, biologic rationale, selectivity, likely safety, and favorable pharmacokinetics can serve as an initial series of filters to weed out combinations that do not merit animal or clinical testing. Given that combination therapies have always been a major basis of success in the treatment of cancer and that the nature of the new generations of drugs that is emerging makes it even less likely that a monotherapy will suffice, it is hoped that what will materialize after applying a series of appropriate *in vitro* filters will be a select and manageable number of combination designs for more advanced testing in a clinical setting.

[COMPETING INTERESTS: Dr. Edward A. Sausville is on the Scientific Advisory Board for Kosan Biosciences and is a consultant for Kosan Biosciences and Keryx Pharmaceuticals. The author declares a competing financial interest.]

## REFERENCES


1. DEVITA, JR., V.T., R.C. YOUNG & G.P. CANELLOS. 1975. Combination versus single agent chemotherapy: a review of the basis for selection of drug treatment of cancer. Cancer **35:** 98–110.
2. ZOLI, W., L. RICOTTI, A. TESEI, *et al.* 2001. In vitro preclinical models for a rational design of chemotherapy combinations in human tumors. Crit. Rev. Oncol./Hematol. **37:** 69–82.
3. HANAHAN, D. & R.A. WEINBERG. 2000. The hallmarks of cancer. Cell **100:** 57–70.
4. VILORIA-PETIT, A., T. CROMBET, S. JOTHY, *et al.* 2001. Acquired resistance to the antitumor effect of epidermal growth factor receptor-blocking antibodies *in vivo*: a role for altered tumor angiogenesis. Cancer Res. **61:** 5090–5101.
5. HURWITZ, H., L. FEHRENBACHER, W. NOVOTNY, *et al.* 2004. Bevacizumab plus irinotecan, fluorouracil, and leucovorin for metastatic colorectal cancer. N. Engl. J. Med. **350:** 2335–2342.
6. RATAIN, M.J., K.T. FLAHERTY, W.M. STADLER, *et al.* 2004. Preliminary antitumor activity of BAY 43-9006 in metastatic renal cell carcinoma and other advanced refractory solid tumors in a phase II randomized discontinuation trial (RDT). 2004 ASCO Annual Meeting Proceedings (post-meeting edit.). J. Clin. Oncol. **22:** 4501.
7. FLAHERTY, K.T., M. BROSE, L. SCHUCHTER, *et al.* 2004. Phase I/II trial of BAY 43-9006, carboplatin (C) and paclitaxel (P) demonstrates preliminary antitumor activity in the expansion cohort of patients with metastatic melanoma. Proc. ASCO **23:** 7507.
8. GERBER, H.P. & N. FERRARA. 2005. Pharmacology and pharmacodynamics of bevacizumab as monotherapy or in combination with cytotoxic therapy in preclinical studies. Cancer Res. **65:** 671–680.
9. GITLER, M.S., A. MONKS & E.A. SAUSVILLE. 2003. Preclinical models for defining efficacy of drug combinations: mapping the road to the clinic. Mol. Cancer Ther. **2:** 929–932.
10. PETERS, G.J., C.L. VAN DER WILT, C.J.A. VAN MOORSEL, *et al.* 2000. Basis for effective combination cancer chemotherapy with antimetabolites. Pharmacol. & Ther. **87:** 227–253.
11. CHOU, T.C. & P. TALALAY. 1984. Quantitative analysis of dose-effect relationships: the combined effects of multiple drugs or enzyme inhibitors. Adv. Enzyme Regul. **22:** 27–55.
12. CARLSON, B., T. LAHUSEN, S. SINGH, *et al.* 1999. Down-regulation of cyclin D1 by transcriptional repression in MCF-7 human breast carcinoma cells induced by flavopiridol. Cancer Res. **59:** 4634–4641.
13. NAHTA, R., J.D. IGLEHART, B. KEMPKES, *et al.* 2002. Rate-limiting effects of cyclin D1 in transformation by erbB2 predicts synergy between herceptin and flavopiridol. Cancer Res. **62:** 2267–2271.
14. KONDAPAKA, S.B., S.S. SINGH, G.P. DASMAHAPATRA, *et al.* 2003. Perifosine, a novel alkylphospholipid, inhibits protein kinase B activation. Mol.Cancer Ther. **2:** 1093–1103.
15. VAN UMMERSEN, L., K. BINGER, J. VOLKMAN, *et al.* 2004. A phase I trial of perifosine (NSC 639966) on a loading dose/maintenance dose schedule in patients with advanced cancer. Clin. Cancer Res. **10:** 7450–7456.

16. Monga, M., R.A. Messmann, D. Headlee, *et al.* 2002. A phase I trial of oral perifosine in patients with refractory neoplasms. Proc. ASCO **21:** 1837.
17. Sato, S., N. Fujita & T. Tsuruo. 2002. Interference with PDK1-Akt survival signaling pathway by UCN-01 (7-hydroxystaurosporine). Oncogene **21:** 1727–1738.
18. Dasmahapatra, G.P., P. Didolkar, M.C. Alley, *et al.* 2004. In vitro combination treatment with perifosine and UCN-01 demonstrates synergism against prostate (PC-3) and lung (A549) epithelial adenocarcinoma cell lines. Clin. Cancer Res. **10:** 5242–5252.
19. Jia, W., C. Yu, M. Rahmani, *et al.* 2003. Synergistic antileukemic interactions between 17-AAG and UCN-01 involve interruption of RAF/MEK- and AKT-related pathways. Blood **102:** 1824–1832.

# Mechanisms of Trastuzumab Resistance and Their Clinical Implications

KENG-HSUEH LAN,[a] CHIEN-HSING LU,[a] AND DIHUA YU[a,b]

*Departments of Surgical Oncology[a] and Molecular and Cellular Oncology,[b] The University of Texas M.D. Anderson Cancer Center, Houston, Texas 77030, USA*

**ABSTRACT: Trastuzumab (Herceptin™) is an excellent model of rationally designed targeted cancer treatment. However, less than 35% of patients with ErbB2-positive breast tumors respond to trastuzumab as a single agent, and 2–5% of trastuzumab-treated patients suffer from severe side effects, including cardiac dysfunction. Recent progress in understanding the mechanisms of trastuzumab antitumor function and cellular defects leading to trastuzumab resistance is summarized. Also explored is the potential of combination therapies for reversing trastuzumab resistance.**

**KEYWORDS: trastuzumab; resistance; ErbB2; breast cancer; PI3K; PTEN**

Therapeutic antibodies have shown great promise as targeted cancer treatment. These rationally designed antibodies possess many potential benefits, including specific binding to cancer cells expressing the targeted antigen, effective antitumor function, and, in the case of conjugated antibodies, preferential delivery of therapeutic cargos to cancer cells.[1] Since 1995, eight therapeutic anticancer antibodies have been approved for the treatment of various human cancers, and 1998 saw the launch of trastuzumab (Herceptin™), the only FDA-approved therapeutic antibody for the treatment of advanced, chemotherapy-refractory metastatic breast cancer.

Trastuzumab is a recombinant, humanized monoclonal antibody (rhMab4D5) that binds to the extracellular domain of the transmembrane receptor tyrosine kinase, ErbB2,[2] alternatively known as HER2 (human EGFR-related) or neu. The development of trastuzumab was inspired by findings that ErbB2 is highly expressed in about 30% of ovarian and breast cancers, and patients with ErbB2 gene amplification/overexpression have a significantly worse prognosis.[3] Overexpression of ErbB2 in breast cancer cells can lead to more malignant phenotypes, including increased metastasis and therapeutic resistance.[4–6] Trastuzumab has proved to be an important option for treating patients with ErbB2-overexpressing breast cancer. It has demonstrated durable responses as a monotherapy,[7] and patients have shown improved survival when trastuzumab was given in combination with other chemotherapeutics such as Taxol.[8,9] Side effects that are commonly observed with

Address for correspondence: D. Yu, Department of Surgical Oncology, The University of Texas M.D. Anderson Cancer Center, Houston, TX 77030. Voice: 713-792-3636; fax: 713-794-4830.
dyu@mdanderson.org

**Ann. N.Y. Acad. Sci. 1059: 70–75 (2005). © 2005 New York Academy of Sciences.
doi: 10.1196/annals.1339.026**

chemotherapy, such as alopecia, mucositis, and neutropenia, are rarely seen.[7] Trastuzumab is a successful example of a rationally designed therapeutic antibody that specifically targets ErbB2-overexpressing breast cancer cells and effectively inhibits ErbB2-mediated malignant phenotypes.

## DRAWBACKS OF TRASTUZUMAB

Breast cancer patients are evaluated for ErbB2 gene amplification based on fluorescence *in situ* hybridization (FISH) before being given trastuzumab therapy. Unfortunately, despite the stringent criteria for patient selection, resistance is quite significant. The response rate for trastuzumab as a single agent remains less than satisfactory at around 35% in patients with high levels of ErbB2 overexpression.[10] This suggests that ErbB2 overexpression, though required, is not the sole determinant of how well breast tumors respond to trastuzumab. It is therefore imperative to investigate mechanisms underlying trastuzumab's antitumor activities other than those related to the inhibition of ErbB2 signaling. It is even more important to understand how some breast cancer cells evade trastuzumab's action despite the overexpression of ErbB2.

Another problem with trastuzumab treatment is that about 2–5% of patients suffer from severe side effects, such as cardiac dysfunction, and 40% suffer from other adverse side effects.[7,10] If the resistance-conferring factors could be identified and their importance established, they could serve as molecular markers for the prediction of patients' responses to trastuzumab, and patients with unfavorable expression profiles of these biomarkers could be spared the unnecessary cost and potential side effects of the treatment.[11] It would further benefit cancer patients if strategies could be developed to target these tumor markers and eventually overcome the resistance to trastuzumab.

## MECHANISMS OF TRASTUZUMAB ACTION AND RESISTANCE

Several molecular mechanisms have been proposed based on trastuzumab's action *in vitro*.[12] In brief, trastuzumab was believed to downregulate the ErbB2 receptor.[13] Trastuzumab can internalize ErbB2 and subsequently inhibit its downstream PI3K/Akt signaling pathway,[14] induce $G_1$ arrest and cyclin-dependent kinase inhibitor $p27^{kip1}$, reduce proliferation,[15] and inhibit ErbB2 ectodomain cleavage.[16] Trastuzumab also induces immune response via the interaction of its Fc domain and reduces vascular endothelial growth factor production.[15,17]

*In vivo* mechanisms of trastuzumab inhibition of ErbB2-overexpressing breast tumor progression have also been demonstrated. Trastuzumab can modulate different pro- and antiangiogenic factors to achieve angiogenesis suppression,[18] and it induces antibody-dependent cellular cytotoxicity.[19] Nevertheless, how trastuzumab executes its antitumor activity is not clearly defined and remains a fundamental question to be addressed.[20]

Several studies have contributed to better understanding of the mechanisms of resistance to trastuzumab treatment. Lu *et al.* reported that activation of the insulin-like growth factor-I receptor (IGF-IR) signaling confers resistance to the anticancer activities of trastuzumab in a human breast cancer cell line model.[21] In a later report, they described that IGF-IR signaling antagonizes the trastuzumab-induced increase of the Cdk inhibitor p27$^{kip1}$, which is an underlying molecular mechanism for IGF-IR-mediated trastuzumab resistance.[22] However, the clinical significance of IGF-IR activation in trastuzumab resistance remains to be validated in patients.

Our lab identified another pivotal ErbB2 downstream tumor-promoting pathway that can be perturbed by trastuzumab to achieve its therapeutic effect.[11] In ErbB2-overexpressing breast cancer cells, non-receptor tyrosine kinase Src is recruited to the autophosphorylated intracellular domain of the ErbB2 dimer. The constitutively activated Src in turn phosphorylates an important lipid phosphatase, PTEN (MMAC1/TEP),[23,24] on tyrosine residues within the PTEN C2 domain, preventing PTEN from translocating to the plasma membrane; thus it inhibits PTEN's phosphatase activity for dephosphorylating the phosphatidylinositol 3,4,5-triphosphate (PIP3) (FIG. 1, left). Therefore, PTEN is unable to antagonize phosphatidylinositol 3-kinase (PI3K) signaling. On the other hand, ErbB2 overexpression leads to sus-

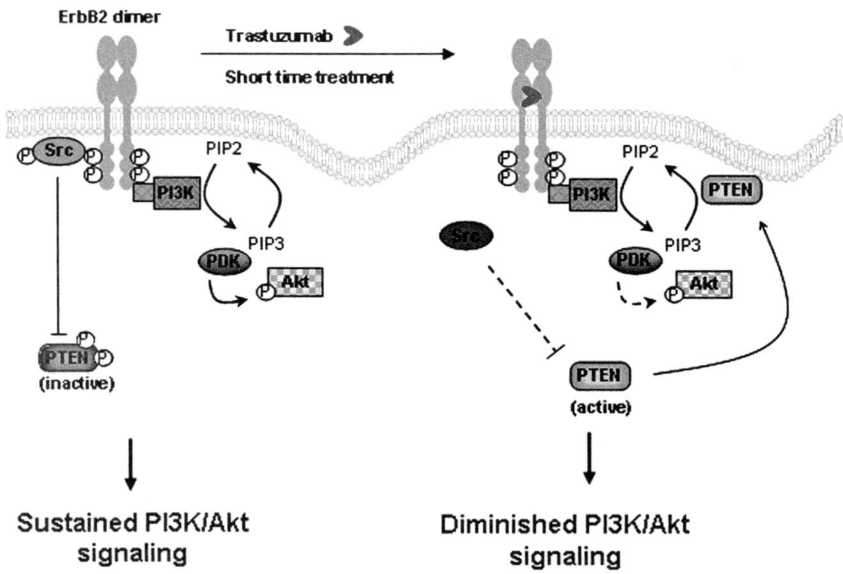


**FIGURE 1.** Mechanisms of trastuzumab's antitumor effect. (*Left*) Overexpression of ErbB2 receptor tyrosine kinase leads to homodimerization and autophosphorylation of tyrosine residues on the cytoplasmic domain. Phosphatidylinositol 3-kinase (PI3K) then associates with these phosphorylated tyrosine residues and activates downstream effectors by phosphorylating PIP2 to form PIP3. Nonreceptor tyrosine kinase Src is also recruited by these phosphorylated tyrosines and activated, which in turn phosphorylates PTEN within the C2 domain, preventing PTEN from translocating to the plasma membrane and dephosphorylating PIP3. Therefore, ErbB2-overexpressing breast tumors manifest a sustained PI3K/Akt signaling. (*Right*) Trastuzumab treatment of ErbB2-overexpressing breast cancer cells quickly dissociates Src from ErbB2, leading to decreased Src kinase activity. PTEN is hypophosphorylated and translocates to the plasma membrane and counteracts the activities of PI3K.

tained PI3K activation that activates Akt signaling, resulting in enhanced protein synthesis, cell proliferation, survival, and motility. Interestingly, trastuzumab treatment rapidly dissociates Src from ErbB2, and the concomitant decrease in Src kinase activity results in reduced PTEN tyrosine phosphorylation, allowing PTEN to translocate to the plasma membrane where it is active and can dephosphorylate PIP3 to antagonize PI3K activity. The downstream effectors of PI3K, for example, Akt and mTOR, are therefore inhibited (FIG. 1, right). This inhibitory effect occurs within minutes of trastuzumab treatment and is independent of either the inhibition of ErbB2, or the inhibition of the kinase activity of PI3K per se, both being later events of trastuzumab signaling.[11]

A functional PTEN has proved to be very important to the efficacy of trastuzumab. Reduction of PTEN protein levels using antisense oligonucleotides renders breast cancer cells resistant to trastuzumab treatment both *in vitro* and *in vivo*.[11] Most importantly, a retrospective analysis of clinical samples from breast cancer patients treated by trastuzumab plus taxane has demonstrated that PTEN deficiency in breast tumors significantly correlates with patients' poor response to trastuzumab-based therapy.[11] In other words, loss of PTEN has been associated with trastuzumab resistance in patients, so PTEN status in patient samples can be a powerful predictor for patients' response to trastuzumab.

## CLINICAL IMPLICATIONS

Loss of PTEN function leads to resistance to the therapeutic effects of trastuzumab on breast cancer cells. Since PTEN functionally antagonizes PI3K, it is highly relevant to study whether inhibiting the PI3K/Akt pathway with inhibitors may improve the anticancer efficacy of and overcome resistance to trastuzumab therapy. Both have been confirmed in our recent study.[11] The trastuzumab resistance induced by PTEN antisense oligonucleotides was overcome with pharmacological inhibitor(s) of PI3K both *in vitro* and *in vivo*. This supports the notion that the PI3K pathway is a critical driving force in breast tumor development and an ideal target of breast cancer treatment.[25] The new insights into mechanisms of action of and resistance to trastuzumab could guide the future development of agents for overcoming trastuzumab resistance and of novel targeted therapies to benefit cancer patients whose tumors overexpress ErbB2 and have loss of PTEN.[11] Indeed, multiple components of the PI3K pathway have been the molecular targets for drug development. Small-molecule compounds are being tested in preclinical studies targeting PI3K, Akt, etc.[25] Rapamycin analogues, such as RAD001 and CCI-779, specifically inhibit mTOR signaling, which is responsible for $G_1$ cell-cycle progression, protein synthesis, and linking mitogen stimulation.[26] Phase I and II clinical trials of CCI-779 and RAD001, respectively, revealed consistent antitumor activity and were well tolerated by patients.[27] Phase II trials of Akt/PKB signaling inhibitor-2, API-2/TCN, have been conducted on advanced carcinomas.[28] With the numerous promising anti-PI3K therapeutics lining up in the pipeline, we stand a good chance of defeating trastuzumab resistance by using combination therapies of trastuzumab plus inhibitors of PI3K signaling pathway. Intensive preclinical and large-scale clinical investigations are needed to develop the strategy of combining an anti-PI3K therapy with trastuzumab to benefit more cancer patients having ErbB2-overexpressing and PTEN-deficient tumors, who are among the patients with worst clinical outcome.

## FUTURE DIRECTIONS

As discussed, multiple signaling pathways contribute to resistance of breast cancers to trastuzumab treatment. The networking nature of the signal transduction makes the development of resistance almost inevitable when a treatment is applied to target certain tumor markers because tumors may readily switch over to alternative treatment-resistant mechanisms/pathways and neutralize the therapeutic effect. It is therefore worthwhile to characterize the expression profiles of the biomarkers involved in determining trastuzumab antitumor activities, for example, PTEN, and IGF-IR, together with the levels of ErbB2, in tumor biopsy specimens from individual patients so that a formulated combination treatment can be delivered accordingly. In order to routinely assess the profiles of molecular markers in tumor tissue, a standardized procedure for sample collection and a validated assay need to be developed. Then, rationally designed targeted therapies would be tailored (as opposed to "one-size-fits-all") based on the tumor expression profiles that potentially are more effective but less toxic, and hold the promise of overcoming the challenge that has existed since the dawn of anticancer treatment, that is, *resistance*.

## ACKNOWLEDGMENTS

We would like to thank Dr. Ming Tan and Dr. Kristine Klos for their valuable suggestions and critical review. We also apologize to those authors whose work is not cited due to space constraints.

## REFERENCES

1. Ross, J.S., D.P. Schenkein, *et al.* 2004. Targeted therapies for cancer 2004. Am. J. Clin. Pathol. **122:** 598–609.
2. Carter, P., L. Presta, *et al.* 1992. Humanization of an anti-p185HER2 antibody for human cancer therapy." Proc. Natl. Acad. Sci. USA **89:** 4285–4289.
3. Slamon, D.J., G.M. Clark, *et al.* 1987. Human breast cancer: correlation of relapse and survival with amplification of the HER-2/neu oncogene. Science **235:** 177–182.
4. Yu, D., T. Jing, *et al.* 1998. Overexpression of ErbB2 blocks Taxol-induced apoptosis by upregulation of p21Cip1, which inhibits p34Cdc2 kinase. Mol. Cell **2:** 581–591.
5. Yu, D. & M.C. Hung. 2000. Overexpression of ErbB2 in cancer and ErbB2-targeting strategies. Oncogene **19:** 6115–6121.
6. Tan, M., T. Jing, *et al.* 2002. Phosphorylation on tyrosine-15 of p34(Cdc2) by ErbB2 inhibits p34(Cdc2) activation and is involved in resistance to Taxol-induced apoptosis. Mol. Cell **9:** 993–1004.
7. Cobleigh, M.A., C.L. Vogel, *et al.* 1999. Multinational study of the efficacy and safety of humanized anti-HER2 monoclonal antibody in women who have HER2-overexpressing metastatic breast cancer that has progressed after chemotherapy for metastatic disease. J. Clin. Oncol. **17:** 2639–2648.
8. Esteva, F.J., V. Valero, *et al.* 2002. Phase II study of weekly docetaxel and trastuzumab for patients with HER-2-overexpressing metastatic breast cancer. J. Clin. Oncol. **20:** 1800–1808.

9. SHAWVER, L.K., D. SLAMON, *et al.* 2002. Smart drugs: tyrosine kinase inhibitors in cancer therapy. Cancer Cell **1:** 117–123.
10. VOGEL, C.L., M.A. COBLEIGH, *et al.* 2002. Efficacy and safety of trastuzumab as a single agent in first-line treatment of HER2-overexpressing metastatic breast cancer. J. Clin. Oncol. **20:** 719–726.
11. NAGATA, Y., K.H. LAN, *et al.* 2004. PTEN activation contributes to tumor inhibition by trastuzumab, and loss of PTEN predicts trastuzumab resistance in patients. Cancer Cell **6:** 117–127.
12. NAHTA, R. & F.J. ESTEVA. 2003. HER-2-targeted therapy: lessons learned and future directions. Clin. Cancer Res. **9:** 5078–5084.
13. HUDZIAK, R.M., G.D. LEWIS, *et al.* (1989). p185HER2 monoclonal antibody has antiproliferative effects in vitro and sensitizes human breast tumor cells to tumor necrosis factor. Mol. Cell. Biol. **9:** 1165–1172.
14. YAKES, F.M., W. CHINRATANALAB, *et al.* 2002. Herceptin-induced inhibition of phosphatidylinositol-3 kinase and Akt Is required for antibody-mediated effects on p27, cyclin D1, and antitumor action. Cancer Res. **62:** 4132–4141.
15. SLIWKOWSKI, M.X., J.A. LOFGREN, *et al.* 1999. Nonclinical studies addressing the mechanism of action of trastuzumab (Herceptin). Semin. Oncol. **26:** 60–70.
16. MOLINA, M.A., J. CODONY-SERVAT, *et al.* 2001. Trastuzumab (herceptin), a humanized anti-Her2 receptor monoclonal antibody, inhibits basal and activated Her2 ectodomain cleavage in breast cancer cells. Cancer Res. **61:** 4744–4749.
17. KLOS, K.S., X. ZHOU, *et al.* 2003. Combined trastuzumab and paclitaxel treatment better inhibits ErbB-2-mediated angiogenesis in breast carcinoma through a more effective inhibition of Akt than either treatment alone. Cancer **98:** 1377–1385.
18. IZUMI, Y., L. XU, *et al.* 2002. Tumour biology: herceptin acts as an anti-angiogenic cocktail. Nature **416:** 279–280.
19. ALBANELL, J., J. CODONY, *et al.* 2003. Mechanism of action of anti-HER2 monoclonal antibodies: scientific update on trastuzumab and 2C4. Adv. Exp. Med. Biol. **532:** 253–268.
20. BASELGA, J. & J. ALBANELL 2001. Mechanism of action of anti-HER2 monoclonal antibodies. Ann. Oncol. **12 Suppl 1:** S35–41.
21. LU, Y., X. ZI, *et al.* 2001. Insulin-like growth factor-I receptor signaling and resistance to trastuzumab (Herceptin). J. Natl. Cancer Inst. **93:** 1852–1857.
22. LU, Y., X. ZI, *et al.* 2004. Molecular mechanisms underlying IGF-I-induced attenuation of the growth-inhibitory activity of trastuzumab (Herceptin) on SKBR3 breast cancer cells. Int. J. Cancer **108:** 334–341.
23. LI, J., C. YEN, *et al.* 1997. PTEN, a putative protein tyrosine phosphatase gene mutated in human brain, breast, and prostate cancer. Science **275:** 1943–1947.
24. STECK, P.A., M.A. PERSHOUSE, *et al.* 1997. Identification of a candidate tumour suppressor gene, MMAC1, at chromosome 10q23.3 that is mutated in multiple advanced cancers. Nat. Genet. **15:** 356–362.
25. MILLS, G.B., E. KOHN, *et al.* 2003. Linking molecular diagnostics to molecular therapeutics: targeting the PI3K pathway in breast cancer. Semin. Oncol. **30:** 93–104.
26. HUANG, S., M.A. BJORNSTI, *et al.* 2003. Rapamycins: mechanism of action and cellular resistance. Cancer Biol. Ther. **2:** 222–232.
27. DANCEY, J.E. 2002. Clinical development of mammalian target of rapamycin inhibitors. Hematol. Oncol. Clin. North Am. **16:** 1101–1114.
28. FEUN, L.G., J.A. BLESSING, *et al.* 1993. A phase II trial of tricyclic nucleoside phosphate in patients with advanced squamous cell carcinoma of the cervix. A Gynecologic Oncology Group Study. Am. J. Clin. Oncol. **16:** 506–508.

# Regulation of Cancer Cell Survival by Par-4

PADHMA RANGANATHAN[a] AND VIVEK M. RANGNEKAR[a,b,c,d]

*Graduate Center for Toxicology,[a] Departments of Radiation Medicine[b] and Microbiology, Immunology and Molecular Genetics,[c] and Markey Cancer Center,[d] University of Kentucky, Lexington, Kentucky 40536, USA*

**ABSTRACT: Prostate apoptosis response-4 (Par-4) is a unique pro-apoptotic protein that selectively induces apoptosis in cancer cells. Moreover, Par-4 sensitizes cells to the action of diverse apoptotic stimuli and causes tumor regression. This review discusses the prominent structural and functional features of Par-4 and the multiple levels of regulation of its apoptotic function, all of which can be utilized to develop targeted cancer therapy.**

**KEYWORDS: Par-4; apoptosis; cancer**

## INTRODUCTION

It was recently reported that cancer has now surpassed heart disease as the leading cause of death in the United States. While a number of therapeutic approaches in clinical trial are yielding success, many treatment strategies are not. The frequency of successful treatment depends upon the suitability of the therapeutic strategy to the type, grade, and stage of the disease. Although tumors of each organ differ widely in their genetic makeup and microenvironment, common features shared by all transformed cells offer potential targets for therapy.

A cell becomes cancerous, or is transformed, when it taps into its potential for uncontrolled cell division. Such unrestricted division can result from the cell responding to promiscuous signals for proliferation and by the cell evading its intrinsic defenses of growth arrest and apoptosis. Although strategies that negate these transforming events may be therapeutically successful, tumor regression and complete therapy could be easily and efficiently achieved if all the cells are able to reinstate a functional apoptotic response. The purpose of this review is to provide an overview of Par-4, a protein that executes apoptosis selectively in cancer cells and is therefore a likely therapeutic candidate for anticancer strategies.

## IDENTIFICATION AND CHARACTERIZATION OF PAR-4

Prostate cancer, one of the most common forms of cancer in the United States, is usually treated by androgen-ablation, which results in tumor regression by

Address for correspondence: Vivek M. Rangnekar, Ph.D., Department of Radiation Medicine, University of Kentucky, Combs Research Building, Rm. 303, 800 Rose Street, Lexington, KY 40536. Voice: 859-257-2677; fax: 859-257-9608.

vmrang01@pop.uky.edu

**Ann. N.Y. Acad. Sci. 1059: 76–85 (2005). © 2005 New York Academy of Sciences.**

**doi: 10.1196/annals.1339.046**

apoptosis. The prostate tumor consists of a mixed population of androgen-dependent and -independent cells. Androgen withdrawal results in the initiation of an apoptotic response in the androgen-dependent cells, which rely on a steady supply of hormones for their survival.

In the androgen-dependent cells, the cell-death program is triggered by the induction of gene expression in response to intracellular calcium elevation on androgen withdrawal; this response is bypassed in the androgen-independent cells and thereby results in the survival of this population of cells. Accordingly, this therapeutic approach, in some cases, generates an aggressive relapse because the few androgen-independent cells, which did not undergo apoptosis, are essentially selected for. The androgen-independent cells can be forced to undergo apoptosis in cell culture paradigms when intracellular calcium levels are increased with the treatment of the calcium ionophore, ionomycin. This apoptotic program can be abolished if transcription or translation inhibitors, such as actinomycin or cyclohexamide, are used, indicating that gene induction is necessary.

Par-4 was first cloned by inducing the rat androgen-independent prostate cells, AT-3, with ionomycin to undergo apoptosis. Using the differential hybridization strategy, Par-4 was identified as a member of a new set of genes that are transcribed in response to calcium elevation. Similarly, Par-4 expression has been observed during the involution of rat ventral prostate by apoptosis following castration, and this Par-4 induction was duly inhibited on pretreatment with the calcium-channel blocker, nifedepine.[1] Par-4 expression was also inhibited by testosterone in the ventral prostate. Neither induction nor repression of Par-4 was observed in the liver, kidneys, or other organs that bear androgen receptors yet do not undergo apoptosis in response to castration. In addition, in the initial studies, Par-4 was induced in cell culture models exclusively by apoptotic signaling and not during necrosis, growth arrest, or serum stimulation.

Par-4 is evolutionarily conserved in vertebrates and is ubiquitously expressed in tissues of ectodermal, mesodermal, and endodermal origin. Par-4, however, is absent from specific cell types (such as lymphocytes, certain smooth muscle cells, the differentiated ductal cells of the prostate, the epithelial cells of the mammary gland, and the terminally differentiated cells of the retina), thus indicating that Par-4 is down-regulated during differentiation.[2] Aligned with the fact that Par-4 is an apoptotic protein, its expression is increased during development in actively dying cells, such as the interdigitating web cells of the mouse embryo and the involuting tadpole tail. Par-4 also plays a key role in neuronal development, where an increase in Par-4 levels results in apoptosis and serves to maintain the number of neurons in the nervous system.[3]

The Par-4 gene produces a 38-kDa protein consisting of 332 amino acids. This protein has a variety of interesting structural domains that allude to its potential mechanism of action. Par-4 has a 42-residue leucine zipper domain in its C-terminus, along with a nuclear export sequence (NES). Two putative nuclear localization sequences (NLS) are present in the amino-terminus, and both NLS are highly conserved in the Par-4 protein among different species. In addition, Par-4 possesses a number of conserved consensus sites for phosphorylation by kinases, such as PKA and PKC, as illustrated in FIGURE 1. Collectively, the presence of these motifs suggests that the function of Par-4 may be tightly regulated by post-translational modification, localization, and dimerization with partners of biological consequence.

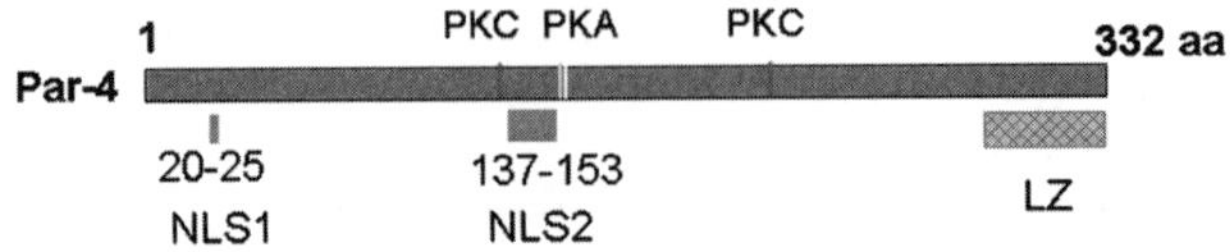


**FIGURE 1.** Schematic representation of the Par-4 protein domain structure and phosphorylation sites. The domains NLS1 (nuclear localization sequence), NLS2, and leucine zipper (LZ) are represented by *bars* underlining the region. Putative PKA and PKC phosphorylation sites are indicated.

## PRO-APOPTOTIC ROLE OF PAR-4

The role of Par-4 in apoptosis has been well studied in cell culture models. Overexpression studies have revealed that an increase in Par-4 level or activity in normal or immortalized cells results in a lowered sensitivity threshold to death stimuli (such as growth factor withdrawal, elevation of intracellular $Ca^{2+}$, TNF-α, IFNγ, or UV, X-ray, and gamma irradiation). In addition, Par-4 has been found to be an essential downstream regulator of cell-death programs initiated by different agents such as TRAIL, vincristine, doxorubicin, and radiation. In transformed cells, Par-4 is capable of initiating the death program in the absence of a second stimulus. Interestingly, strong oncogenic or growth-promoting factors render tumor cells susceptible to Par-4–induced apoptosis. This ability of Par-4 to effect apoptosis exclusively in cancer cells is intriguing and indicates that Par-4 has merit as a potent therapeutic tool.

While most studies have focused on ectopic overexpression of Par-4, under specific conditions endogenous Par-4 expression is also powerful as an apoptotic agent. Beyond the aforementioned role of Par-4 in the tadpole tail and interdigitating web, Par-4 plays a role in neuronal apoptosis during embryonic development and serves to prevent hyperproliferation of nerve tissue.[3] This is achieved by the asymmetric distribution of Par-4 protein during the mitosis of neuronal progenitor cells; the daughter cells lacking Par-4 differentiate into neurons, while those with high levels of Par-4 undergo apoptosis.[4] A recent study demonstrated that this function of Par-4 can be exploited during neural transplant to beget selective apoptosis of pluripotent stem cells and enrich the neuronal precursors among this population of embryonic stem cells.[5]

It is well established that normal physiological processes can become skewed during the onset of a disease and thereby augment the disease process. Several observations support the fact that Par-4 is also involved in the development of neurodegenerative disorders by increasing the apoptosis of healthy neurons. First, elevated levels of Par-4 mRNA and protein have been observed in the apoptotic neurons of patients, animal models, and cell culture models of diseases such as Alzheimer's, Parkinson's, Huntington's chorea, amyotrophic lateral sclerosis (ALS), and ischemic brain injury or stroke.[3,6] Second, Par-4 is also thought to facilitate the development of such degenerative conditions by inhibiting the uptake of choline at the cholinergic synapse.[7] Finally, it was recently reported that Par-4 is involved in the regulation of the protease that cleaves the amyloid beta precursor protein to give Aβ peptide, the key pathogenic protein in Alzheimer's.[8]

In addition to apoptosis, Par-4 has been identified as playing a non-apoptotic role in various cell types. One such example is the role of Par-4 in the modulation of immune response by keeping in check the secretion of IL-2 and other important immunomodulatory cytokines.[9] Because this role of Par-4 is beyond the scope of this review, it will not be discussed further.

## MECHANISM OF APOPTOSIS BY PAR-4

Programmed cell death usually occurs through one of the two major signaling pathways, known as the extrinsic and the intrinsic pathway. The extrinsic pathway proceeds through death receptors while the intrinsic pathway is mediated by the mitochondria. The extrinsic pathway is initiated at the cell surface via the activation of transmembrane death receptors of the CD95 (Apo-1 or Fas)/TRAIL/tumor-necrosis factor (TNF) receptor 1 family. Engagement of these receptors with their cognate ligand triggers the assembly of a multiprotein complex that activates the upstream caspase 8. In the intrinsic pathway, reception of a stress/death signal is transduced to the mitochondria, which in turn release cytochrome ***c*** into the cytosol; this results in the formation of the apoptosome complex to activate caspase 9. Caspases 8 and 9 both activate downstream effector caspases that carry out the final steps of apoptosis, such as release of the endonuclease CAD (caspase-activated DNAase) from its inhibitor iCAD and cleavage of key cellular enzymes and proteins[10] Although the intrinsic and extrinsic pathways ultimately converge at the level of the effector caspases, molecular cross talk between the two pathways is known to exist. A number of factors—both pro-apoptotic factors that drive the cell toward suicide and pro-survival proteins that protect the cell from death—are involved in regulating apoptosis at each level of this signaling cascade.

Since Par-4 is a pro-apoptotic protein, it sets the cell-death program in motion by acting at two levels: the activation of molecular components of the cell-death machinery and the inhibition of pro-survival factors. Par-4, as characterized to date, appears to act through the extrinsic pathway by enabling the trafficking of Fas and Fas ligand to the plasma membrane. Fas (CD95) is a member of the TNF-R family and is activated by binding to Fas ligand. Such binding leads to the formation of a complex consisting of trimeric Fas, the adaptor protein FADD (Fas-associated death domain) and pro-caspase 8; this complex is called the death-inducing signaling complex, or DISC. The formation of DISC in turn leads to the cleavage and activation of the zymogen, pro-caspase 8, to its active caspase form. Interestingly, Par-4 translocates Fas and FasL to the plasma membrane in androgen-independent cancer cells, in which overexpression of Par-4 leads directly to death. However, the same effect is not observed in the androgen-dependent cancer cells, wherein Par-4 serves only to sensitize. The mechanism of apoptosis when Par-4 has a sensitizing effect may involve the intrinsic pathway or may vary depending on the second signal.[11]

As previously mentioned, in addition to its effect on the extrinsic pathway, Par-4 also plays a very important role in antagonizing the pro-survival/anti-apoptotic factors that present a major obstacle to the apoptosis cascade. One of the most important anti-apoptotic factors active in a cell is the transcription factor NF-κB. NF-κB is a heterodimer consisting of p65 (RelA) and p50 subunits. This dimer is held inactive in the cytoplasm as a result of being bound to the inhibitory protein IκB, which on the appropriate signal is phosphorylated by IKKβ, ubiquitinated, and ultimately degraded to release an active NF-κB. Following other phosphorylation events and translocation into the nucleus, the active NF-κB transcription factor binds to the promoter of its target genes and regulates transcription. One of the very important anti-apoptotic targets of NF-κB is the XIAP (X-linked inhibitor of apoptosis), which hinders the activity of both upstream and effector caspases.[12,13] Par-4 inhibits NF-κB activity and this Par-4–mediated inhibition of NF-κB is carried out without disrupting the DNA-binding capacity of the NF-κB complex. It is proposed that Par-4 acts in the nucleus to inhibit phosphorylation of NF-κB by IKKβ or PKCζ,which would otherwise confer maximal activity to NF-κB. In addition, interference with IKKβ phosphorylation of the IκB complex in the cytoplasm acts as another molecular safeguard against the activation of NF-κB.[14] This ability of Par-4 to inhibit pro-survival factors might be essential to its apoptosis-sensitizing function.

## CANCER ANTAGONISM BY PAR-4

Consistent with its role in apoptosis, Par-4 has a tumor-suppressive function. Although the function of Par-4 in apoptosis is an important component of a cell's anti-transformation surveillance,[15] Par-4 also exerts considerable influence in its tumor-suppressive role. In support of its role in tumor suppression, Par-4 is downregulated in a variety of cancers, such as renal-cell carcinomas, neuroblastoma, acute lymphoblastic leukemia, and chronic lymphocytic leukemia.[16,17] Moreover, Par-4 mRNA and protein are downregulated by oncogenic Ras in a variety of cell types through the MEK-ERK pathway.[18,19] This downregulation is necessary for Ras to initiate transformation because ectopic overexpression of Par-4 in Ras-transformed cells impedes formation of colonies in a soft agar assay.[18] This anti-transformation effect may be attributed to the fact that Par-4 antagonizes the Ras–MAPK pathway by repressing ERK, an essential downstream kinase in this pathway.[18] This function of Par-4 is independent of its pro-apoptotic ability although oncogenic Ras is known to sensitize cells to apoptosis by Par-4.[20]

In addition to inhibiting transformation, Par-4 plays a role in tumor regression; hence, Par-4 is antagonistic to both tumor formation and tumor maintenance. Subcutaneous tumors, which were generated in nude mice using PC-3 cells, regressed in less than 3 weeks after a single injection of Par-4 adenovirus.[11] In another study, Par-4 overexpression decreased tumor development in xenotransplants of A375-C6 melanoma cells in mice; tumor reduction was due to an increase in apoptosis.[21] This effect of Par-4 is due to its pro-apoptotic function because both activation of the Fas pathway and inhibition of NF-κB are essential for tumor regression.[11] Tumors expressing either dn-FADD (an inhibitor of the Fas pathway) or RelA (resulting in an active NF-κB) are resistant to the tumor-regressive effects of Par-4.[11] Par-4 has been recently implicated in the suppression of tumors in hematopoietic stem cells by disrupting the BCR-Abl signaling pathway.[22] In addition, Par-4 may be a player in the control of metastasis as well because Par-4 inhibited the migration of B16F1 melanoma cells by acting as a negative regulator of PKC kinase activity.[23] Collectively, the data discussed above validate Par-4 as a viable target for therapeutic intervention in cancer treatment.

## REGULATION OF PAR-4 FUNCTION

Given the pro-apoptotic function of Par-4, it is essential for the cell to tightly regulate its activity, thereby keeping Par-4 in a dormant state and activating it only when necessary. Consequently, regulation is managed by localizing Par-4 to distinct cellular compartments. It was observed during Par-4 overexpression studies that Par-4 is translocated to the nucleus well before the cell undergoes apoptosis. Inhibition of nuclear entry abrogated the apoptotic potential of Par-4. As mentioned earlier, Par-4 contains two putative NLS at its amino-terminus. A deletion mutant that lacks both of these nuclear localization sequences is incapable both of nuclear entry and promoting apoptosis. Additional deletion analysis indicated that the first NLS (NLS1) was not necessary for nuclear entry and that the second NLS (NLS2) plays an important role in nuclear translocation. Consistent with these results, it was observed that in androgen-dependent cancer cells (in which Par-4 is unable to induce apoptosis), Par-4 is predominantly localized in the cytoplasm. In contrast, nuclear localization of Par-4 is the norm in androgen-independent cancer cells, as well as many other cancer cells; in these cells, Par-4 has a lethal effect. The functional role of the nuclear export sequence present in the C-terminus has yet to be elucidated. Furthermore, there are substantial data indicating the presence of Par-4 in the PML bodies (promyelocytic leukemia bodies) of the nucleus. Although the significance of this localization remains to be clarified, it is possible that the Par-4 mechanism of apoptosis specifically resides in the PML bodies.[17] Control of Par-4 function cannot be ascribed to the regulation of its localization alone and, as explained below, there are additional mechanisms through which its activity is monitored.

Par-4 that is present in the cytoplasm is partnered with various proteins, and many of the functions of Par-4 can be attributed to the effect of these interactions. One of the very important and extensively studied partners of Par-4 is the kinase, PKCζ. [24] Par-4 binds to PKCζ and inhibits its major functions, not the least among them being activation of NF-κB. PKCζ-induced activation of NF-κB is lost in the presence of equal or excess amounts of Par-4. This effect on PKCζ is the key to NF-κB inhibition by Par-4, although this does not preclude the existence of other mechanisms. To add further complexity to this equation, another protein, p62, is sometimes bound to the Par-4/ PKCζ complex. When p62 interacts with the Par-4/ PKCζ complex, the effect of Par-4 on PKCζ is lost and, as a result, cell survival is promoted.[25]

Another important partner for Par-4 is the Wilms' tumor protein, WT-1.[26] WT-1 is a transcription factor that possesses a zinc finger and acts as either an activator or repressor for many growth factor genes. WT-1 protein is expressed during development in the kidney, testis, and ovary and plays an important role in the development of Wilms' tumor, as its name suggests. WT-1 induces the transcription of the anti-apoptotic protein Bcl2; this transcriptional activity is inhibited when Par-4 is bound to WT-1. Par-4, along with WT-1, binds to the promoter of Bcl2, inhibits transcription, and thereby promotes apoptosis.[27] Par-4 regulates the function of WT-1 during the transcription of other genes as well; however, the significance of these regulations has yet to be studied.

Par-4 also binds to ZIP kinase (also known as ZIPK or DLK) in the PML bodies. This interaction is necessary for ZIPK-induced apoptosis[28] because Par-4 promotes interactions between ZIPK and DAXX, which is a regulator of apoptosis. In addition, Par-4 complexes with THAP-1, a pro-apoptotic protein that is also associated with the PML subnuclear bodies.[29] These Par-4 interactions with ZIPK, DAXX, and THAP-1 all function to catalyze apoptosis, and it is likely that these associations are mediated by the C-terminal leucine zipper domain of Par-4, which is essential for the pro-apoptotic function of this protein.[30] Beyond the binding interactions detailed here, there may be other binding partners of Par-4 for which identity and function are yet to be elucidated.

## CANCER-SELECTIVE APOPTOSIS

Since Par-4 is subject to regulation at multiple levels, a study was undertaken to identify the minimum region of Par-4 essential for apoptosis induction, and this search ultimately led to the discovery of Par-4's remarkably unique property of cancer-selective apoptosis. Deletion analysis was used to identify the minimum essential domain that would facilitate apoptosis and yet be free of inhibitory interactions. Par-4, which contains 332 amino acids, was progressively and selectively pared to make a variety of small mutants. In the course of this study, a mutant comprising the region spanning amino acids 137–195 was identified as the core domain that orchestrates the apoptotic function of Par-4. Upon further deletion up to the amino acid 187 (thus a fragment consisting of amino acids 137–187), the apoptotic function was lost. It was also observed that the small 137–195 domain was constitutively nuclear and caused selective apoptosis of cancer cells upon overexpression. Therefore, this 137–195 mutant is now called SAC for selective apoptosis of cancer cells.[31]

SAC, which localized to the nucleus both in normal and cancer cells, caused apoptosis only in cancer cells when overexpressed. This led to the conclusion that, in addition to nuclear entry, an activating event that is present only in cancer cells is necessary for Par-4 to attain its full apoptotic potential. The SAC region contains a few phosphorylation sites, and so the possibility of phosphorylation as a potential regulator was studied. Two amino acids, a serine at 154 and a threonine at 155 are consensus sites for PKA (protein kinase A). PKA is a universal kinase that phosphorylates a wide range of substrates that are involved in the regulation of metabolism, cell growth, and differentiation. Elevation of intracellular levels of cAMP (cyclic adenosine monophosphate) results in the activation of PKA and the transduction of a signal downstream via phosphorylation. PKA occurs in two isoforms, I and II, depending on the regulatory subunit that is associated with the kinase. Isoform I is overexpressed in human cancer cells and primary tumors and, consequently, the PKA enzymatic activity is higher in transformed cells than in normal or immortalized cells.[32] This enhanced PKA activity may explain the cancer-specific activation of Par-4. Indeed, further studies revealed that phosphorylation by PKA is a crucial event that triggers the apoptotic function of Par-4; in the absence of this phosphorylation, Par-4 completely lost it ability to effect apoptosis.

To further clarify the regulation of Par-4, the PKA consensus serine (154) and threonine (155) were individually mutated to alanine in order to eliminate phosphorylation at these sites. It was found that a mutation at the 155 residue abolished-apoptosis by Par-4, while the Par-4-154A mutant retained its apoptotic ability. SAC with 155 mutated, although still nuclear in localization, was unable to kill transformed and androgen-independent cell types such as NIH3T3/Ras, lung cancer cells

A549, H460, H157, and H838 and breast cancer cells MCF-7, MDAMB-231, and MDAMB-435. Phosphorylation of ectopically expressed Par-4 by PKA has been confirmed by metabolic labeling, while phosphorylation of endogenous Par-4 has been established using an antibody raised against the phospho-threonine residue at 155. These experiments reveal that Par-4 is phosphorylated in its active state and that this phosphorylation event is very common in cancer cells when compared to normal cells. Additional experiments, including the inhibition of phosphorylation of Par-4 (and thus apoptosis) with an inhibitory peptide and the provision of cAMP to normal cells in order to make them susceptible to apoptosis by Par-4, support the fact that Par-4 is controlled at several levels in the cell.[33]

Par-4–inducible apoptosis can now be explained by the model that Par-4 requires two distinct events—specifically, nuclear entry and phosphorylation by PKA—for activation. Both regulating events are present and active in cells that display sensitivity to Par-4. In cells that are resistant to Par-4, such as hormone-dependent cancer cells and normal or immortalized cells, one or both of these activating events are absent, and, despite the presence of substantial amounts of Par-4, the cells remain resistant to apoptosis. This activation scheme is illustrated in FIGURE 2.

Although studies so far have revealed much about the regulation and the mechanism of action of Par-4, it is likely that Par-4 acts in more complex ways than can be

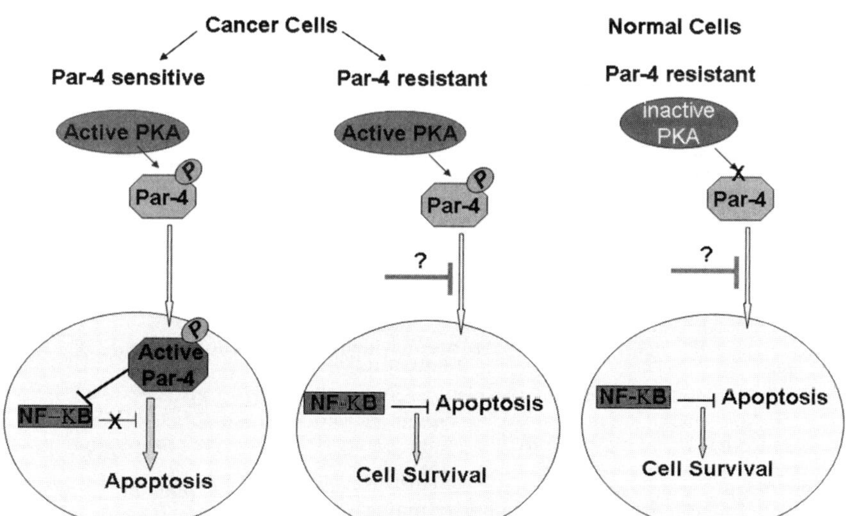


**FIGURE 2.** Model for cancer-selective apoptosis by Par-4. Two independent events are necessary to activate Par-4—nuclear entry and phosphorylation by PKA. In normal or immortalized cells, owing to low levels of active PKA, Par-4 is not phosphorylated at the T155 residue; in addition, it is retained in the cytoplasm by an unknown mechanism, and hence Par-4 is inactive. In cancer cells that are resistant to apoptosis by Par-4, despite phosphorylation at the T155 residue, Par-4 is inhibited from entering the nucleus by pro-survival factors. In cancer cells sensitive to Par-4, it is phosphorylated by PKA at T155 and the inhibition by pro-survival factors is absent. Par-4, which is thus activated by phosphorylation and nuclear entry, causes apoptosis of cancer cells.

accounted for by the pathways detailed thus far. Studies are ongoing to examine systems that might inactivate the high levels of endogenous Par-4 present in cancer cells and to dissect the mechanism of tumor antagonism. Based on knockout data with regard to immunological relevance and our own studies with tumor regression in mice, it can be safely reasoned that Par-4 has several functions in addition to apoptosis; attempts are being made to delineate these functions as well. Par-4 is clearly emerging as a tumor suppressor that would be ideal for therapeutic intervention strategies, keeping in mind that each small effort, as is the case with all cancer research, takes us one step closer to understanding the genesis of cancer and the ultimate goal of developing a superior oncotherapy.

## ACKNOWLEDGMENTS

This study was supported by Grants CA60872, CA105453, and CA84511 from the National Institutes of Health/National Cancer Institute (to V.M.R.).

## REFERENCES

1. SELLS, S.F. *et al.* 1994. Commonality of the gene programs induced by effectors of apoptosis in androgen-dependent and -independent prostate cells. Cell Growth Differ. **5:** 457–466.
2. BOGHAERT, E.R. *et al.* 1997. Immunohistochemical analysis of the proapoptotic protein Par-4 in normal rat tissues. Cell Growth Differ. **8:** 881–890.
3. EL-GUENDY, N. & V.M. RANGNEKAR. 2003. Apoptosis by Par-4 in cancer and neurodegenerative diseases. Exp. Cell Res. **283:** 51–66.
4. BIEBERICH, E. *et al.* 2003. Regulation of cell death in mitotic neural progenitor cells by asymmetric distribution of prostate apoptosis response 4 (PAR-4) and simultaneous elevation of endogenous ceramide. J. Cell Biol. **162:** 469–479.
5. BIEBERICH, E. *et al.* 2004. Selective apoptosis of pluripotent mouse and human stem cells by novel ceramide analogues prevents teratoma formation and enriches for neural precursors in ES cell-derived neural transplants. J. Cell Biol. **167:** 723–734.
6. MATTSON, M.P. *et al.* 1999. Par-4: an emerging pivotal player in neuronal apoptosis and neurodegenerative disorders. J. Mol. Neurosci. **13:** 17–30.
7. XIE, J. & Q. GUO. 2004. Par-4 inhibits choline uptake by interacting with CHT1 and reducing its incorporation on the plasma membrane. J. Biol. Chem. **279:** 28266–28275.
8. XIE, J. & Q. GUO. 2005. Par-4 is involved in regulation of beta-secretase cleavage of the Alzheimer's amyloid precursor protein. J. Biol. Chem. **280**: 13824–13832.
9. LAFUENTE, M.J. *et al.* 2003. Regulation of mature T lymphocyte proliferation and differentiation by Par-4. EMBO J. **22:** 4689–4698.
10. STRASSER, A., L. O'CONNOR & V.M. DIXIT. 2000. Apoptosis signaling. Annu. Rev. Biochem. **69:** 217–245.
11. CHAKRABORTY, M. *et al.* 2001. Par-4 drives trafficking and activation of Fas and Fasl to induce prostate cancer cell apoptosis and tumor regression. Cancer Res. **61:** 7255–7263.
12. BALDWIN, A.S., JR. 1996. The NF-kappa B and I kappa B proteins: new discoveries and insights. Annu. Rev. Immunol. **14:** 649–683.
13. BARKETT, M. & T.D. GILMORE. 1999. Control of apoptosis by Rel/NF-kappaB transcription factors. Oncogene **18:** 6910–6924.
14. DIAZ-MECO, M.T. *et al.* 1999. Inactivation of the inhibitory kappaB protein kinase/nuclear factor kappaB pathway by Par-4 expression potentiates tumor necrosis factor alpha-induced apoptosis. J. Biol. Chem. **274:** 19606–19612.
15. HANAHAN, D. & R.A. WEINBERG. 2000. The hallmarks of cancer. Cell **100:** 57–70.

16. BOEHRER, S. *et al.* 2001. Deregulated expression of prostate apoptosis response gene-4 in less differentiated lymphocytes and inverse expressional patterns of par-4 and bcl-2 in acute lymphocytic leukemia. Hematol. J. **2:** 103–107.
17. GURUMURTHY, S. & V.M. RANGNEKAR. 2004. Par-4 inducible apoptosis in prostate cancer cells. J. Cell. Biochem. **91:** 504–512.
18. QIU, S.G. *et al.* 1999. Negative regulation of Par-4 by oncogenic Ras is essential for cellular transformation. Oncogene **18:** 7115–7123.
19. BARRADAS, M. *et al.* 1999. The downregulation of the pro-apoptotic protein Par-4 is critical for Ras-induced survival and tumor progression. EMBO J. **18:** 6362–6369.
20. NALCA, A. *et al.* 1999. Oncogenic Ras sensitizes cells to apoptosis by Par-4. J. Biol. Chem. **274:** 29976–29983.
21. LUCAS, T. *et al.* 2001. Differential expression levels of Par-4 in melanoma. Melanoma Res. **11:** 379–383.
22. KUKOC-ZIVOJNOV, N. *et al.* 2004. Prostate apoptosis response gene-4 (par-4) abrogates the survival function of p185(BCR-ABL) in hematopoietic cells. Exp. Hematol. **32:** 649–656.
23. SANZ-NAVARES, E. *et al.* 2001. Atypical protein kinase Czeta suppresses migration of mouse melanoma cells. Cell Growth Differ. **12:** 517–524.
24. DIAZ-MECO, M.T. *et al.* 1996. The product of par-4, a gene induced during apoptosis, interacts selectively with the atypical isoforms of protein kinase C. Cell **86:** 777–786.
25. CHANG, S., J.H. KIM & J. SHIN. 2002. p62 forms a ternary complex with PKCzeta and PAR-4 and antagonizes PAR-4-induced PKCzeta inhibition. FEBS Lett. **510:** 57–61.
26. JOHNSTONE, R.W. *et al.* 1996. A novel repressor, par-4, modulates transcription and growth suppression functions of the Wilms' tumor suppressor WT1. Mol. Cell. Biol. **16:** 6945–6956.
27. QIU, G. *et al.* 1999. Mutually exclusive expression patterns of Bcl-2 and Par-4 in human prostate tumors consistent with down-regulation of Bcl-2 by Par-4. Oncogene **18:** 623–631.
28. PAGE, G. *et al.* 1999. Interaction partners of Dlk/ZIP kinase: co-expression of Dlk/ZIP kinase and Par-4 results in cytoplasmic retention and apoptosis. Oncogene **18:** 7265–7273.
29. ROUSSIGNE, M. *et al.* 2003. THAP1 is a nuclear proapoptotic factor that links prostate-apoptosis-response-4 (Par-4) to PML nuclear bodies. Oncogene **22:** 2432–2442.
30. SELLS, S.F. *et al.* 1997. Expression and function of the leucine zipper protein Par-4 in apoptosis. Mol. Cell. Biol. **17:** 3823–3832.
31. EL-GUENDY, N. *et al.* 2003. Identification of a unique core domain of Par-4 sufficient for selective apoptosis induction in cancer cells. Mol. Cell. Biol. **23:** 5516–5525.
32. TORTORA, G. & F. CIARDIELLO. 2002. Protein kinase A as target for novel integrated strategies of cancer therapy. Ann. N.Y. Acad. Sci. **968:** 139–147.
33. GURUMURTHY, S. *et al.* 2005. Phosphorylation of Par-4 by protein kinase A is critical for apoptosis. Mol. Cell. Biol. **25:** 1146–1161.

# *Morphogenics* as a Tool for Target Discovery and Drug Development

NICHOLAS C. NICOLAIDES, WOLFGANG EBEL, BRAD KLINE, QIMIN CHAO, ERIC ROUTHIER, PHILIP M. SASS, AND LUIGI GRASSO

*Morphotek Inc., Exton, Pennsylvania 19342, USA*

ABSTRACT: **Mutations in DNA mismatch repair (MMR) genes lead to genetically hypermutable cells. Germline mutations in MMR genes in man have been linked to the genetic predisposition to hereditary nonpolyposis colon cancer and a number of other inherited and sporadic malignancies. The ability to modulate the MMR process (referred to as *morphogenics*) in model systems offers a powerful tool for generating functional diversity in cells and multicellular organisms via the perpetual genomewide accumulation of randomized point and slippage mutation(s). *Morphogenics* is a platform process that employs a dominant negative MMR gene to create genetic diversity within defined cellular systems and results in a wide range of phenotypes, thus enabling the development and improvement of pharmaceutical products and the discovery of new pharmaceutical targets. Libraries of *morphogenics*-derived siblings are generated through random mutagenesis from naturally occurring DNA polymerase-induced mutations that occur during DNA replication. Morphogenic cells are screened in high-throughput assays to identify subclones with desired phenotypes for pathway discovery and/or product development. *Morphogenics* has been successfully applied to a wide range of hosts, including mammalian cells, transgenic mice, plants, yeast, and bacteria. Manipulation of these systems via *morphogenics* has led to the discovery of novel disease-associated phenotypes in targeted model systems. Moreover, *morphogenics* has been successfully applied to antibody-producing cell lines to yield subclones producing antibodies with enhanced binding affinities for therapeutic use, as well as to derive subclones with enhanced titers that are suitable for scaleable manufacturing. The selective manipulation of the MMR process via *morphogenics* is a platform technology that offers many advantages for the discovery of druggable targets, as well as for the development of novel pharmaceutical products.**

KEYWORDS: **mismatch repair; mutagenesis; PMS2; MORPHOGENE; *morphogenics;* systems biology**

## THE MISMATCH REPAIR DNA SPELL-CHECKING SYSTEM

Mismatch repair (MMR) is a ubiquitous, evolutionarily conserved DNA repair process whose function is the post-replicative correction of misincorporated base pairs introduced by DNA polymerase during replication. The process involves a

Address for correspondence: Nicholas C. Nicolaides, Morphotek Inc., 210 Welsh Pool Road, Exton, PA 19342. Voice: 610-423-6100; fax: 610-423-6199.
nicolaides@morphotek.com

**Ann. N.Y. Acad. Sci. 1059: 86–96 (2005). © 2005 New York Academy of Sciences.**
**doi: 10.1196/annals.1339.029**

group of gene products, including the *mutS* homologues *MSH2, MSH3,* and *MSH6/GTBP* and the *mutL* homologues *MLH1*, *MLH3, PMS1*, and *PMS2* that work in concert to correct mispaired mono-, di-, and trinucleotides and point mutations that occur during DNA synthesis.[1,2] FIGURE 1 shows a schematic diagram of the MMR process. Several reports have documented that a recessive germline mutation(s) in any of the MMR genes results in defective MMR, leading to genomewide point mutations and instability of mono-, di- and trinucleotide repeats, a feature referred to as microsatellite instability (MI). In humans, genetic defects in the MMR machinery results in a mutator phenotype and predisposition to hereditary nonpolyposis colon

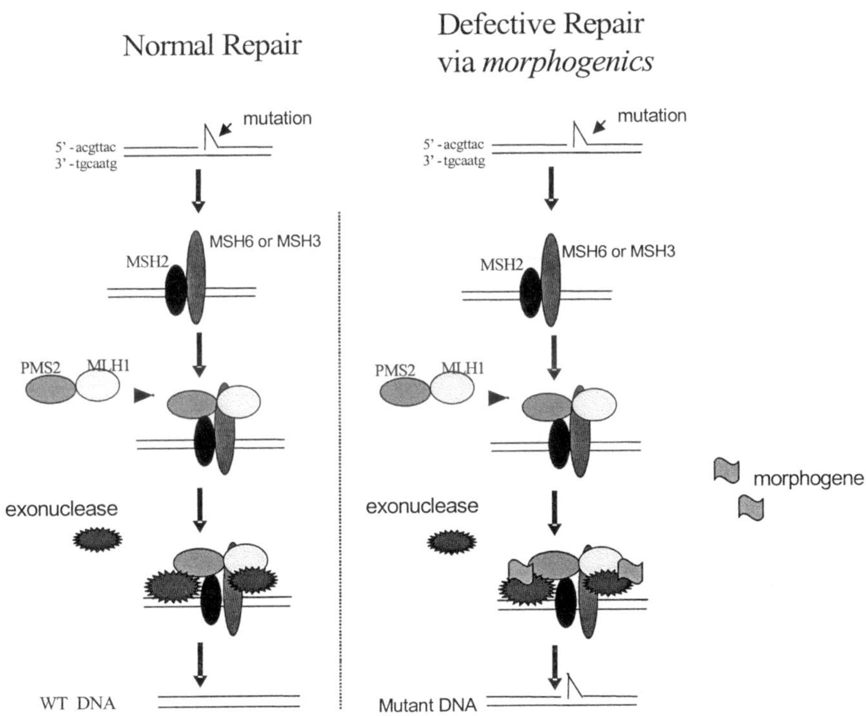


**FIGURE 1.** The mismatch repair system. MMR corrects single base-pair mismatches and larger loops of mismatched DNA that result from polymerase-induced mutations during DNA replication. The MSH2 subunit surveys newly replicated DNA for mismatched base pairs. It forms a complex with either the MSH6 or MSH3, depending on the number of mismatched nucleotides. A second heterodimeric complex (MLH1/PMS2) then binds to the complex and recruits exonuclease to excise the mispaired nucleotides and the lesion is repaired by DNA polymerase. *Morphogenics* employs a dominant negative MMR protein, referred to as the MORPHOGENE, to inhibit MMR activity within a target cell host. The MORPHOGENE is a truncated mutant of PMS2 that is able to dominantly interfere with the MMR activity allowing for the inheritance of mutations to daughter cells.

cancer (HNPCC), a disease in which tumors retain a diploid genome but have widespread point mutations and MI.[3] Though the mutator defect that arises from MMR deficiency can affect any DNA sequence, microsatellite sequences are particularly sensitive to defective MMR.[4] MI is therefore a useful indicator for monitoring MMR activity in cells. In addition to its occurrence in virtually all tumors arising in patients with HNPCC, MI is found in a fraction of sporadic tumors with distinctive molecular and phenotypic properties that has been attributed to defective MMR.[5] Interestingly, karyotypic analysis of tumors arising from MMR deficiency have found that these tumors retain a pseudodiploid genome in contrast to the highly aneuploid genomes observed in the majority of sporadic cancers. This observation suggests that defective MMR-occurring mutagenesis can effect transformation without incorporating gross aberrations into the genome of the cell.

The genome of MMR-defective cells exhibits a wide spectrum of mutations (point mutations, insertions, deletions, recombination, etc.) as shown by genetic analysis of a diverse array of organisms ranging from but not limited to unicellular microbes such as bacteria and yeast to more complex organisms such as drosophila, plants, and mammals.[6–10] Inhibiting MMR in a targeted host cell or organism can lead to the generation of genetically altered offspring or sib cells exhibiting *de novo* phenotypes. The ability to reversibly regulate MMR offers the potential to generate genetic diversity within a model host organism. The diverse phenotypes exhibited by the offspring of MMR-deficient organisms are useful for studying molecular pathways of disease for target discovery and systems biology, as well as for developing cell hosts producing improved biological pharmaceuticals, including antibodies.

Here we characterize a method called *morphogenics* that reversibly regulates MMR function in mammalian cells to yield genetically evolved sibs exhibiting *de novo* phenotypes for gene discovery and product development. The process involves the use of a dominant negative MMR gene, referred to as the MORPHOGENE, which can inhibit endogenous MMR activity across a wide array of organisms (N. Nicolaides, personal observation). The MORPHOGENE is a truncated version of the full-length PMS2 MMR gene product. PMS2 was identified in a subset of kindreds that developed HNPCC (unpublished data).[11] The molecular structure of the MORPHOGENE comprises the first 133 amino acids of human PMS2 and represents the most conserved domain of the mutL family of proteins. The highly conserved nature of the aminoterminus among different species has been noted for organisms as disparate as bacteria and mammals, suggesting an important role of the N-terminal domain in exerting MMR functions.[11–12] TABLE 1 shows the homology of the MORPHOGENE with the amino-terminal regions of mutL proteins from different species. A key feature of *morphogenics* is the reversible nature of this process, whereby genetic hypermutability is induced by expressing the MORPHOGENE and then suppressed by removing the MORPHOGENE in selected sibs once the desired phenotype has been selected. We have engineered vectors that allow the regulated expression of the MORPHOGENE in targeted host cells, thereby increasing genetic diversity within these cells and consequently yielding a genetically diverse pool of sib cells that can be functionally screened to identify those exhibiting desirable phenotypes. *Morphogenics* offers a robust method for creating genetic diversity in virtually any cell host to develop model systems to study target pathways involved in normal or diseased states, as well as the use of cell hosts for the discovery and manufacturing of biologically based drugs.

**TABLE 1. Homology of MORPHOGENE to other mutL proteins**

| Organism | Accession No. | % Identity to the MORPHOGENE |
|---|---|---|
| *Mus musculus* | NP_032912 | 89 |
| *Rattus norvegicus* | XP_213712 | 88 |
| *Drosophila melanogaster* | AAC19245 | 71 |
| *Arabidopsis thaliana* | AAL01156 | 58 |
| *Schizosaccharomyces pombe* | NP_594417 | 59 |
| *Plasmodium yoelii* | EAA20769 | 58 |
| *Danio rerio* | AAH55651 | 50 |
| *Xenopus laevis* | AAH44098 | 49 |
| *Caenorhabditis elegans* | NP_505933 | 44 |
| *Escherichia coli* | NP_418591 | 42 |
| *Staphylococcus aureus* | NP_374412 | 42 |

NOTE: A list of proteins with amino-terminal homology to the MORPHOGENE and percent identity are provided. Corresponding accession number is provided for reference to the NCBI database.

## REGULATING MISMATCH REPAIR TO INCREASE GENETIC DIVERSITY IN MAMMALIAN CELL HOSTS FOR TARGET DISCOVERY AND PRODUCT DEVELOPMENT

The reversible regulation of MMR via *morphogenics* results in an accelerated rate of genetic evolution within a host organism due to the ability of the process to obtain a wide spectrum of mutations within virtually any gene or genes. Genetic stability of the evolved host is established by restoring the MMR activity within a selected sib cell. This is accomplished by utilizing expression vectors that can reversibly control the intracellular expression of the MORPHOGENE gene product. Several expression vectors were evaluated for their ability to regulate MORPHOGENE expression. Surprisingly, most inducible systems were found to be "leaky" in the uninduced state and resulted in low-level expression of the MORPHOGENE which was sufficient to perturb MMR activity. In order to avoid the "leaky" phenomenon, we engineered a mammalian expression vector that produced robust levels of MORPHOGENE and has the ability to be negatively selected out from the genome of sibs exhibiting a desired phenotype(s). Removing the MORPHOGENE from the genome is critical to avoid further genetic drifting of the cell carrying the phenotype of interest. For example, the expression vector (p-MOR) was engineered to contain a neomycin-resistance gene as a positive selection marker plus a bicistronic gene containing the MORPHOGENE linked to the herpes simplex virus–thymidine kinase (HSV-tk), which serves as a negative selection marker. FIGURE 2 shows a schematic diagram of the salient features of this vector. Transfection of the p-MOR plasmid into mammalian cells has demonstrated the ability to generate robust MORPHOGENE expression in all cell lines tested from a variety of species (FIG. 2B).

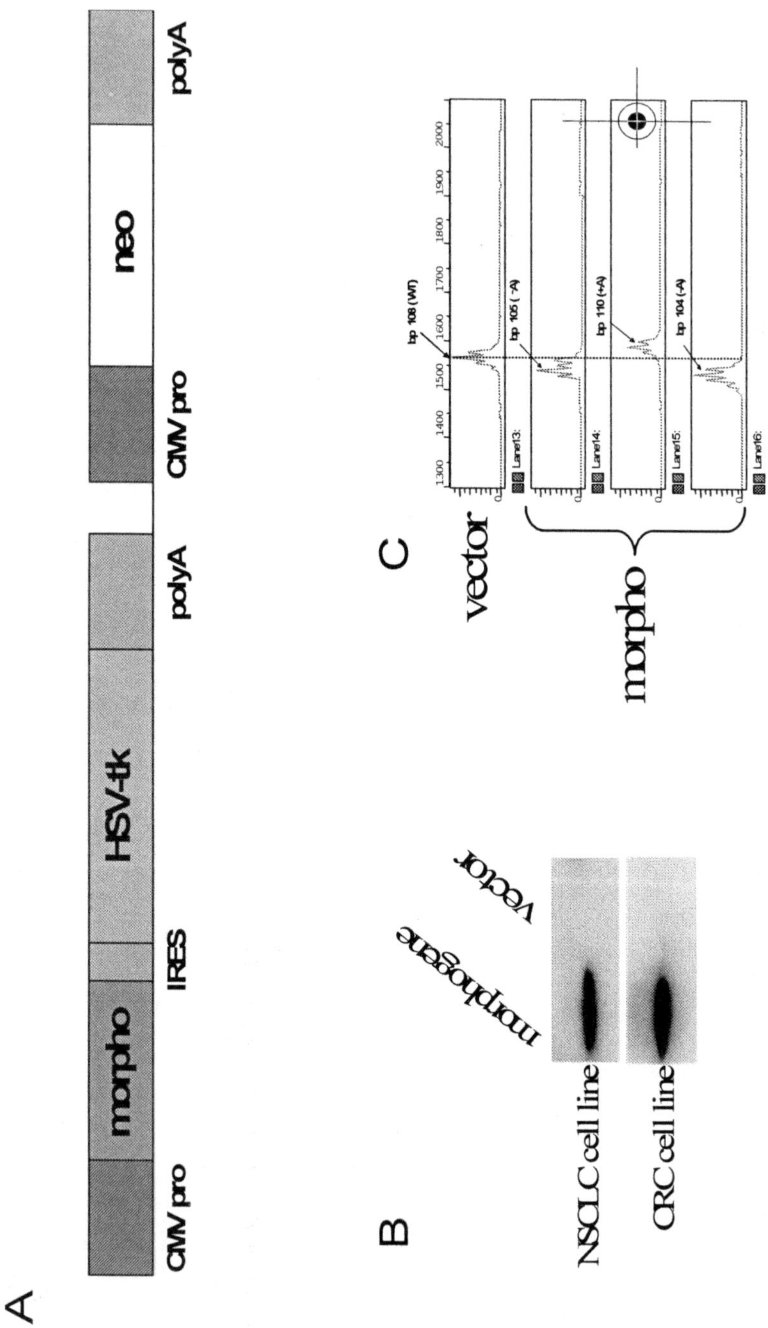


**FIGURE 2.** *See following page for legend.*

Furthermore, expression of the MORPHOGENE by the p-MOR vector was shown to enhance genetic hypermutation as determined by the induction of MI in p-MOR–containing cells as compared to the parental wild-type cell line (FIG. 2C). Genetic stability in evolved sibs is restored using negative selection to identify sib cells that are MORPHOGENE null due to intragenic homologous recombination. Ganciclovir is a prodrug that is converted into a cytotoxic agent by HSV-tk. Therefore, MORPHOGENE and HSV-tk–expressing cells die in the presence of ganciclovir while those cells that have lost the MORPHOGENE vector survive. Negatively selected ("cured") clones are then validated for stability by assaying for the MORPHOGENE message by reverse transcriptase-polymerase chain reaction (RT-PCR) and the MORPHOGENE vector by PCR analysis of genomic DNA. The elimination of the MORPHOGENE from the genome of selected sib cells is demonstrated by the analyses shown in FIGURE 3. RT-PCR was carried out using primers specific for the MORPHOGENE message, while amplification of the endogenous actin mRNA served as an internal control. Similarly, genomic analysis was performed by PCR using primers that are specific for the MORPHOGENE and the endogenous actin gene. The absence of contraction or expansion in microsatellite markers demonstrated the restoration of genetic stability of the cell host after curing of the MORPHOGENE (data not shown).

To demonstrate the utility of *morphogenics* to enhance mammalian cell evolution, two cellular systems were employed. The first system involved the use of a recombinant mammalian cell line expressing an MMR-sensitive reporter gene target while the second cellular system explored the ability of *morphogenics* to mutate an endogenous gene locus within a mammalian cell host. The p-MOR vector was introduced into the MMR-proficient human embryonic kidney 293 (HEK293) cell line contain-

---

**FIGURE 2.** Regulated mammalian expression vectors to reversibly control MMR. **Panel A:** A mammalian expression vector (p-MOR) was constructed that contains the PMS134–dominant negative MMR gene (MORPHOGENE, referenced as morpho) linked to the herpes simplex virus thymidine kinase (HSV-tk) gene as a negative selection marker. An internal ribosome entry site (IRES) was inserted between the morpho and HSV-tk genes to ensure efficient translation of the bicistronic message. The gene was cloned into a plasmid containing the neomycin resistance (neo) gene for positive selection. A number of human and rodent cell lines have been transfected and shown by Western blot to produce detectable amounts of the MORPHOGENE gene product. A control vector (p-VEC) contains all of the same elements of p-MOR except for the MORPHOGENE. **Panel B** is a representative example of MORPHOGENE expression in two different human cancer cell lines. Cells were transfected with p-MOR or p-VEC and screened for plasmid uptake of the linked neo gene by G418 selection. Neo-resistant clones were then analyzed for MORPHOGENE expression by Western blotting using a monoclonal antibody that is specific to the MORPHOGENE gene product (L. Grasso, personal observation). As shown in **panel B**, p-MOR cells expressed robust steady-state levels of the MORPHOGENE product. **Panel C** shows a representative genetic analysis of cells expressing the MORPHOGENE whereby MI is observed in cells transfected with the p-MOR vector that is not observed in parental wild-type or p-VEC transfected cells. MI is a hallmark of MMR deficiency and is characterized by the shifting of mono-, di-, and trinucleotide repeats in the genome of the cell. For MI analysis, the BAT-26 marker was used to assess stability in a MMR-proficient cancer cell line as described.[18] Cells transfected with the p-MOR vector showed altered BAT-26 alleles differing by as much as two added or three subtracted nucleotides (FIG. 2C). The *black line* represents the marker size of the parent cell.

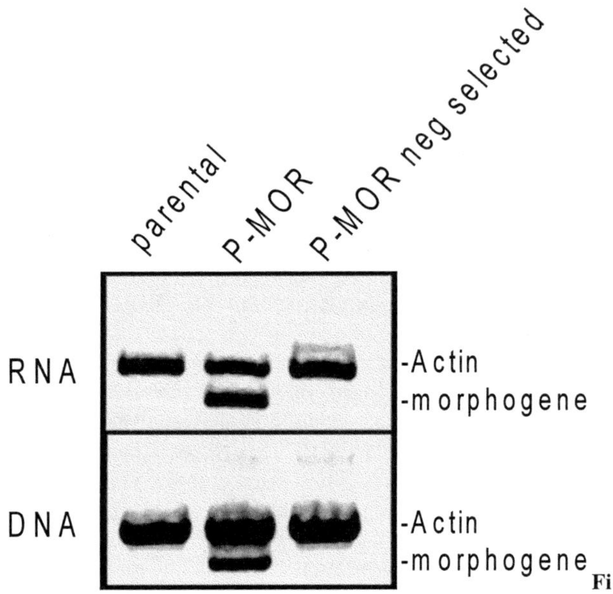


**FIGURE 3.** Restoring MMR via negative selection. Morphogenic sib cells exhibiting *de novo* phenotypes are genetically stabilized by negatively selecting ("curing") subclones that have spontaneously lost the p-MOR vector via recombination. To carry out negative selection, $4 \times 10^7$ cells are grown in the presence of 40 μM of the prodrug ganciclovir, which is converted into the toxin ganciclovir triphosphate by the HSV-tk gene product. Cells that no longer contain the p-MOR vector or lose expression of the HSV-tk gene are able to grow in the presence of the nontoxic prodrug, while those expressing the HSV-tk gene die due to the cytotoxic effect of the converted compound. In **panel A,** MORPHOGENE steady-state RNA expression is shown in parental cells, sib-selected p-MOR cells, and negatively selected p-MOR cells. RNA was isolated from cells and analyzed for MORPHOGENE expression by RT-PCR as described.[11] Actin was used as a positive control to ensure integrity of materials and proper reaction conditions. DNA was isolated from cells and analyzed for presence of MORPHOGENE by PCR as described.[11] As shown, robust MORPHOGENE expression was observed in p-MOR transfected cells while no expression was observed in the parental wild-type or the cured p-MOR cells. Genomic analysis revealed loss of MORPHOGENE from the genome of the cured cell. Microsatellite analysis of morphogenic and cured clones found the ability of these cells to retain their selected phenotype while the cured clones no longer exhibit MI (not shown).

ing the pCAR-OF reporter gene vector that allows monitoring of the MMR activity within a living cell.[11] The pCAR-OF reporter (out-of-frame) contains a hygromycin-resistance gene plus a β-galactosidase gene containing a 58-bp out-of-frame poly(C-A) tract at the 5′ end of its coding region. The pCAR-OF reporter does not generate β-galactosidase activity unless a frame-restoring mutation (i.e., insertion or deletion) arises due to defective MMR activity. The reporter construct pCAR-IF (in-frame) is identical to pCAR-OF with the exception that the poly(C-A) tract is 54 bp and therefore does not disrupt the β-galactosidase translational reading frame and serves as a positive control. Cells transfected with the p-MOR or p-VEC vectors were selected

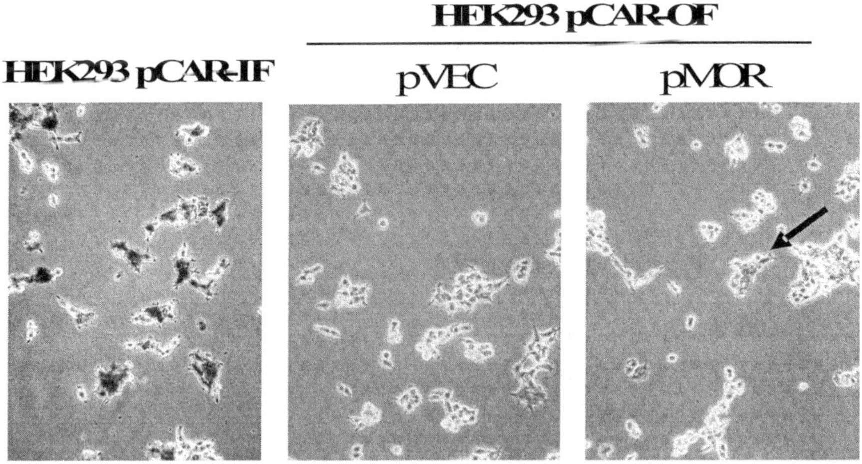


**FIGURE 4.** *Morphogenics* evolves recombinant genes in mammalian cells. HEK293 cells expressing the pCAR-OF (out-of-frame β-galactosidase) or pCAR-IF (in-frame β-galactosidase) were transfected with the p-MOR or p-VEC (same as p-MOR but does not contain the MORPHOGENE) vectors by electroporation and were selected for p-MOR or p-VEC uptake. At 17 days after transfection, cells were analyzed *in situ* for β-galactosidase activity to assay for frame-restoring mutations within the pCAR-OF reporter gene in p-MOR or p-VEC transfected cells as described.[11] In brief, cells were washed in PBS and fixed in 1% glutaraldehyde in phosphate-buffered saline and incubated in 0.15 M NaCl 1 mM, $MgCl_2$ 3.3 mM, $K_4Fe(CN)_6$ 3.3 mM, $K_3Fe(CN)_6$ 0.2% 4-chloro-3-bromo-2-indolyl-β–D-galactopyranoside (X-Gal) for 2 h at 37°C and visualized by microscopy. Shown above is a representative sampling of data showing the presence of frame-restoring mutations in the β-galactosidase (*arrows*) in p-MOR transfected cells that are not observed in p-VEC cells. As control, HEK293 cells expressing the pCAR-IF (HEK293 pCAR-IF) are used to ensure robustness of the assay.

for neomycin drug resistance and screened *in situ* for β-galactosidase activity 17 days after transfection. FIGURE 4 shows representative data whereby restoration of β-galactosidase activity was observed after MORPHOGENE transfection in contrast to control vector-transfected cells. Molecular analysis of endogenous polynucleotide repeats within the reporter vector found these elements to be hypermutable as confirmed by the presence of insertion and deletions within the C-A repeat (data not shown).

A second cellular system was used to show the applicability of *morphogenics* to evolve endogenous gene loci of a cell host. The p-MOR vector was introduced into an MMR-proficient Chinese hamster ovary (CHO) cell line to monitor for mutations within the X-chromosome-linked hypoxanthine phosphoribosyltransferase (HPRT) locus. The frequency with which mutants arise in cell cultures provides an indication of the mutation rate.[13] HPRT-null mutants are conveniently identified by their ability to grow in the presence of the purine analogue, 6-thioguanine (6-TG). CHO cells were first positively selected for HPRT expression in HAT medium (selects for functional HPRT activity) to remove any HPRT-null sibs that arise from spontaneous mu-

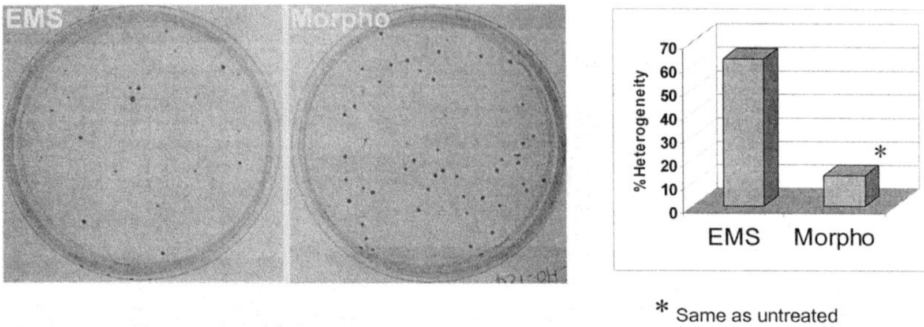


**FIGURE 5.** *Morphogenics* can evolve endogenous genes in mammalian cells. To demonstrate the ability of *morphogenics* to evolve endogenous gene loci, MMR-proficient Chinese hamster ovary (CHO) cells were transfected with the p-MOR or p-VEC vectors. Stable cultures were then plated at 100,000 cells/mL in the presence of 7 μg/mL 6-TG and scored for HPRT mutations by the presence of foci at day 10. As a control, CHO cells were also treated with ethanemethylsulfonate (EMS) to ensure the ability of the assay to detect HPRT mutants and to compare the mutagenesis activity of *morphogenics* to chemical mutagenesis. As shown above, *morphogenics* (morpho) treatment yielded similar numbers of resistant foci as observed using EMS; however, the foci established via *morphogenics* appeared hardier and more homogeneous in morphology and size in contrast to the more heterogeneous morphology of the foci derived using the chemical mutagen. While genotoxicity made the expansion of HPRT mutant colonies obtained via EMS treatment problematic, the mutant clones obtained via *morphogenics* were genetically stable and could be expanded with virtually no loss of cell viability.

tations after extended culturing.[14] HAT-selected CHO cells were then transfected with p-MOR or p-VEC and stable cultures were selected for null-mutations within the HPRT locus by screening for survival in the presence of the 6-TG prodrug, which is converted to toxic thioguanine by active HPRT. FIGURE 5 shows a representative HPRT assay whereby the presence of HPRT-null cells are observed in MORPHOGENE-expressing CHO in contrast to control vector-transfected cells (not shown). Typical assays found a 100–500-fold increase in HPRT-null foci from morphogenic cultures as compared to vector control. We next compared the mutagenic activity of *morphogenics* to a standard chemical mutagenesis approach using the HPRT screen in CHO cells. For chemical mutagenesis, CHO cells were exposed to ethanemethylsulfonate (EMS) as previously described.[14] After initial mutagenesis, equal numbers of EMS-treated and morphogenic CHO cells were cultured in the presence of 6-TG to select for those cells that lack HPRT activity. Quantitative analysis of selected cultures identified a similar number of HPRT-null CHO foci in both treatments; however, a qualitative difference was observed among foci from the two treatments. A homogeneous population of large, hardy foci were present in the *morphogenics*-derived cultures in contrast to the EMS-treated cultures, which contained foci that were heterogeneous in morphology and size (FIG. 5). High-power microscopy revealed that the morphology of the cellular foci derived using *morphogenics* resembled that of clones derived by subcloning the parental cells, while those resulting after EMS treatment appeared fragmented. In contrast to *morphogenics*-derived HPRT-null CHO cells, a number of clones obtained using EMS had a short, finite growth profile upon clonal expansion. These differences are likely due to the genotoxicity (i.e., chromosomal aberrations) affecting EMS-treated cells, whereas *morphogenics* results in a nontoxic mutagenic effect from polymerase-induced, misincorporated base pairs during DNA replication.[15,16]

These data demonstrate the ability of *morphogenics* to induce robust mutagenesis at recombinant and endogenous gene loci. Importantly, *morphogenics* provides a nontoxic, perpetual mutagenesis process that is in stark contrast to standard chemical mutagenesis methods and offers the ability to generate hardy, genetically diverse cells for discovery and product development.

## MANIPULATING MMR IN TARGET CELLS FOR RESEARCH AND COMMERCIAL APPLICATIONS

The use of *morphogenics* offers several advantages over current methods used to create genetic and functional diversity within host cells for discovery and product development. Because of the high degree of conservation between the MORPHOGENE and mutL proteins from other species, this system is applicable for enhancement of genomewide mutagenesis across a wide array of biological systems including mammalian cells, plants,[10] yeast, and a variety of bacterial strains (N. Nicolaides, personal observation). In light of the high degree of genetic diversity obtained via *morphogenics* and the ability to generate hardy, genetically stable sib cells, this technology offers an efficient method for developing evolved cells for target discovery as well as for developing cells suitable for the manufacturing of biologically based industrial and pharmaceutical products. One such example comes from the recent work by Grasso *et al.*[17] that demonstrates the utility of *morphogenics* to evolve antibody-producer cells to yield subclones generating higher titers of antibody for scaleable manufacturing. In addition, the authors showed that *morphogenics* can also evolve immunoglobulin genes to yield sibs containing mutant light or heavy chain immunoglobulins with enhanced binding affinity to target antigen as compared to the parent molecule. Yet another application of *morphogenics* is to evolve cancer cells to become more susceptible or resistant to chemotherapeutic agents. Isogenic cancer cells that respond differently to chemotherapeutic drugs can be used to identify genes and pathways involved in drug response employing a variety of discovery methods.[19] Several examples have been developed using *morphogenics* to derive human cancer cell lines that are resistant to FDA-approved chemotherapies. These cells have been analyzed via genomic and proteomic techniques to map pathways responsible for resistance/susceptibility and offer the ability to rationally design new drugs to treat chemoresistant tumors. These are but a few of many examples of how the reversible manipulation of MMR can be applied to yield novel hosts organisms suitable to study systems biology as well as for use in target discovery and product development.

[COMPETING INTERESTS: Drs. Nicholas C. Nicolaides, Philip M. Sass, and Luigi Grasso, officers of Morphotek, a biotechnology company, declare potential competing financial interests.]

## REFERENCES

1. MODRICH, P. 1994. Mismatch repair, genetic stability, and cancer. Science **266:** 1959–1960.
2. JIRICNY, J. 1998. Replication errors: challenging the genome. EMBO J. **17:** 6427–6436.
3. GHADIMI, B.M., D.L. SACKETT, M.J. DIFILIPPANTONIO, *et al.* 2000. Centrosome amplification and instability occurs exclusively in aneuploid, but not in diploid colorectal cancer cell lines, and correlates with numerical chromosomal aberrations. Genes Chromosomes & Cancer **27:** 183–190.
4. STRAND, M., T.A. PROLLA, R.M. LISKAY & T.D. PETES. 1993. Destabilization of tracts of simple repetitive DNA in yeast by mutations affecting DNA mismatch repair. Nature **365:** 274–276.
5. GOEL, A., C.N. ARNOLD, D. NIEDZWIECKI, *et al.* 2003. Characterization of sporadic colon cancer by patterns of genomic instability. Cancer Res. **63:** 1608–1614.
6. LEONARD, J.M., S.R. BOLLMANN & J.B. HAYS. 2003. Reduction of stability of arabidopsis genomic and transgenic DNA-repeat sequences (microsatellites) by inactivation of AtMSH2 mismatch-repair function. Plant Physiol. **133:** 328–338.
7. HALL, M.C., P.V. SHCHERBAKOVA, J.M. FORTUNE, *et al.* 2003. DNA binding by yeast Mlh1 and Pms1: implications for DNA mismatch repair. Nucleic Acids Res. **31:** 2025–2034.
8. PEDRAZA-REYES, M. & R.E. YASBIN. 2004. Contribution of the mismatch DNA repair system to the generation of stationary-phase-induced mutants of *Bacillus subtilis.* J Bacteriol. **186:** 6485–6491.
9. FLORES, C. & W. ENGELS. 1999. Microsatellite instability in Drosophila spellchecker1 (MutS homolog) mutants. Proc. Natl. Acad. Sci. USA **96:** 2964–2969.
10. CHAO, Q., C. SULLIVAN, J. GETZ, *et al.* 2005. Rapid generation of plant traits via regulation of DNA mismatch repair. Plant Biotech. J. **3:** 399–407.
11. NICOLAIDES, N.C., S.J. LITTMAN, P. MODRICH, *et al.* 1998. A naturally occurring hPMS2 mutation can confer a dominant negative mutator phenotype. Mol. Cell. Biol. **18:** 1635–1641.
12. NICOLAIDES, N.C., K.C. CARTER, B.K. SHELL, *et al.* 1995. Genomic organization of the human PMS2 gene family. Genomics **30:** 195–206.
13. LITTLEFIELD, J.W. 1964. Selection of hybrids from matings of fibroblasts in vitro and their presumed recombinants. Science **145:** 709.
14. BRANDA, R.F., A.R. LAFAYETTE, J.P. O'NEILL & J.A. NICKLAS. 1999. The effect of folate deficiency on the HPRT mutational spectrum in Chinese hamster ovary cells treated with monofunctional alkylating agents. Mutat. Res. **427:** 79–87.
15. PARSONS, R., M. LONGLEY, P. MODRICH, *et al.* 1995. Mismatch repair deficiency in phenotypically normal human cells. Science **268:** 738–740.
16. WAGNER, E.D., D. ANDERSON, A. DHAWAN, *et al.* 2003. Evaluation of EMS-induced DNA damage in the single cell gel electrophoresis (Comet) assay and with flow cytometric analysis of micronuclei. Teratog. Carcinog. Mutagen Suppl. **2:** 1–11.
17. GRASSO, L., J.B. KLINE, Q. CHAO, *et al.* 2004. Enhancing therapeutic antibodies and titer yields of mammalian cell lines. BioProcess. Intl. **10:** 58–65.
18. CAI, K.Q., C. ALBARRACIN, D. ROSEN, *et al.* 2004. Microsatellite instability and alteration of the expression of hMLH1 and hMSH2 in ovarian clear cell carcinoma. Hum. Pathol. **35:** 552–559.
19. FRANCIA, G., S. MAN, B. TEICHER, *et al.* 2004. Gene expression analysis of tumor spheroids reveals a role for suppressed DNA mismatch repair in multicellular resistance to alkylating agents. Mol. Cell. Biol. **24:** 6837–6849.

# A Comprehensive Strategy to Combat Colon Cancer Targeting the Adenomatous Polyposis Coli Tumor Suppressor Gene

EUGENE W. GERNER, NATALIA A. IGNATENKO, PETER LANCE, AND LAURENCE H. HURLEY

*The University of Arizona, Arizona Cancer Center, Tucson, Arizona 85724, USA*

**ABSTRACT: Somatic cells in the majority of colorectal polyps and cancers contain mutations/deletions in the adenomatous polyposis coli (APC) tumor suppressor gene. APC is involved in normal intestinal development and acts to influence a variety of cellular processes. Loss of APC function leads to intestinal neoplasia in both mice and humans. APC influences expression of specific genes, including the c-Myc oncogene, which functions as a transcriptional activator. Loss of APC function leads to alterations in c-Myc-regulated genes including ornithine decarboxylase (ODC), the first enzyme in polyamine synthesis. A single nucleotide polymorphism (SNP) in the ODC promoter affecting c-Myc-dependent expression has been associated with risk of colorectal and other cancers. Pharmaceuticals that target structural features of the c-Myc promoter, and suppress expression of c-Myc and other genes regulated by similar promoter elements, are being developed as potential colorectal cancer chemotherapies. Difluoromethylornithine (DFMO), a selective inhibitor of ODC, is under clinical evaluation as a colorectal cancer chemopreventive agent. APC and APC-dependent genes, such as c-Myc and ODC, may be useful as genetic markers of risk and as targets for chemoprevention and therapy for colorectal cancer.**

**KEYWORDS: adenomatous polyposis coli (APC) tumor suppressor gene; c-Myc; ornithine decarboxylase (ODC); colon cancer; cancer chemoprevention; chemotherapy; aspirin; difluoromethylornithine (DFMO)**

## A COMPREHENSIVE APPROACH TO PREVENTING DEATH DUE TO COLON CANCER

Colorectal cancer (CRC) mortality rates in the United States have been decreasing over the past two decades in males, and over the past five decades in females. Therapy for CRC is very effective for early, but not late, stages of this disease. Despite these advances, CRC continues to be the second leading cause of cancer deaths in the U.S.[1] Our Gastrointestinal Cancer Program at the University of Arizona has

Address for correspondence: Eugene W. Gerner, The University of Arizona, Arizona Cancer Center, 1515 North Campbell Avenue, Tucson, AZ 85724. Voice: 520-626-2197; fax: 520-626-4480.

egerner@azcc.arizona.edu

**Ann. N.Y. Acad. Sci. 1059: 97–105 (2005).** 
**doi: 10.1196/annals.1339.033**

developed a strategy to address the problem of CRC that involves a coordinated effort of risk assessment, screening, prevention, and treatment. We are optimistic that we can reduce mortality due to CRC *in the foreseeable future* because of specific factors that are unique to this disease. These factors include current knowledge of genetic risk factors for CRC and availability of effective methods for CRC screening, chemoprevention, and treatment of early invasive cancers.

Our approach to risk assessment includes development of genetic tests that can determine an individual's risk of developing CRC. Such genetic tests will include measurement of rare alleles, such as those occurring in the adenomatous polyposis coli (APC) tumor suppressor gene[2] or in genes responsible for hereditary nonpolyposis colon cancers (HNPCC).[3] APC is responsible for the genetic syndrome familial adenomatous polyposis (FAP). Individuals afflicted with FAP have an elevated risk of developing CRC. We also anticipate that genetic measures of risk assessment in germline cells will include more common alleles, such as single nucleotide polymorphisms (SNPs) in pathways downstream of APC.[4] We are working to develop both biological and physical methods for colon cancer screening and subsequent surveillance, and to expand the application of these procedures in populations at risk for this disease. Risk groups include people over age 50 and those with a family history of cancer. This latter group of people with family history of cancer includes individuals with one or more first-degree relatives with CRC, especially with disease development at age 55 years or younger, and who are distinct from those with FAP and HNPCC. Even though the largest risk group is easily identified (i.e., those over age 50), less than half of this group is currently screened even though screening is known to reduce CRC incidence. An important research goal in the near term is to identify barriers to adherence with screening recommendations, and then to institute simple, inexpensive measures to overcome the barriers. Our group has been in the forefront of those developing and testing novel strategies to prevent CRC.[5,6] Prevention strategies are now being targeted to those individuals in high-risk groups, identified by either family history and/or a previous colon polyp.[7] Target-directed therapies are being developed[8] to treat patients who are identified in screening programs and who have failed prevention strategies. Early detection of cancer is crucial to this strategy because it is already known that early-stage CRCs respond, while advanced disease is quite resistant, to therapeutic interventions. Finally, we are establishing programs to manage treatment sequelae, in order to improve quality of life for patients who benefit from treatment that eradicates their cancer, but suffer from the consequences of the same therapy on normal physical and cognitive functions. FIGURE 1 depicts the relative sizes of groups in the U.S. that are relevant to our overall strategy to reduce colon cancer deaths, by the combination of risk assessment, screening, prevention, and treatment.

The U.S. currently has a population of nearly 300 million people. This total number is our target for CRC risk assessment. Within a few years, the percentage of the population 50 years or older is estimated to be near 60 million in number. About half this number will develop colon polyps during their lifetime. Nearly 10% of this latter group will develop large adenomas or early invasive cancers, and about one-third of this group will have a family history of colon cancer. The group of 60 million people over age 50 years, along with individuals with family history of colon cancer, defines our target for CRC screening. A subset of the group of 30 million people who have or will develop colon polyps, specifically those with large polyps, along with indi-

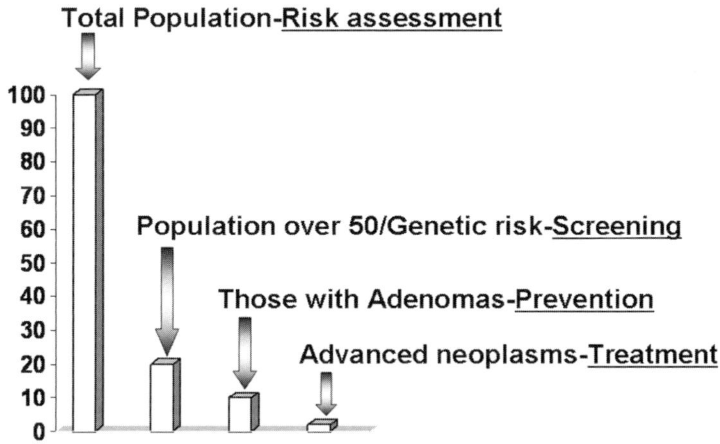


**FIGURE 1.** Target group sizes for an overall strategy to prevent colon cancer deaths. The ordinate is presented as percentage. Improvements in risk assessment, screening, chemoprevention, and treatment should lead to reductions in cancer incidence and subsequent mortality.

viduals with family history of colon cancer, defines our potential target population for chemoprevention. Since the majority of people in this latter group are in good health, it is imperative that chemoprevention strategies be both effective and safe. Efficacy of several chemopreventive agents, including aspirin and calcium, has been established in randomized clinical trials of intermediates in the development of invasive CRC.[9,10] Implementation of effective screening and chemoprevention strategies could render CRC a largely preventable disease in the foreseeable future. In order to accomplish this goal, a two-pronged attack is required. Optimized screening needs to be delivered to the entire at-risk population, and then mechanism-based combination chemoprevention strategies that are more effective than single-agent approaches need to be identified in experimental models and tested for safety and efficacy in human clinical trials. We recognize that optimal application of risk assessment, screening, and prevention strategies will not prevent CRC completely. Thus, we are committed to finding therapeutic methods that will effectively treat those individuals for whom other health-care strategies fail.

## APC AND APC-REGULATED GENES

FAP is an autosomal dominant inherited syndrome associated with increased risk of colon cancer. FAP, which accounts for only a small fraction of colon cancers, is caused by inheritance of a defective form of the APC gene. The majority of colon adenomas and adenocarcinomas in humans, without FAP or a family history of colon cancer, contain defective copies of the APC gene. APC is a component of the Wnt signaling pathway. Wnt and other developmental pathways, including hedgehog, are now understood to play important roles in both genetic and sporadic forms of human epithelial cancers.[11] Studies in genetically modified rodents and human cells have identified APC-regulated genes and genes that modify APC-dependent intestinal carcinogenesis. We have used DNA microarray technologies to identify patterns of APC-dependent gene expression in human colon tumor cells conditionally expressing wild-type APC and in intestinal mucosa obtained from multiple intestinal neoplasia (Min) mice, which are heterozygous for a germline amber mutation at codon 850 in the murine homologue of the APC gene.[12–15] These investigations have caused us to focus on one specific pathway, depicted in FIGURE 2, that appears to be causatively associated with APC-dependent intestinal and colonic carcinogenesis. Wild-type APC suppresses the expression of the E-box transcriptional activator c-Myc[14] and increases expression of the transcriptional repressor Mad1.[12] The APC-dependent regulation of c-Myc is mediated by β-catenin, which interacts with a member of the Lef/Tcf family of nuclear transcription factors.[14] This interaction promotes binding of complexes of these proteins to specific sequences in the c-Myc promoter and subsequent transcription of the c-Myc gene. Using a human cell culture model, we showed that wild-type APC suppressed ODC protein expression in a manner that depended on an intact E-box consensus sequence in the ODC promoter and that antisense inhibition of c-MYC suppressed ODC enzyme activity.[12] Loss of wild-type APC, as occurs in the majority of sporadic colorectal adenomas and cancers, leads to an increase in c-Myc expression, a subsequent increase in ODC transcription and polyamine synthesis associated with an increase in expression of genes associated with cell proliferation, cell survival, and tissue remodeling/invasion, and decreased apoptosis.[7] Expression of wild-type APC, as occurs in the nonproliferat-

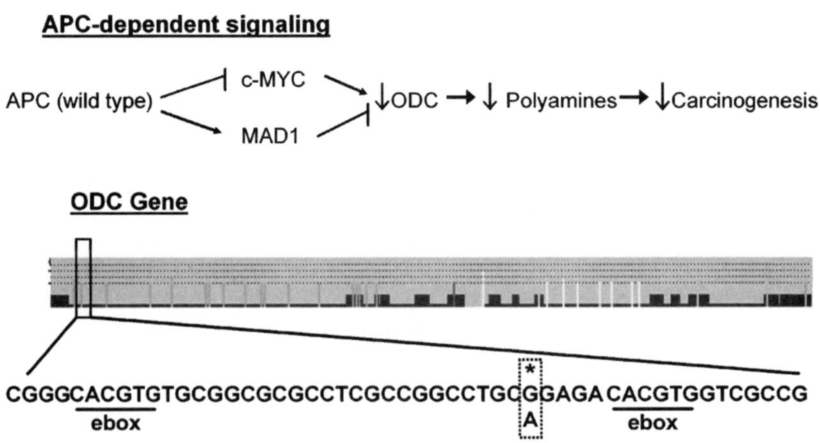


**FIGURE 2.** Relationship between APC, APC-dependent genes, and carcinogenesis. Wild-type APC suppresses the expression of the E-box transcriptional activator c-MYC, while promoting the expression of the c-MYC antagonist MAD1. MAD1 represses, while c-MYC activates, the expression of ODC, the first enzyme in polyamine synthesis. Polyamines promote normal growth and development and epithelial cancers, including CRC. The *lower panel* depicts the ODC gene structure, along with the location of numerous single nucleotide polymorphisms (SNPs) identified by *vertical bars*. One regions is expanded and shows the sequence of one SNP, for which frequency and functional studies suggest a role in colon carcinogenesis.[4] See text for details.

ing cells of the colonic epithelium, reverses these processes. These findings provided a mechanistic basis for results reported by us for the Min mouse model[16] and for humans with FAP,[17] which indicated that ODC and polyamine contents were elevated in intestinal mucosa of both mice and humans expressing mutant APC.

## RISK ASSESSMENT BASED ON APC AND APC-DEPENDENT GENES

Germline mutations in APC cause FAP, and these mutations are being used as potential markers of CRC risk.[2] While FAP accounts for only a small fraction of total CRC, the majority of sporadic CRC adenomas and cancers contain APC mutations in somatic cells.[18] Thus, APC mutations appear to be a selection criterion for CRC development in colorectal epithelial cells. Several SNPs in APC have been associated with CRC risk,[19–21] and these also become potential markers of gene risk. We have recently obtained evidence for the association of genetic variability in a common allele with risk of colon polyp recurrence.[4] We evaluated the relationship of a SNP affecting ODC promoter activity to risk of colon polyp recurrence in a human colon polyp prevention study. The ODC SNP occurs 316 nucleotides downstream of the ODC transcriptional start site and is located between two consensus E-boxes in the promoter region, as shown in FIGURE 2. The transcriptional activator c-Myc and the transcriptional repressor Mad1 bind to these elements. The frequency of this SNP has been measured in several groups of people, including participants in one colorectal cancer prevention trial. Fifty-five percent of participants in this trial, all of whom previously had a colon polyp, were homozygous G at this locus; 35% were heterozygous G/A and 10% were homozygous A. The SNP was shown to have functional consequences for ODC expression. The transcriptional repressor Mad1, a c-Myc antagonist, selectively repressed ODC transcription in an A-allele–specific manner. Finally, it was found that the A-allele was associated with a statistically significant reduction in risk of colorectal polyp recurrence. This SNP has been associated with risk of prostate cancer in a case control study.[22]

## CHEMOPREVENTION TARGETING APC-DEPENDENT GENES

Nonsteroidal anti-inflammatory drugs (NSAIDs), which act by both cyclooxygenase-dependent and -independent mechanisms, and inhibitors of ODC suppress APC-dependent intestinal carcinogenesis in APC-deficient mice and chemical carcinogen-treated rodents. In our evaluation of the association of the ODC SNP and risk of polyp recurrence, we noted that this risk was lowest in participants who were homozygous for the minor ODC SNP allele and who reported taking aspirin regularly. Aspirin use did not affect ODC allele-specific transcription, but did affect polyamine catabolism by inducing the transcription of SSAT.[4] The ODC A-allele therefore appears to be a potential prognostic factor for polyp risk in humans and allele number may be a predictor of human response to aspirin as a colon cancer preventive agent. The ODC A-allele favors binding of the transcriptional repressor Mad1. Thus, the ODC A-allele may work in concert with aspirin to lower tissue polyamine levels and, thus, risk of colon polyp recurrence. A potential mechanism for this coordinate action may involve the spermidine/spermine $N^1$-acetyltransferase

(SSAT), a polyamine catabolic enzyme. SSAT is a transcriptional target for several nonsteroidal anti-inflammatory drugs (NSAIDS). The nonselective COX-1 and -2 inhibitor sulindac activates the peroxisomal proliferator activated receptor gamma (PPARγ), a member of the steroid hormone family of transcriptional activators, which recognizes a unique DNA sequence in the SSAT promoter to induce transcription of this gene.[23] NSAIDS structurally unrelated to sulindac, like aspirin, also induce SSAT transcription.[23] Aspirin, sulindac and several other structurally diverse NSAIDS act to promote SSAT transcription by both COX-dependent and -independent mechanisms. One mechanism of the chemopreventive and therapeutic effects of certain NSAIDS is their ability to induce apoptosis. NSAID-induced apoptosis can be reversed, in part, by exogenous polyamines,[23] suggesting that NSAID-induced SSAT induction and subsequent polyamine export are causatively involved in NSAID-induced apoptosis. Consequently, NSAIDS act as inducers of polyamine catabolism and export, and they complement inhibitors of polyamine synthesis in acting to lower tissue polyamine contents. Thus, ODC inhibitors and NSAIDS counter the effects of mutation of tumor suppressor genes, such as APC and PPARγ, and oncogenes, such as c-Myc and K-ras, which act to increase tissue polyamine contents in cancer. Combinations of DFMO and NSAIDS work at least additively in several models of colon and intestinal carcinogenesis,[24,25] corroborating the model depicted in FIGURE 3. Strategies evaluating combinations of NSAIDs and agents that disrupt normal polyamine homeostasis are currently under evaluation in clinical colon cancer prevention and treatment trials.

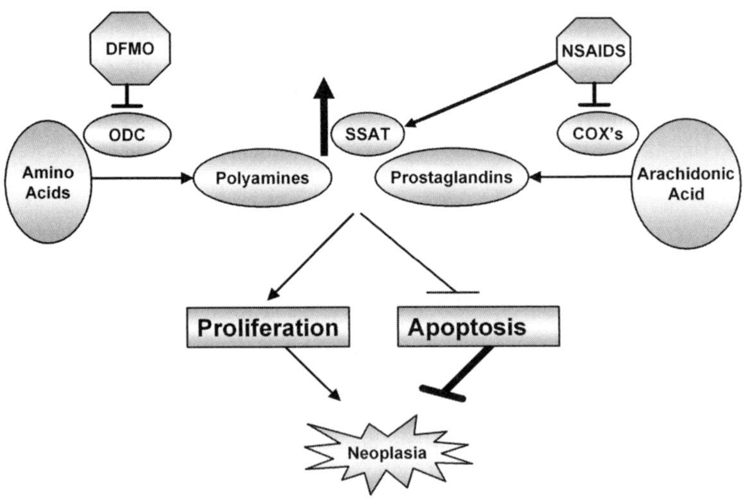


**FIGURE 3.** Rationale for combination chemoprevention with inhibitors of polyamine synthesis and nonsteroidal anti-inflammatory drugs (NSAIDS). Difluoromethylornithine (DFMO) inhibits ODC, the first enzyme in polyamine synthesis, while NSAIDS inhibit cyclooxygenases, which produce prostaglandins. Polyamines and prostaglandins promote cell proliferation and suppress apoptosis, thus enhancing carcinogenesis. Certain NSAIDS activate SSAT, the first enzyme in polyamine catabolism via cyclooxygenase-dependent and -independent mechanisms.

## CHEMOTHERAPY TARGETING C-MYC

In order to determine whether c-Myc is a relevant therapeutic target for colorectal cancer, we have developed a mouse model in which c-Myc is selectively deleted in regions of the intestinal tract of Min mice (E. Gerner, unpublished results). Lack of c-MYC protein expression was associated with regions of aberrant intestinal development (e.g., shortened crypts, lack of intestinal villi) and a reduced number of intestinal adenomas. These data support the hypothesis that c-Myc is a relevant target for intestinal cancer treatment strategies. One of us (L.H.H.) has focused on targeting the G-quadruplex in the c-MYC promoter, as depicted in FIGURE 4, and achieving selectivity for the c-MYC G-quadruplex over other DNA structures. Cationic porphyrins are known to bind to and stabilize different types of G-quadruplexes.[26] Recent studies have shown the biological relevance of the intramolecular parallel G-quadruplex as a transcriptional silencer in the c-MYC promoter.[27, 28] TMPyP4 also binds to this G-quadruplex and most likely converts it to a mixed parallel/antiparallel G-quadruplex with two external lateral loops and one internal propeller loop, suppressing c-MYC transcriptional activation.[27] To achieve therapeutic selectivity by targeting G-quadruplexes, it is necessary to synthesize drugs that can differentiate among the different types of G-quadruplexes. A core-modified expanded porphyrin analogue, 5,10,15,20-[tetra-(*N*-methyl-3-pyridyl)]-26,28-diselena sapphyrin chlo-

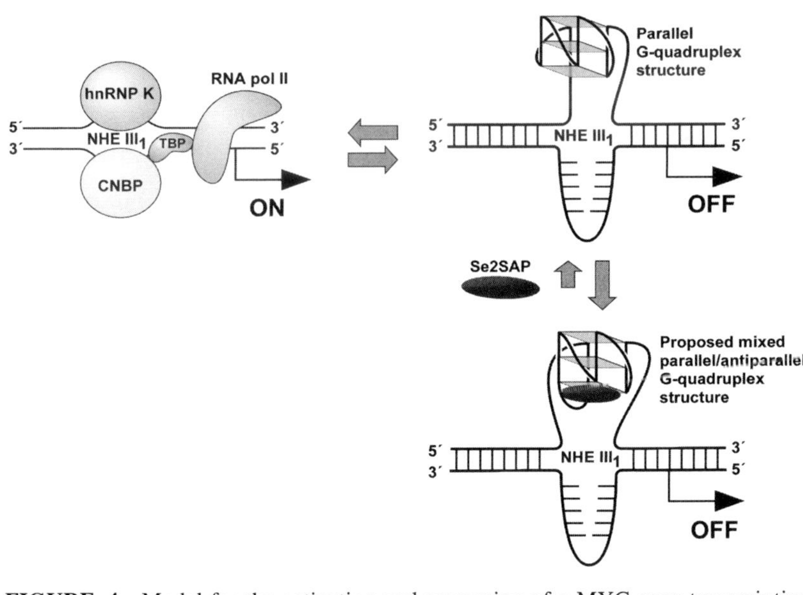


**FIGURE 4.** Model for the activation and repression of c-MYC gene transcription involving the conversion of the paranemic secondary DNA structures (gene off) to purine and pyrimidine single-stranded DNA forms for transcriptional activation. hnRNP K and CNBP are single-stranded DNA binding proteins involved in transcriptional activation. Interaction of the parallel G-quadruplex structure with Se2SAP stabilizes the gene-off form by conversion to the proposed single-loop hybrid G-quadruplex structures that stabilize the silencer element and results in transcriptional repression.[29]

ride (Se2SAP) has been designed and synthesized.[29] Se2SAP converts the parallel c-MYC G-quadruplex into a mixed parallel/antiparallel G-quadruplex with one external lateral loop and two internal propeller loops, resulting in strong and selective binding to this G-quadruplex. A *Taq* polymerase stop assay was used to evaluate the binding of TMPyP4 and Se2SAP to G-quadruplex DNA.

Compared to TMPyP4, Se2SAP showed a greater selectivity for and a 40-fold increase in stabilization of the single lateral-loop hybrid. Surface plasmon resonance and competition experiments with duplex DNA and other G-quadruplexes further confirmed the selectivity of Se2SAP for the c-MYC G-quadruplex. Se2SAP was a more potent inhibitor of c-MYC transcriptional activation than TMPyP4, although longer cellular incubation times were required. Significantly, Se2SAP was found to be less photoactive and noncytotoxic in comparison to TMPyP4. In cooperation with Cylene Pharmaceuticals, a drug (CX-3543) targeted to the G-quadruplex in the c-MYC promoter, is in advanced preclinical evaluation. This drug has efficacy in colon and pancreatic cancer cell models. Studies in mice, rats, and dogs have confirmed a desirable pharmacokinetic profile and therapeutic index. Phase I and II trials in patients with CRC and other cancers are planned.

## SUMMARY AND FUTURE DIRECTIONS

Our group has established a comprehensive strategy to eliminate death due to CRC. Key elements of this strategy include risk assessment, screening, prevention, and treatment. Specific features of our strategy focus on the APC tumor suppressor gene and APC-regulated genes. Genetic variability in one APC-regulated gene, ODC, has prognostic value for colon polyp recurrence and may have relevance in CRC and other epithelial cancers. ODC and other polyamine metabolic genes are targets for chemoprevention strategies in patients at risk for CRC. Clinical studies, including Phase III clinical trials to test this hypothesis, are in progress. A SNP in the ODC promoter may have additional utility as a predictive factor for the protective effects of aspirin against CRC development. Finally, our group, along with private industry, is developing pharmaceuticals to target genetic elements affecting the expression of c-MYC and other genes. Clinical trials for such agents are planned for the near future.

## REFERENCES

1. Jemal, A., R.C. Tiwari, *et al.* 2004. Cancer statistics, 2004. CA Cancer J. Clin. **54:** 8–29.
2. Childs, O. 2004. In the news: UK approves screening embryos for cancer. Nat. Rev. Cancer **4:** 926.
3. Burke, W., G. Petersen, *et al.* 1997. Recommendations for follow-up care of individuals with an inherited predisposition to cancer. I. Hereditary nonpolyposis colon cancer. Cancer Genetics Studies Consortium. JAMA **277:** 915–919.
4. Martinez, M.E., T.G. O'Brien, *et al.* 2003. Pronounced reduction in adenoma recurrence associated with aspirin use and a polymorphism in the ornithine decarboxylase gene. Proc. Natl. Acad. Sci. USA **100:** 7859–7864.
5. Alberts, D.S., M.E. Martinez, *et al.* 2000. Lack of effect of a high-fiber cereal supplement on the recurrence of colorectal adenomas. Phoenix Colon Cancer Prevention Physicians' Network. N. Engl. J. Med. **342:** 1156–1162.

6. ALBERTS, D.S., M.E. MARTINEZ, *et al.* 2005. Phase III trial of ursodeoxycholic acid to prevent colorectal polyp recurrence. J. Natl. Cancer Inst. **97:** 846–853.
7. GERNER, E.W. & F.L. MEYSKENS, JR. 2004. Polyamines and cancer: old molecules, new understanding. Nat. Rev. Cancer **4:** 781–792.
8. WELSH, S.J., R.R. WILLIAMS, *et al.* 2003. The thioredoxin redox inhibitors 1-methylpropyl 2-imidazolyl disulfide and pleurotin inhibit hypoxia-induced factor 1alpha and vascular endothelial growth factor formation. Mol. Cancer Ther. **2:** 235–243.
9. BARON, J.A., M. BEACH, *et al.* 1999. Calcium supplements for the prevention of colorectal adenomas. Calcium Polyp Prevention Study Group. N. Engl. J. Med. **340:** 101–107.
10. BARON, J.A., B.F. COLE, *et al.* 2003. A randomized trial of aspirin to prevent colorectal adenomas. N. Engl. J. Med. **348:** 891–899.
11. TAIPALE, J. & P.A. BEACHY. 2001. The hedgehog and Wnt signalling pathways in cancer. Nature **411:** 349–54.
12. FULTZ, K.E. & E.W. GERNER. 2002. APC-dependent regulation of ornithine decarboxylase in human colon tumor cells. Mol. Carcinog. **34:** 10–18.
13. IGNATENKO, N.A., H. ZHANG, *et al.* 2004. The chemopreventive agent [alpha]-difluoromethylornithine blocks K-ras dependent tumor formation and specific gene expression in Caco-2 cells. Mol. Carcinog. **39:** 221–233.
14. HE, T.C., A.B. SPARKS, *et al.* 1998. Identification of c-MYC as a target of the APC pathway. Science **281:** 1509–1512.
15. SU, L.K., K.W. KINZLER, *et al.* 1992. Multiple intestinal neoplasia caused by a mutation in the murine homolog of the APC gene. Science **256:** 668–670.
16. ERDMAN, S.H., N.A. IGNATENKO, *et al.* 1999. APC-dependent changes in expression of genes influencing polyamine metabolism, and consequences for gastrointestinal carcinogenesis, in the Min mouse. Carcinogenesis **20:** 1709–1713.
17. GIARDIELLO, F.M., S.R. HAMILTON, *et al.* 1997. Ornithine decarboxylase and polyamines in familial adenomatous polyposis. Cancer Res. **57:** 199–201.
18. IWAMOTO, M., D.J. AHNEN, *et al.* 2000. Expression of beta-catenin and full-length APC protein in normal and neoplastic colonic tissues. Carcinogenesis **21:** 1935–1940.
19. JORDE, L.B., W.S. WATKINS, *et al.* 1994. Linkage disequilibrium predicts physical distance in the adenomatous polyposis coli region. Am. J. Hum. Genet. **54:** 884–898.
20. HAMPEL, H. & P. PELTOMAKI. 2000. Hereditary colorectal cancer: risk assessment and management. Clin. Genet. **58:** 89–97.
21. SLATTERY, M.L., W. SAMOWITZ, *et al.* 2001. A molecular variant of the APC gene at codon 1822: its association with diet, lifestyle, and risk of colon cancer. Cancer Res. **61:** 1000–1004.
22. VISVANATHAN, K., K.J. HELZLSOUER, *et al.* 2004. Association among an ornithine decarboxylase polymorphism, androgen receptor gene (CAG) repeat length and prostate cancer risk. J. Urol. **171:** 652–655.
23. BABBAR, N., N.A. IGNATENKO, *et al.* 2003. Cyclooxygenase-independent induction of apoptosis by sulindac sulfone is mediated by polyamines in colon cancer. J. Biol. Chem. **278:** 47762–47775.
24. MEYSKENS, F.L., JR. & E.W. GERNER. 1999. Development of difluoromethylornithine (DFMO) as a chemoprevention agent. Clin. Cancer Res. **5:** 945–951.
25. BABBAR, N. & E.W. GERNER. 2003. Polyamines as modifiers of genetic risk factors in human intestinal cancers. Biochem. Soc.Trans. **31:** 388–392.
26. SIDDIQUI-JAIN, A., C.L. GRAND, *et al.* 2002. Direct evidence for a G-quadruplex in a promoter region and its targeting with a small molecule to repress c-MYC transcription. Proc. Natl. Acad. Sci. USA **99:** 11593–11598.
27. SEENISAMY, J., E.M. REZLER, *et al.* 2004. The dynamic character of the G-quadruplex element in the c-MYC promoter and modification by TMPyP4. J. Am. Chem. Soc. **126:** 8702–8709.
28. PHAN, A.T., Y.S. MODI, *et al.* 2004. Propeller-type parallel-stranded G-quadruplexes in the human c-myc promoter. J. Am. Chem. Soc. **126:** 8710–8716.
29. SEENISAMY, J., S. BASHYAM, *et al.* 2005. Design and synthesis of an expanded porphyrin that has selectivity for the c-MYC G-quadruplex structure. J. Am. Chem. Soc. **127:** 2944–2959.

# External Imaging of *CCND1*, *MYC*, and *KRAS* Oncogene mRNAs with Tumor-Targeted Radionuclide-PNA-Peptide Chimeras

XIAOBING TIAN,[a,c] ATIS CHAKRABARTI,[a,c] NARIMAN V. AMIRKHANOV,[a,c] MOHAN R. ARUVA,[b] KAIJUN ZHANG,[b] BOBY MATHEW,[b] CHRISTOPHER CARDI,[b,c] WENYI QIN,[d] EDWARD R. SAUTER,[d] MATHEW L. THAKUR,[b,c] AND ERIC WICKSTROM[a,c]

*Departments of Biochemistry and Molecular Biology[a] and Radiology,[b] and Kimmel Cancer Center,[c] Thomas Jefferson University, Philadelphia, Pennsylvania 19107, USA*

*[d]Department of Surgery, University of Missouri, Columbia, Missouri 65212, USA*

**Abstract: In 2005, breast cancer will kill approximately 40,410 women in the U.S., and pancreatic cancer will kill approximately 31,800 men and women in the U.S. Clinical examination and mammography, the currently accepted breast cancer screening methods, miss almost half of breast cancers in women younger than 40 years, approximately one-quarter of cancers in women aged 40–49 years, and one-fifth of cancers in women over 50 years old. Pancreatic cancer progresses rapidly, with only 1% of patients surviving more than 5 years after diagnosis. However, if the disease is diagnosed when it is localized, the 5-year survival is approximately 20%. It would be beneficial to detect breast cancer and pancreatic cancer at the earliest possible stage, when multimodal therapy with surgery, radiotherapy, and chemotherapy have the greatest chance of prolonging survival. Human estrogen receptor–positive breast cancer cells typically display elevated levels of Myc protein due to overexpression of *MYC* mRNA, elevated cyclin D1 protein due to overexpression of *CCND1* mRNA, and elevated insulin-like growth factor 1 receptor (IGF1R) due to overexpression of *IGF1R* mRNA. We hypothesized that scintigraphic detection of *MYC* or *CCND1* peptide nucleic acid (PNA) probes with an IGF1 peptide loop on the C-terminus, and a Tc-99m-chelator peptide on the N-terminus, could measure levels of *MYC* or *CCND1* mRNA noninvasively in human *IGF1R*-overexpressing MCF7 breast cancer xenografts in immunocompromised mice. Similarly, human pancreatic cancer cells typically display elevated levels of *KRAS* mRNA and elevated IGF1R. Hence, we also hypothesized that a *KRAS* Tc-99m-chelator PNA-peptide probe could detect overexpression of *KRAS* mRNA in pancreatic cancer xenografts by scintigraphic imaging, or by positron emission tomography (PET) with a *KRAS* Cu-64-chelator PNA-peptide. Human MCF7 breast cancer xenografts in immunocompromised mice were imaged scintigraphically 4–24 h after tail-vein administration of *MYC* or *CCND1* Tc-99m-chelator PNA-peptides, but not after administration of mismatch controls. Similarly, human Panc-1 pancreatic cancer cells xenografts were imaged**

Address for correspondence: Eric Wickstrom, Department of Biochemistry and Molecular Biology, Thomas Jefferson University, 233 S. 10th Street, Suite 219, Philadelphia, PA 19107-5541. Voice: 215-955-4578; fax: 215-955-4580.
eric@tesla.jci.tju.edu

**Ann. N.Y. Acad. Sci. 1059: 106–144 (2005). © 2005 New York Academy of Sciences. doi: 10.1196/annals.1339.038**

**scintigraphically 4 and 24 h after tail-vein administration of a *KRAS* Tc-99m-chelator PNA-peptide, and AsPC1 xenografts were imaged by PET 4 and 24 h after tail-vein adminstration of a *KRAS* Cu-64-chelator PNA-peptide. The radioprobes distributed normally to the kidneys, livers, tumors, and other tissues. External molecular imaging of oncogene mRNAs in solid tumors with radiolabel-PNA-peptide chimeras might in the future provide additional genetic characterization of pre-invasive and invasive breast cancers.**

KEYWORDS: **antisense; breast cancer; chelators; conjugates; gene expression; hybridization; imaging; noninvasive; oligonucleotides; oncogenes; pancreatic cancer; peptides; positron emission; radionuclides; scintigraphy; tumors**

## INTRODUCTION

Cancerous cells overexpress normal or mutated proteins derived from one or more of the 5,000 genes involved in cell proliferation.[1] Such genes are called proto-oncogenes.[2] The implication is that the targets that must be attacked in breast cancer cells are normal cellular genes that have sustained an activating lesion. There are hundreds of different cancer types, and it was recently shown that at least five genes were mutated in each tumor,[3] confirming Knudson's original statistical model for adult cancers.[4] Based on these data, it was subsequently estimated that there are approximately 200 different genes that are mutated in different cancers.[5] Furthermore, each gene can be mutated at different locations within the gene. We may presume, then, that every cancer will be unique, and every tumor will be heterogeneous. Using clinical symptoms to classify tumors therefore cannot provide all the needed information. With high-throughput microarray transcript profiling techniques, it is possible to screen a sample and determine the genes that are expressed. Therefore, expression profiling has attracted great interest in cancer biology because of its potential to revolutionize cancer diagnosis[6,7] by using cluster analysis to identify genes that characterize the transformed cell.[8,9] Expression profiling has also been used to classify cutaneous malignant melanoma,[8] breast cancer,[10] and to identify genes that are important for metastasis.[9] While imaging of oncogenic marker expression from outside the body could precisely direct clinicians to appropriate molecular intervention at the onset of disease, no such method exists currently. This represents a critical issue for breast and pancreatic cancers, among others.

Breast cancer, despite advances in detection and treatment, is the second leading cause of cancer death in U.S. women. In 2005, approximately 40,410 women in the U.S. will die from breast cancer.[11] Clinical examination and mammography, the currently accepted breast cancer screening methods, miss almost half of breast cancers in women younger than 40 years, approximately one-quarter of cancers in women aged 40–49 years, and one-fifth of cancers in women over 50 years old.[12] The breast is the most common site of noncutaneous cancer in U.S. women.[14] Moreover, if an abnormality is found, an invasive diagnostic procedure must still be performed to determine whether the breast contains atypia or cancer, even though at least two-thirds of the abnormalities are benign. Despite recent improvements in Breast Imaging Reporting and Data System (BIRADS) standardization of mammography (including the use of two views of the breast rather than one, spot compression, and digital images) that have improved sensitivity and specificity,[13] 66–85% of women with suspicious mammograms who undergo surgery are found to have a benign abnormality.[14] In many other patients recently determined to have a benign mammogram, clinical examination reveals a mass found to be malignant.

Similarly, cancer of the exocrine pancreas (pancreatic cancer) will kill an estimated 31,800 Americans in 2005.[11] Pancreatic cancer occurs more frequently in African Americans than in European Americans. The disease progresses rapidly, and is usually refractory to treatment, with a median survival time of 12 months. Overall, only 1% of patients live more than 5 years after diagnosis. However, if the disease is diagnosed when it is localized, the 5-year survival is approximately 20%.[15] It would be beneficial to detect pancreatic cancer at an early stage, when combination therapy with surgery, radiotherapy, and chemotherapy might permit survival.

At the oncogene level, *CCND1*, *HER2*, and *MYC* oncogenes, as well as the tumor suppressor p53, are frequently mutated or overexpressed in breast cancer cells. The same oncogenes are found active in pancreatic cancer cells, and, in addition, 90% of patients with pancreatic cancer carry activating mutations in their *KRAS* oncogenes. Oncogene-targeted oligonucleotide sequences have specifically downregulated *CCND1,*[16,17] *HER2,*[18,19] *IGF1R,*[20] *MYC,*[21–24] *KRAS,*[9, 25–29] and p53,[30,31] inhibiting cancer cell proliferation. Therefore, we hypothesized that mutated or overexpressed *CCND1*, *HER2*, *MYC*, *KRAS*, and p53 mRNAs are significant markers of oncogenic transformation that we could use to identify cancerous masses in breast and pancreatic xenografts by external single photon emission computerized tomography (SPECT) or positron emission tomography (PET) imaging.

F-18-fluorodeoxyglucose,[32] F-18-fluoroguanine derivatives,[33] F-18-2′-fluoro-5′-iodo-uridine,[34] and F-18-fluorothymidine[35] enable PET imaging of sites of cellular proliferation. Similarly, [I-123]VIP has been used for imaging pancreatic cancer sites,[36] as well as [In-111]PAM4 monoclonal antibody against mucin-1.[37] However, none of these imaging methods provides the identities of overexpressed genes. To measure overexpressed oncogene mRNAs directly, we hypothesized that radiolabeled oligonucleotide derivatives with ligands specific to malignant cells would permit noninvasive imaging of transformed foci.

Normal DNA (FIG. 1) would not be a good choice for imaging mRNA because it is metabolized and cleared rapidly,[38] enters all cells nonspecifically,[39] and activates RNase H attack on hybridized mRNA,[40] thereby destroying its intended analyte. Phosphorothioate DNA (FIG. 1) is metabolized more slowly, but binds nonspecifically to proteins, and similarly destroys its target.[41] Peptide nucleic acids (PNAs) (FIG. 1) show promise as a diagnostic tool for detecting gene expression because they resist both proteases and nucleases,[42] they do not interact with cellular proteins that normally bind negatively charged macromolecules,[43] and they hybridize more strongly and specifically to RNA and DNA than do normal oligonucleotides.[44] PNA probe hybridization does not induce RNase H degradation of bound mRNA.[45]

On the other hand, mammalian cells take up PNA 10 times less efficiently than phosphorothioates.[39] To return cellular uptake to the level of phosphorothioates, but only for metastatic cells, we add a peptide analogue of insulin-like growth factor 1 (IGF1) that binds to the insulin-like growth factor 1 receptor (IGF1R), which is amplified in ≈70% of human tumors, particularly in metastatic cells.[46] A small cyclic peptide analogue of IGF1, D(Cys-Ser-Lys-Ala-Pro-Lys-Leu-Pro-Ala-Ala-Tyr-Cys), whose Cys thiols are bridged to form a loop with limited flexibility that favors receptor binding, inhibits the growth of certain cancer cell lines and competes with the

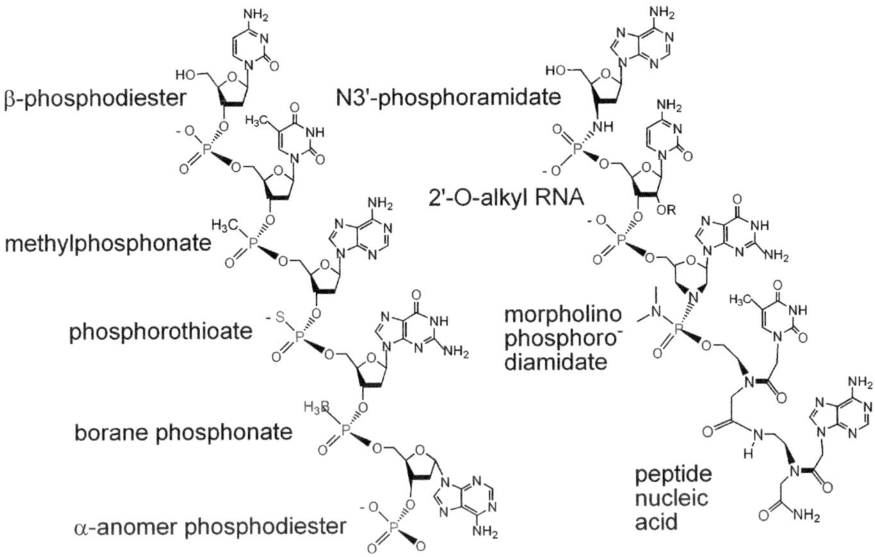


**FIGURE 1.** Oligonucleotide backbone derivatives.

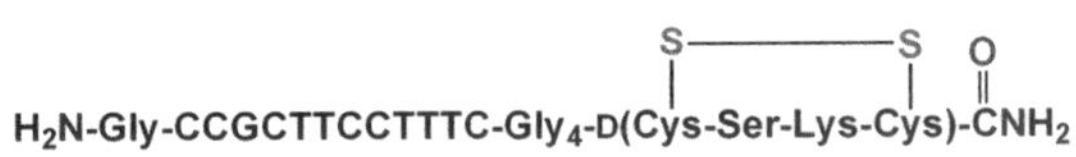


**FIGURE 2.** PNA-peptide specific for *IGF1R* mRNA and IGF1 receptor.

natural ligand for binding to the IGF1R.[47] The use of D-amino acids gave the peptide stability against cellular proteases. A reverse sequence was synthesized with respect to the normal L-amino acid sequence to account for the reversal of chirality. This is the "retro-inverso" approach.

To reduce the complexity of ligand synthesis, a smaller version, D(Cys-Ser-Lys-Cys) [D(CSKC)], was selected for conjugation with the PNA. Extension of an antisense PNA against *IGF1R* mRNA from the N-terminus of the D-peptide IGF1 analogue (FIG. 2) provided specificity to cells overexpressing IGF1R and boosted cellular uptake by those cells 5–10-fold, back to the level of phosphorothioates.[48] Cellular uptake of a PNA-peptide control sequence with two D-Ala residues in the peptide in place of D-Ser-Lys and a control PNA without a peptide adduct were negligible.

For external imaging, we previously developed technology to label peptides with Tc-99m for SPECT imaging by conjugating an $N_4$ chelating peptide, Gly-D-Ala-Gly-Gly-aminobutanoate (GDAGGB).[49,50] We have radiolabeled several peptides, such as GDAGGB-vasoactive intestinal peptide (VIP), with Tc-99m and applied them with success *in vitro*, in experimental animals, and in humans.[49,50] Recently, we have observed that labeling VIP with Cu-64 chelated by an $N_2S_2$ chelator, N,N′-bis(S-benzoyl-thioglycoloyl)diaminopropanoate ($SBTG_2DAP$) for PET imaging, instead of Tc-99m chelated by GDAGGB, increased MCF7 xenograft uptake by >75-fold.[51]

We postulated that solid-phase synthesis on a single resin support could be extended to continuous Fmoc coupling of all GDAGGB chelating amino acids, antisense PNA monomers, and IGF1 analogue amino acids during a single, continuous solid-phase synthesis on an automated synthesizer.[52] A single solid-phase run would eliminate the need for post-synthetic conjugation of purified chelator peptides and purified ligand peptides with purified PNA, and further purification and characterization of the resulting conjugate. Fmoc coupling was used for the synthesis because Fmoc reaction conditions are much milder than those for Boc coupling and deprotection.

That (development enabled us to label GDAGGB-PNAs with Tc-99m.[53] We have now succeeded in labeling GDAGGB-PNA-peptides with Tc-99m for SPECT imaging of *MYC* mRNA (FIG. 3)[54] and *CCND1* mRNA[17] in breast cancer xenografts. Furthermore, we have prepared $SBTG_2DAP$-PNA-peptides FIG. 4) with Cu-64 for PET imaging of *KRAS* mRNA in pancreatic cancer xenografts.[55]

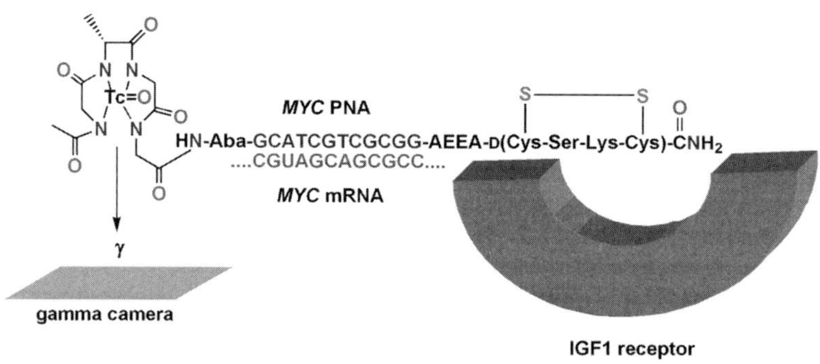


**FIGURE 3.** Tc-99m-GDAGGB-PNA-peptide specific for *MYC* mRNA and IGF1 receptor, designed to bind to the receptor for IGF1, internalize, and hybridize with *MYC* mRNA.[54] Scintigraphic imaging of γ-particles emitted upon decay of Tc-99m might identify sites of high *MYC* mRNA expression. Aba, aminobutanoate; AEEA, aminoethoxyethoxyacetate.

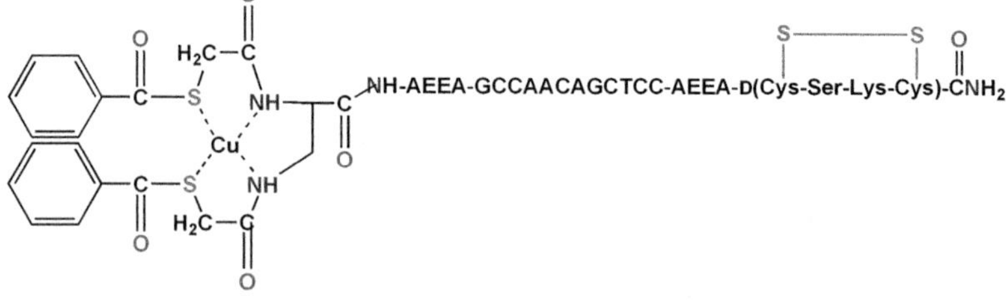


**FIGURE 4.** Cu-64-$SBTG_2DAP$-PNA-peptide specific for *KRAS* mRNA and IGF1 receptor.[55]

**TABLE 1. GDAGGB-PNA-peptide chimera characterization**

| Name | Sequence | Label | Yield | Calculated mass | Measured mass |
|---|---|---|---|---|---|
| PNA-free | GDAGGB-$(Gly)_4$-D(CSKC) | WT990 | 19.0% | 990.0 Da | 992.0 Da |
| *MYC* PNA mismatch | AcGDAGGB-GCAT-GTCTGCGG-AEEA-D(CSKC) | WT4235 | 30.6% | 4235.0 Da | 4234.7 Da |
| *MYC* PNA antisense | AcGDAGGB-GCATCGTCGCGG-AEEA-D(CSKC) | WT4219 | 27.2% | 4219.0 Da | 4221.6 Da |
| *CCND1* PNA mismatch | AcGDAGGB-CTGGA-CAACCAT-AEEA-D(CSKC) | WT4172 | 39.1% | 4172.0 Da | 4174.1 Da |
| *CCND1* peptide mismatch | AcGDAGGB-CTGGTGT-TCCAT-AEEA-D(CysAlaAlaCys) | WT4113 | 34.0% | 4113.0 Da | 4113.7 Da |
| *CCND1* PNA antisense | AcGDAGGB-CTGGTGT-TCCAT-AEEA-D(CSKC) | WT4185 | 30.6% | 4185.0 Da | 4187.2 Da |
| Fl-*CCND1* peptide mismatch | SFX-AEEA-CTGGTGT-TCCAT-AEEA-D(CysAlaAlaCys) | WT4361 | 3.0% | 4361.0 Da | 4360.6 Da |
| Fl-*CCND1* PNA antisense | SFX-AEEA-CTGGTGT-TCCAT-AEEA-D(CSKC) | WT4433 | 2.8% | 4433.0 Da | 4433.8 Da |
| *KRAS* PNA antisense | $SBTG_2$-DAP-AEEA-GCCAACAGCTCC-AEEA-D(CSKC) | WT4351 | 40% | 4351.1 Da | 4350.5 Da |

## SYNTHESIS

The chelator-PNA-peptide chimeras (TABLE 1) were assembled (SCHEME 1), purified, and characterized as described previously.[52] In brief, the IGF1 analogue D(CSKC), or the mismatch control D(CysAlaAlaCys), was assembled by coupling of Fmoc-D-amino acids (Novabiochem, San Diego, CA) activated by O-(7-azabenzotriazole-1-yl)-1,1,3,3-tetramethyluronium hexafluorophosphate (HATU) (Applied Biosystems, Foster City, CA) onto 9-Fmoc-amino-xanthen-3-yloxy TG resin (NovaSyn TG Sieber resin) (0.2–0.3 mmol/g) (Novabiochem) using an Applied Biosystems 430A peptide synthesizer. Then the linker Fmoc-AEEA and PNA monomers (Applied Biosystems, Foster City, CA) were sequentially coupled to the N-terminus of the peptide-resin on an Applied Biosystems 8909 DNA synthesizer, running the manufacturer's PNA 2 μmol protocol. Finally, the chelator peptide Fmoc-GDAGGB (Novabiochem) was coupled to the N-terminus of the PNA-peptide using a long coupling cycle protocol,[52] then acetylated. The cysteine residues were cyclized on solid phase with 10 equivalents of $I_2$ in $Me_2NCHO$ for 4 h at room temperature.[52]

The chimeras were cleaved and deprotected with 85% $CF_3CO_2H$, 5% $CH_2Cl_2$, 9.5% m-cresol, and 0.5% $Et_3SiH$ for 2 h at room temperature,[53] then purified by re-

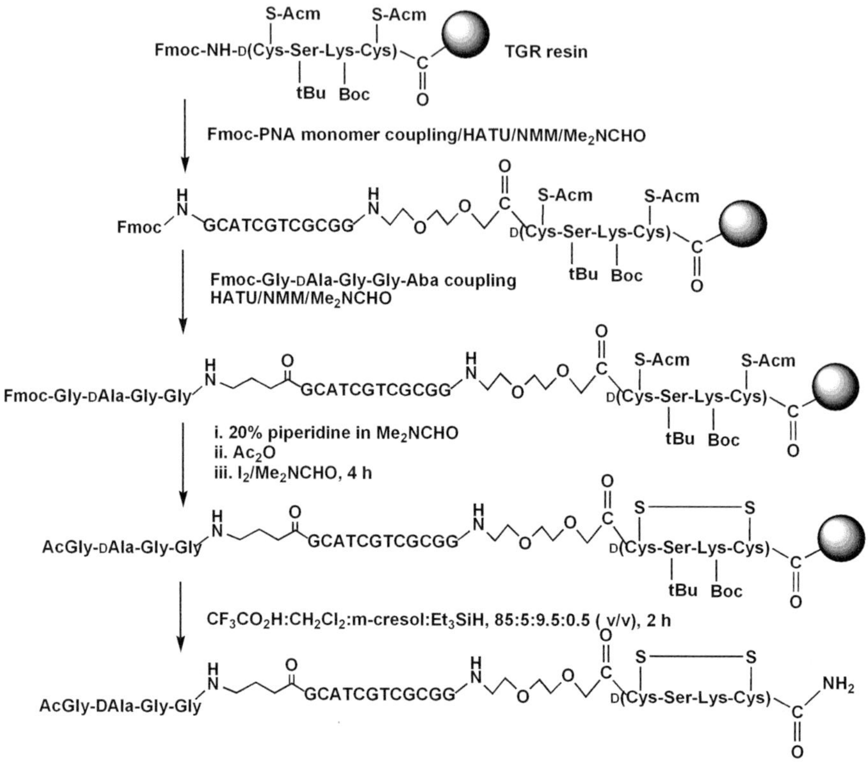


SCHEME 1.

versed phase liquid chromatography on a 10 × 250 mm Alltima $C_{18}$ column eluted with a gradient linear 25 min from 5% to 45% $CH_3CN$ in aqueous 0.1% $CF_3CO_2H$, at 1 mL/min, at 50°C, monitored at 260 nm. Matrix-assisted laser desorption/ionization time of flight mass spectrometry (MALDI-TOF MS, Ciphergen Corp., Fremont, CA) was carried out from an α-cyano-hydroxycinnamic acid matrix excited at 338 nm, and calibrated with porcine neuropeptide Y.

We prepared a cyclized chelator-PNA-peptide chimera AcGDAGGB-GCATCGTCGCGG-AEEA-D(CSKC), WT4219, specific for *MYC* mRNA and the IGF1 receptor (FIG. 3).[54] Preparative RP-HPLC of the crude product yielded a main peak containing 98.05% of the absorbance at 260 nm (FIG. 5A). The overall yield following preparative RP-HPLC was 27.2%. MALDI-TOF MS confirmed the identity of the main product peak at 4221.6 Da (FIG. 5B). Similarly, we prepared a *MYC* PNA 4-mismatch control, AcGDAGGB-GCATGTCTGCGG-AEEA-D(CSKC), WT4235, with 30.6% overall yield following preparative RP-HPLC (FIG. 6A), and MALDI-TOF mass of 4234.7 Da (FIG. 6B).

We also prepared a probe specific for oncogene *CCND1* mRNA and the IGF1 receptor.[16,17] The probe is a cyclized peptide-PNA-peptide chimera AcGDAGGB-

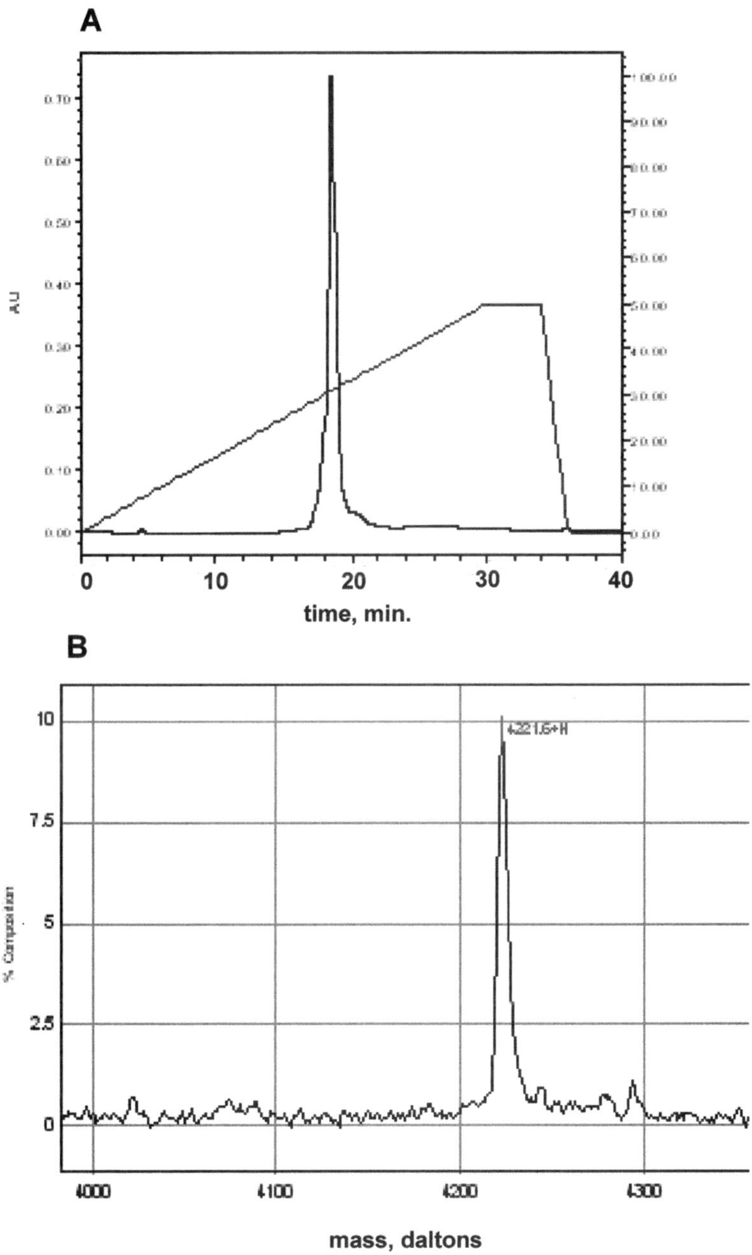


**FIGURE 5.** Characterization of cyclized *MYC* antisense chimera AcGDAGGB-GCATCGTCGCGG-AEEA-D(CSKC), WT4219.[54] (**A**) Analytical reversed phase liquid chromatography of cyclized chimera on a 10 × 250 mm Alltima $C_{18}$ column eluted with a linear 30-min gradient from 5% to 45% $CH_3CN$ in aqueous 0.1% $CF_3CO_2H$, at 1 mL/min, at 50°C, monitored at 260 nm. (**B**) MALDI-TOF mass spectrum of chimera in a matrix of α-cyano-hydroxycinnamic acid. Experimental mass: 4221.6 Da; calculated mass: 4219.0 Da.

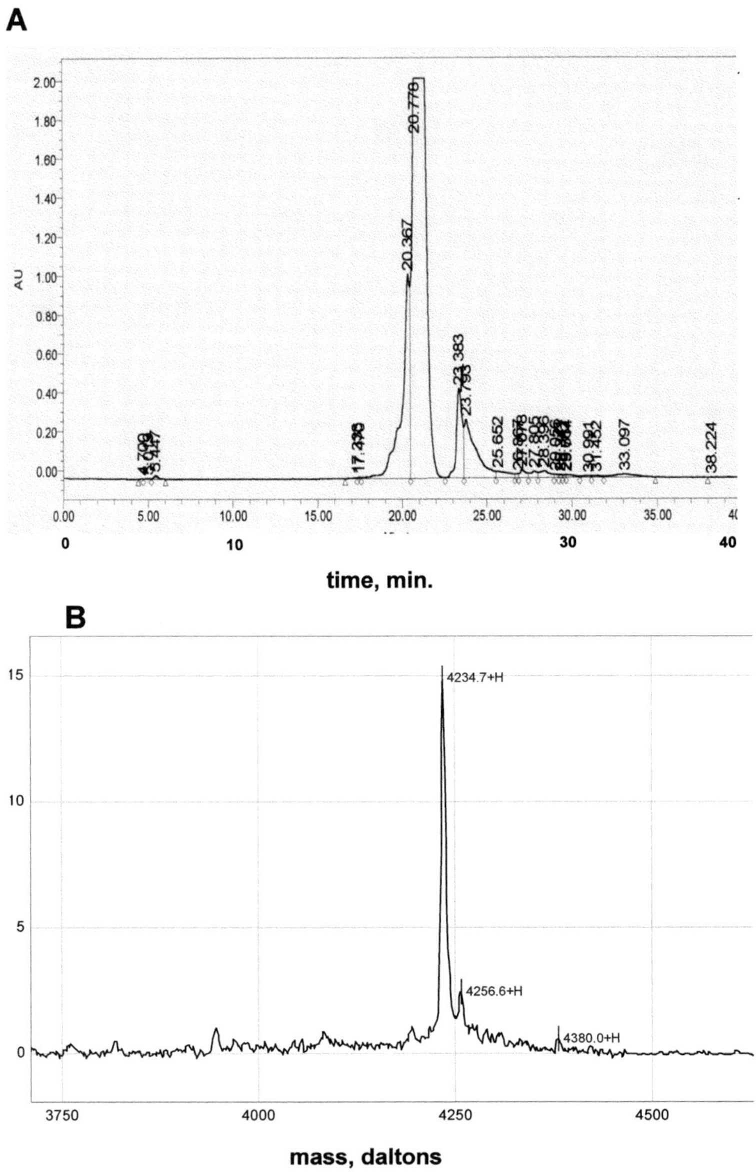


**FIGURE 6.** Characterization of cyclized *MYC* mismatch chimera AcGDAGGB-GCAT-GTCTGCGG-AEEA-D(CSKC), WT4235.[54] (**A**) Preparative $C_{18}$ HPLC of cyclized chimera as in FIGURE 5. (**B**) MALDI-TOF mass spectrum of chimera as in FIGURE 5. Experimental mass: 4234.7 Da; calculated mass: 4235.0 Da.

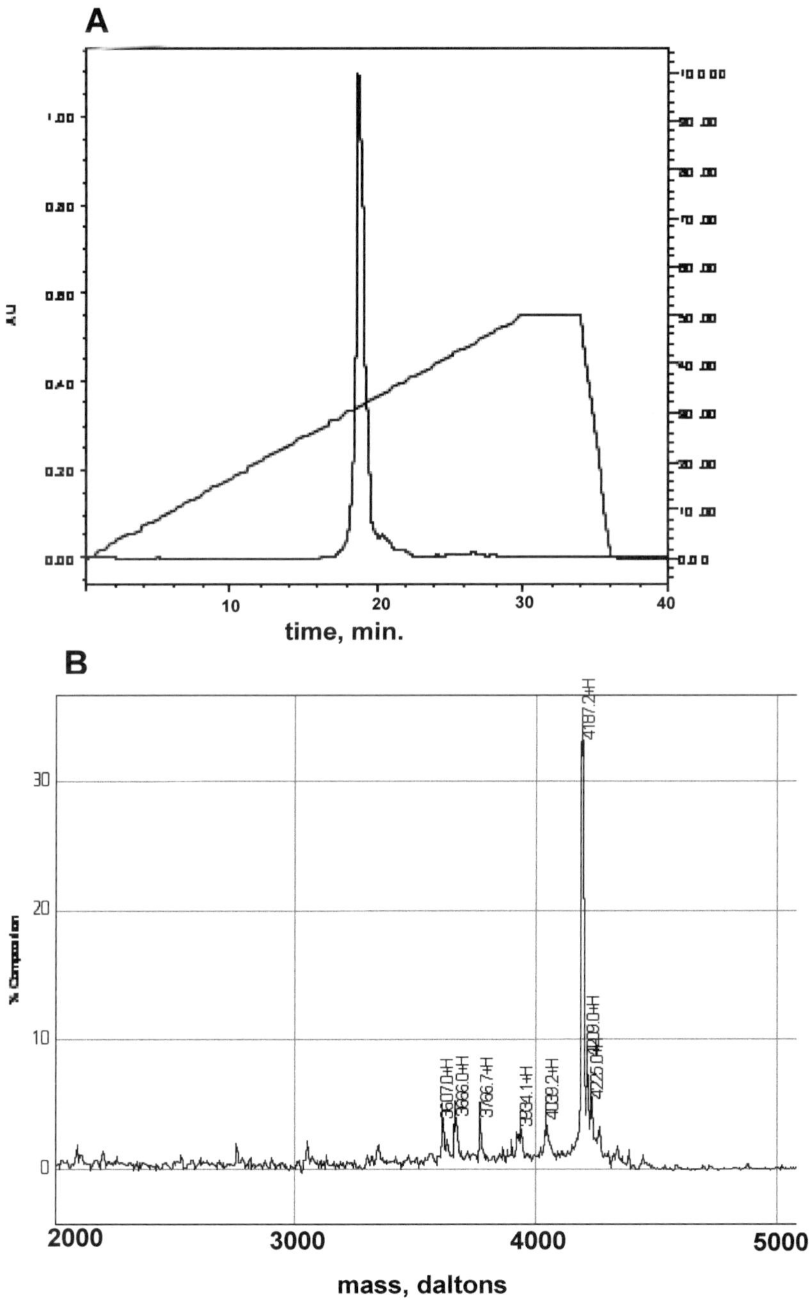


**FIGURE 7.** *See following page for legend.*

CTGGTGTTCCAT-AEEA-D(CSKC), WT4185. Preparative RP-HPLC of the crude product yielded a main peak containing 95% of the absorbance at 260 nm (FIG. 7A). The overall yield of the HPLC-purified chimera relative to the initial solid support was 30.6%. MALDI-TOF MS of the purified chimera confirmed the identity of the main product peaks at 4187.2 Da (FIG. 7B). Similarly, we prepared a *CCND1* PNA 4-mismatch control, AcGDAGGB-CTGGACAACCAT-AEEA-D(CSKC), WT4172, an IGF1 peptide alanine substitution control, AcGDAGGB-CTGGTGTTCCAT-AEEA-D(CysAlaAlaCys), WT4113, and a PNA-free control, AcGDAGGB-$(Gly)_4$-D(CSKC), WT990. TABLE 1 displays the characteristics of the peptide-PNA-peptide chimeras.

For Cu-64 PET probes, the route was modified slightly (SCHEME 2).[55] The IGF1 peptide analogue D(CSKC) was extended from C to N by Fmoc coupling,[52] using a PS3 peptide synthesizer (Protein Technologies, Phoenix, AZ) for all amino acid, PNA, and chelator coupling steps. AEEA was coupled, then Fmoc-PNA monomers (Applied Biosystems) to create the *KRAS* V12 mutant sequence N-GCCAC-CAGCTCC-C, followed by two AEEA spacers, then diaminopropanoate (DAP). The chelator moiety S-benzoyl thioglycolic acid (SBTG) was synthesized, recrystallized from ethyl acetate, and characterized by melting point analysis.[56] SBTG was then coupled on solid phase to both amines of deprotected DAP to yield a $SBTG_2DAP$ $N_2S_2$ chelator.[57] The cysteine thiols of D(CSKC) were cyclized and the products were cleaved and purified as described above.[52] High-performance liquid chromatography (HPLC) analysis of the crude $SBTG_2DAP$-PNA-peptide chimera (FIG. 4) yielded a main product peak (FIG. 8A) with a mass of 4350.5 Da (calculated 4351.09 Da) (FIG. 8B).[55]

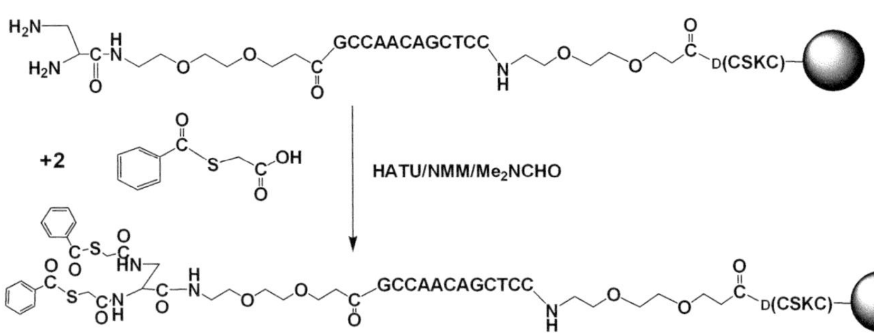


**SCHEME 2.**

**FIGURE 7.** Characterization of cyclized *CCND1* antisense chimera AcGDAGGB-CTGGTGTTCCAT-AEEA-D(CSKC), WT4185.[17] (**A**) Preparative $C_{18}$ HPLC of cyclized chimera as in FIGURE 5. (**B**) MALDI-TOF mass spectrum of chimera as in FIGURE 5. Experimental mass: 4187.2 Da; calculated mass: 4185.0 Da.

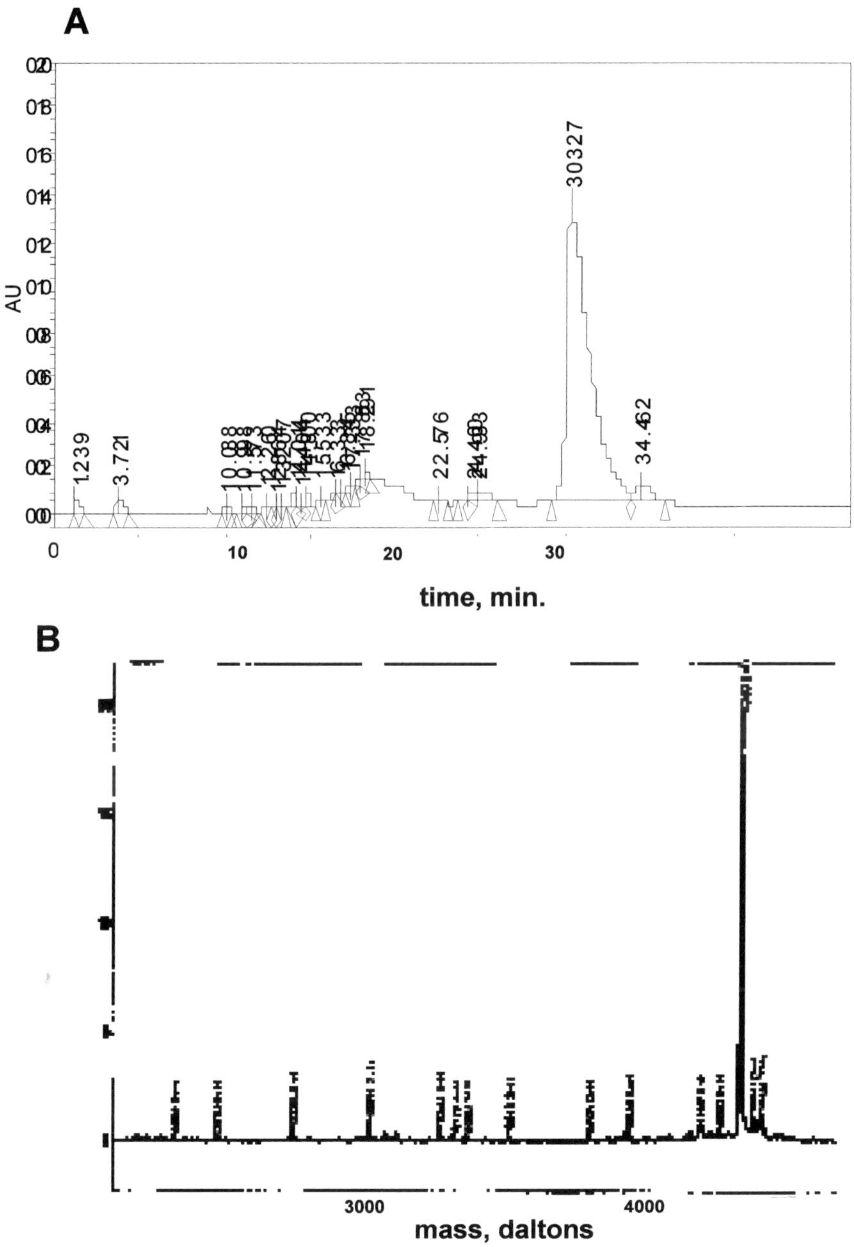


**FIGURE 8.** Characterization of cyclized *KRAS* antisense chimera SBTG$_2$DAP-AEEA-GCCAACAGCTCC-AEEA-D(CSKC), WT4351.[55] (**A**) Preparative $C_{18}$ HPLC of cyclized chimera as in FIGURE 5. (**B**) MALDI-TOF mass spectrum of chimera as in FIGURE 5. Experimental mass: 4350.5 Da; calculated mass: 4351.09 Da.

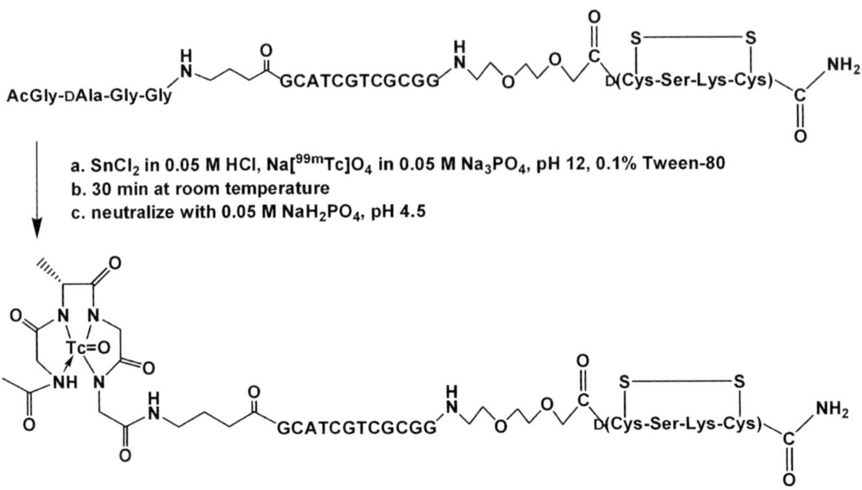


SCHEME 3.

## RADIOLABELING

Purified GDAGGB-PNA-peptide chimeras were labeled with Tc-99m (SCHEME 3), essentially as described previously.[50] In brief, 20 µg of GDAGGB-PNA-peptide chimera and 45–60 µg of $SnCl_2 \cdot 2H_2O$ were vortexed in 20 µL of 50 mM HCl. Next, 12 mCi of $Na^{99m}TcO_4$, freshly eluted from the Tc-99m generator with 200 µL of 0.15 M NaCl, were vortexed with 600 µL of 50 mM $Na_3PO_4$, pH 12, 0.1% Tween 80. The radionuclide mixture was then added to the GDAGGB-PNA-peptide/$SnCl_2$ solution and incubated for 30 min at room temperature. Finally, the solution was neutralized by the addition of 1 mL of 50 mM $NaH_2PO_4$, pH 4.5.

Reaction mixtures were analyzed to determine free Tc-99m and chelated Tc-99m by reversed phase liquid chromatography on a 4.5 × 250 mm reversed phase $C_{18}$ microbond HPLC column (Rainin, Emeryville, CA) coupled to a UV detector, NaI (Tl) radioactivity monitor, and a rate meter. The column was eluted with a 28-min gradient from 10% to 100% $CH_3CN$ in aqueous 0.1% $CF_3CO_2H$, at 1 mL/min, at 25°C. Unchelated free Tc-99m (Rf 1.0) was also determined by instant thin layer chromatography on silica gel (ITLC-SG, Gelman Sciences, Ann Arbor, MI) developed with methylethyl ketone. Colloid formation (Rf 0.0) was determined on ITLC-SG developed with pyridine/HOAc/$H_2O$ (3:5:1.5). These preparations were stable at 22°C for more than 4 h, as determined by HPLC, and were stable to challenges with 100-fold molar excesses of diethylenetriaminepentaacetic acid, human serum albumin, or cysteine. Specific activities of the preparations were approximately 2 Ci/µmol.[54]

Aliquots (20 µg) of the *MYC* GDAGGB-PNA-peptide antisense probe, WT4219, labeled well at 22°C (FIG. 9A).[54] Free Tc-99m was only 0.36%, and colloids were only 4.84%. The PNA mismatch, WT4235, also labeled well (FIG. 9B). Free Tc-99m was 0.99%, and colloids were 4.84%. Similarly, the *CCND1* probe labeled well (FIG. 10A).[16,17] Free Tc-99m was only 1.5%, and colloids were only 2.5%. The PNA mis-

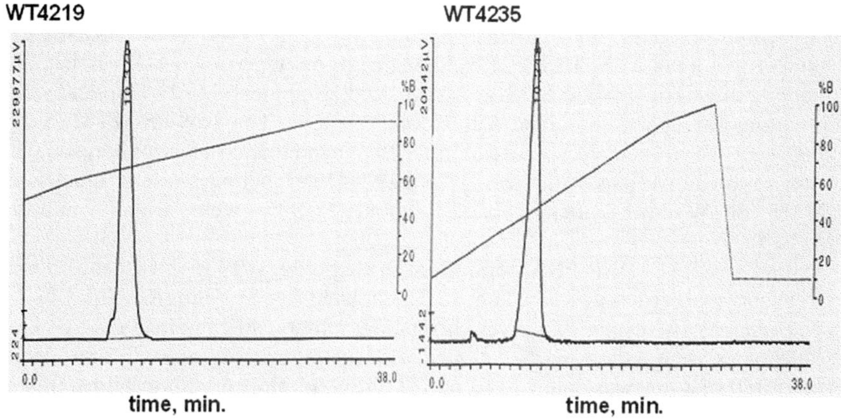


**FIGURE 9.** Analysis of *MYC* antisense probe Tc-99m-AcGDAGGB-GCATCGTCGCGG-AEEA-D(CSKC), WT4219, and *MYC* mismatch probe Tc-99m-AcGDAGGB-GCATGTCTGCGG-AEEA-D(CSKC), WT4235.[54] An aliquot of each labeling reaction was analyzed on a 10 × 250 mm Rainin Microbond $C_{18}$ column eluted with a 28- min gradient from 10% to 100% $CH_3CN$ in aqueous 0.1% $CF_3CO_2H$, at 1 mL/min, at 25°C. %B ($CH_3CN$) is shown on the *right y-axis*, and NaI (Tl) radiometric gamma emission is shown on the *left y-axis*. *Left*: antisense probe, WT4219. The single labeled peak eluted at 10.37 min. *Right*: mismatch probe, WT4235. The single labeled peak eluted at 10.25 min.

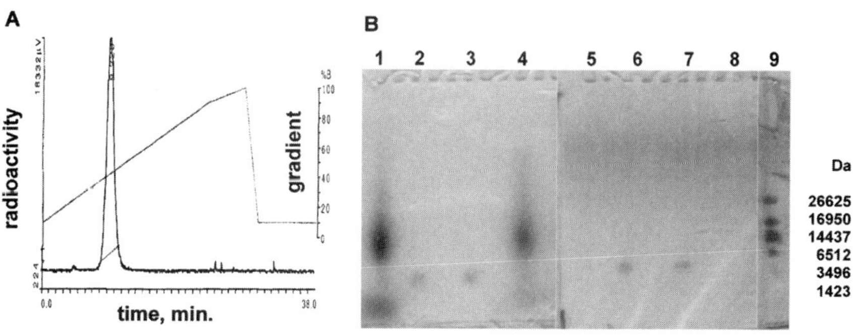


**FIGURE 10.** Analysis of *CCND1* antisense probe Tc-99m-AcGDAGGB-CTGGTGT-TCCAT-AEEA-D(CSKC), WT418517 (**A**) An aliquot of the labeling reaction was analyzed by $C_{18}$ HPLC as in FIGURE 9. The single labeled peak eluted at 9.3 min. (**B**) Denaturing gel electrophoresis on 10–20% polyacrylamide Tris-Tricine SDS gels (Bio-Rad). The *left side* is an autoradiogram, while the *right side* was stained with Coomassie blue. Lanes 1and5, Tc-99m labeling reaction; lanes 2 and 6, mock reaction without Tc-99m; lanes 3 and 7, purified WT4185; lanes 4 and 8, 9.3 min. Tc-99m peak from **panel A**; lane 9, peptide mass standards.

match, WT4172, peptide mismatch, WT4113, and PNA-free, WT990, controls labeled similarly (data not shown). Radiolabeled chimeras and mock-treated unlabeled chimeras were analyzed by denaturing gel electrophoresis on 10–20% polyacrylamide Tris-Tricine SDS gels (Bio-Rad, Hercules CA).[48] Duplicate gels were autoradiographed or stained with Coomassie blue. The Tc-99m-WT4185 9.3-min peak from FIGURE 10A showed a radioactive band that co-electrophoresed with the main radioactive band from the Tc-99m-WT4185 labeling mixture; unchelated WT4185 or WT4185 mock-chelated without Tc-99m were slightly retarded (FIG. 10B).

The *KRAS* SBTG$_2$DAP-PNA-peptide antisense probe, WT4351, was labeled with Tc-99m and analyzed as described above. Unchelated free Tc-99m ($R_f$ 1.0) of 14.1% was determined by instant thin layer chromatography on silica gel (ITLC-SG, Gelman Sciences, Ann Arbor, MI) developed with methylethyl ketone. Colloid formation ($R_f$ 0.0) of 4.4% was determined on ITLC-SG developed with pyridine/HOAc/$H_2O$ (3:5:1.5). A 34 μCi aliquot was analyzed by $C_{18}$ HPLC (FIG. 11), showing a single labeled chimera peak at 12 min.[55]

The *KRAS* SBTG$_2$DAP-PNA-peptide antisense probe, WT4351, was also labeled with Cu-64 for PET imaging. WT4351 (20 μg), dissolved in 15 μL of water, were added to 200 μL of 0.1 M ammonium acetate, pH 5.5 and vortexed; then 2 μL of $^{64}CuCl_2$ (100 μCi) in 0.1 M HCl were added. The reaction mixture was incubated for 30 min at 90°C. The *KRAS* Cu-64-SBTG$_2$DAP-PNA-peptide probe was analyzed as described above (FIG. 12), eluting at 6.8 min with only approximately 10% labeling efficiency in the first attempt. Unchelated free Cu-64 ($R_f$ 1.0) of 1.22% was determined by instant thin layer chromatography on silica gel (ITLC-SG, Gelman

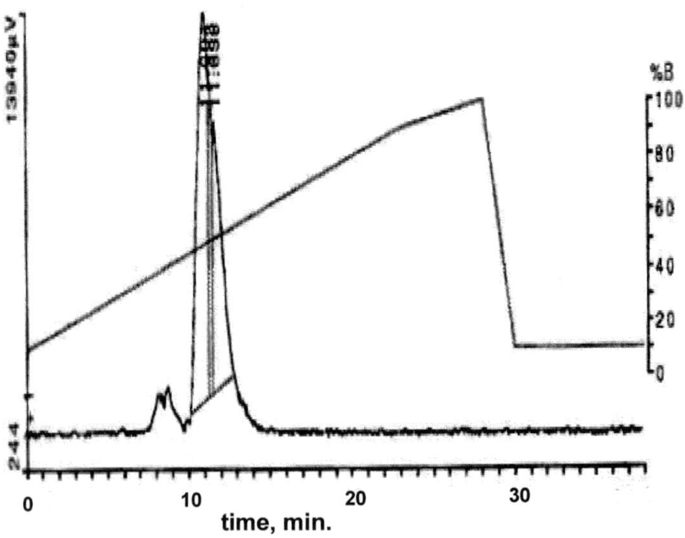


**FIGURE 11.** Analysis of *KRAS* antisense probe Tc-99m-SBTG$_2$DAP-AEEA-GCCAA-CAGCTCC-AEEA-D(CSKC), WT4351, as in FIGURE 9 above.[55]

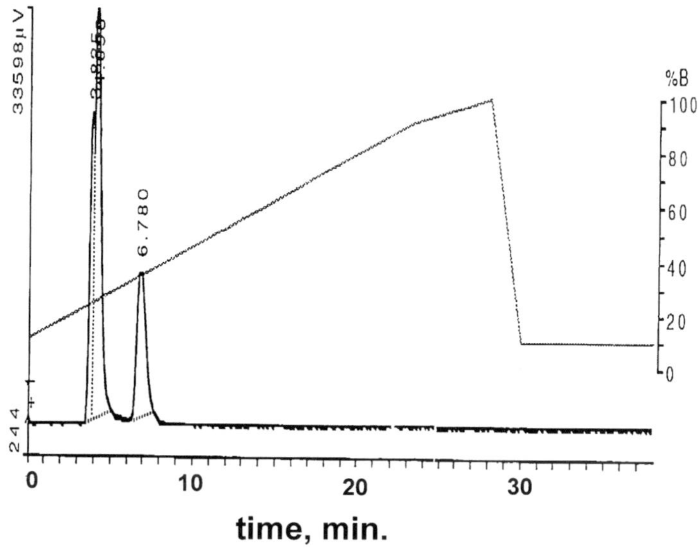


**FIGURE 12.** Analysis of *KRAS* antisense probe Cu-64-SBTG$_2$DAP-AEEA-GCCAA-CAGCTCC-AEEA-D(CSKC), WT4351, as in FIGURE 9 above.

Sciences) developed with methylethyl ketone. Colloid formation ($R_f$ 0.0) of 0.58% was determined on ITLC-SG developed with pyridine/HOAc/$H_2O$ (3:5:1.5).[55]

## CELLULAR INTERACTIONS

Human MCF7:IGF1R estrogen receptor–positive breast cancer cells, clone 17, transformed to express $1 \times 10^6$ IGF1R/cell constitutively from a cytomegalovirus promoter[58] were maintained in DMEM plus 5% calf serum, 50 U/mL penicillin, 5 μg/mL streptomycin, 2 mM glutamine, and 7.5 nM 17-β-estradiol (Sigma, St. Louis, MO) at 37°C under 5% $CO_2$. Internalization of fluoresceinyl-PNA-peptide chimeras by MCF7:IGF1R cells was analyzed essentially as described for p6 cells.[48] In brief, MCF7:IGF1R cells were grown in DMEM/F12 (1:1) (Sigma) containing 5% calf serum, 100 U/mL penicillin, 10 μg/mL streptomycin, and 2 mM glutamine. Cells were detached from their flasks with 0.02% EDTA solution (Sigma) and plated in LabTek 8-well chamber slides (Nalge Nunc International Corp., Naperville, IL) at a concentration of $1.5 \times 10^4$ cells/well. Cells were allowed to attach and were grown to 50% confluence, then synchronized in phenol red-free and serum-free DMEM (Life Technologies, Inc., Gaithersburg, MD) containing 0.1% bovine serum albumin, 50 g/mL holo-transferrin (Sigma), 100 U/mL penicillin, 10 μg/mL streptomycin, and 2 mM glutamine (PRF-SFM) for 24 h. After synchronization, the cells were stimulated with 10 nM 17-β-estradiol for 24 h.

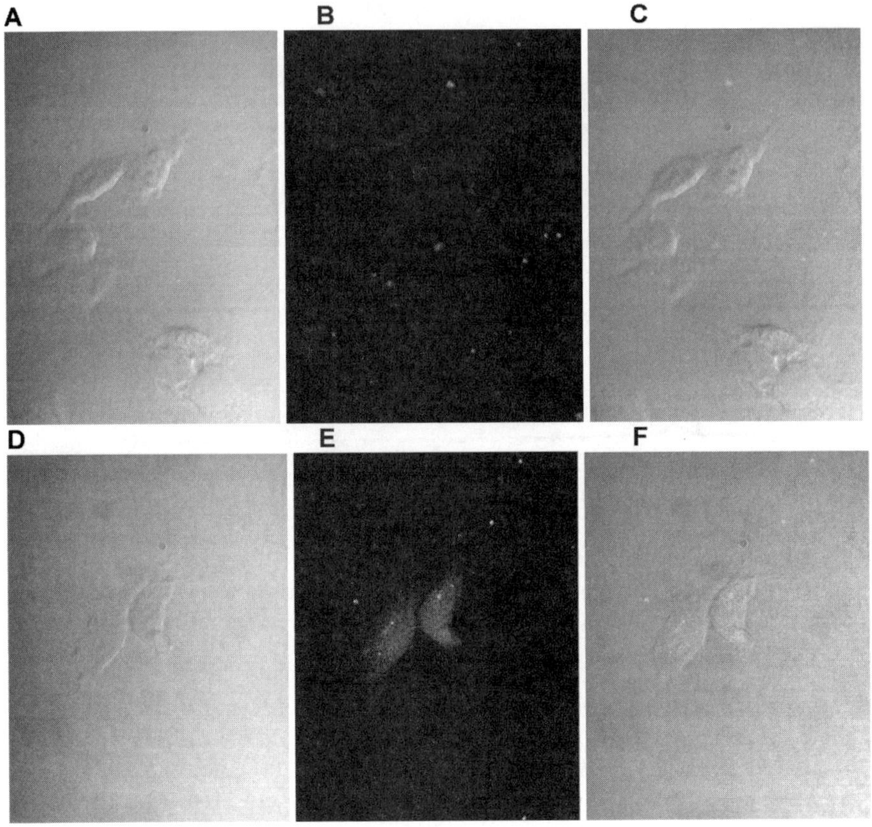

**FIGURE 13.** MCF7:IGF1R cell uptake of the *CCND1* fluoresceinyl-PNA-mismatch peptide probe, WT4361 (**A–C**), and the *CCND1* fluoresceinyl-PNA-IGF1 peptide probe, WT4433 (**D–F**).[1 7]Cells were incubated in 1 μM fluoresceinyl-PNA-peptide for 8 h at 37°C in PRF-SFM, then fixed and examined by confocal microscopy. *Left*: phase contrast; *middle*: fluorescence; *right*: overlay.

The cells were washed once with PRF-SFM and then incubated for 4 or 8 h with 1 μM or 5 μM fluoresceinyl-*CCND1* PNA-peptide in PRF-SFM.[16,17]At the end of the incubation, the cells were washed three times with PBS. Then the cells were fixed with 1% paraformaldehyde in PBS for 1 h at 37°C and washed three times with PBS. The chamber superstructure was removed, and 40 μL of ProLong Antifade reagent (Molecular Probes, Eugene, OR) was applied to cover the fixed cells in each well on the slide. A coverslip was then applied and sealed to the slide. The fixed slides were examined on a Bio-Rad MRC-600 laser scanning confocal microscope, interfaced to an Axiovert 100 inverted microscope (Zeiss) with a PlanApo 63× 1.40NA oil-immersion lens (Zeiss). Eight hours after exposure of MCF7:IGF1R cells to 1 μM of the fluorescent peptide mismatch chimera, SFX-AEEA-CTGGT-GTTCCAT-AEEA-D(CysAlaAlaCys), WT4361, no cellular uptake was apparent (FIG. 13A–C). On the other hand, significant uptake of the fluorescent PNA anti-

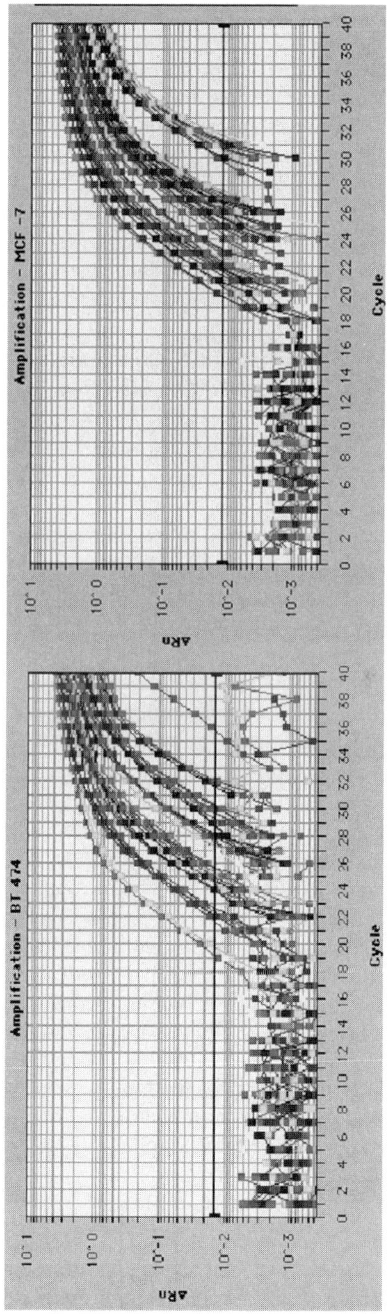


**FIGURE 14.** Cellular oncogene mRNA levels. BT474 (*left*) and MCF7:IGF1R (*right*) breast cancer cell mRNAs (10, 1, 0.1 ng) were analyzed by QRT-PCR on the ABI Prizm 7700 to determine expression levels of *HER2* (black [blue online]), *CCND1* (light gray [green online]), *IGF1R* (dark gray [red online]), *MYC* (medium gray [pink online]), and *TBP* (white [yellow online]).[17]

sense chimera, SFX-AEEA-CTGGTGTTCCAT-AEEA-D(CSKC), WT4433, was observed throughout the cells (FIG. 13D–F). These results agree with those reported previously for p6 cells.[48]The same results were seen in cells treated with 5 μM fluorescent probes for 4 h (not shown).

We then measured oncogene expression levels in untreated cells by quantitative reverse transcription-polymerase chain reaction (QRT-PCR). For QRT-PCRs, cells were lysed with Trizol (Sigma) and RNA was extracted with phenol/chloroform. From each sample, 0.5 μg of RNA was amplified and analyzed as described previously.[59] We compared BT474 human breast cancer cells, which overexpress *HER2* and *MYC* oncogenes, but not the estrogen receptor, with MCF7:IGF1R human breast cancer cells, which overexpress the estrogen receptor, IGF1 receptor, and *CCND1* and *MYC* oncogenes (FIG. 14).[16,17] Comparison of threshold cycle numbers for *MYC* mRNA with those for TATA-box binding protein mRNA yielded an average ratio of 8 for MCF7:IGF1R cells over two logs of RNA template. Similarly, comparison of threshold cycle numbers for *CCND1* mRNA with those for TATA-box binding protein mRNA yielded ratios of 32 for BT474 cells and 8 for MCF7:IGF1R cells. Based on the previously reported TATA-box binding protein mRNA copies per breast cancer cell of 1000–2000,[60] we estimated approximately 8,000 *MYC* mRNAs and 8,000 *CCND1* mRNAs per MCF7:IGF1R cell.

For an independent measure of cellular oncogene mRNA levels by binding of Tc-99m probes, MCF7:IGF1R cells were grown to 80% confluency, detached using trypsin-EDTA (Sigma), and washed with DMEM medium. For uptake of Tc-99m-AcGDAGGB-PNA-peptide probes, aliquots of $11.5 \pm 0.5 \times 10^6$ cells were dispensed in 0.5 mL of culture medium in test tubes. To each tube 2.8 pmol ($1.66 \times 10^{12}$ molecules) of Tc-99m-AcGDAGGB-PNA-peptide was added, mixed, and incubated at 22°C for 30 min. Cells were then centrifuged at $450 \times g$ for 5 min, and the supernatant was saved for counting. Cells were then washed twice with DMEM. The three supernatants were combined. Radioactivity associated with the supernatants and with the cell pellets was then determined. Knowing the % Tc-99m taken up by the cells (A = cell pellet counts/total counts) and assuming that one Tc-99m atom is bound per AcGDAGGB-PNA-peptide molecule, the number of PNA probes bound was calculated ($B = A \times 1.66 \times 10^{12}$). The number of Tc-99m-AcGDAGGB-PNA-peptides bound per cell ($C = B/11.5 \times 10^6$ cells) yields the number of *CCND1* mRNAs per cell, assuming that all molecules were uniformly distributed per cell, internalized, and hybridized. Assuming that each Tc-99m-AcGDAGGB-PNA-peptide molecule was internalized and hybridized, we used the specific activity of Tc-99m to calculate *CCND1* mRNAs/cell. For 12 cell suspensions measured on three different days, *CCND1* mRNA copy number was estimated at $6089 \pm 2000$ per cell for the antisense probe, Tc-99m-WT4185, compared with only $2388 \pm 615$ for the PNA mismatch control, Tc-99m-WT4172, measured on 8 cell suspensions.[16,17] The difference of $3701 \pm 2615$ *CCND1* mRNAs/cell is the same order of magnitude as that estimated by qRT-PCR above.

Similarly, we used the *KRAS* probe Tc-99m-SBTG$_2$DAP-AEEA-GCCAA-CAGCTCC-AEEA-D(CSKC), WT4351, and the *CCND1* probe Tc-99m-GDAAGB-AEEA-CTGGTGTTCCAT-AEEA-D(CSKC), WT4185, to measure pancreatic cancer cell binding of the two oncogene probes. The human pancreatic cancer cell line AsPC1 (American Type Culture Collection, Rockville, MD), which was isolated from ascites of a female patient with invasive pancreatic adenocarcinoma,[61] expresses a 12th codon GGT-GAT mutant *KRAS* oncogene.[62] AsPC1 cells were maintained in log phase at 37°C in DMEM supplemented with 2 mM glutamine, 5000 U/mL penicillin, 50 μg/mL streptomycin, and 10% fetal bovine serum (Sigma Chemical Co.). We found that after a 30-min incubation at 37°C, Tc-99m-WT4351 binding was 3235 ± 316 probes/cell versus Tc-99m-WT4185 binding of 1151 ± 132 probes/cell. The latter result probably represents nonspecific binding, implying a *KRAS* mRNA copy number of about 2000/AsPC1 cell.

## IMAGING

For breast cancer xenograft induction, 5–6 × $10^6$ MCF7:IGF1R cells in 0.2 mL of culture medium were implanted intramuscularly through a sterile 27-gauge needle into the thighs of female Balb/c nude mice obtained from the National Institutes of Health (NIH). Tumors were allowed to grow to no more than 0.5 cm in diameter. Each injection included 10 mg of Matrigel (Becton Dickinson). A pellet that releases 4.5 mg of 17-β-estradiol over 60 days (Innovative Research of America) was implanted subdermally in each mouse. Tumors were allowed to grow to about 0.5 cm in diameter. All animal studies were conducted in accordance with federal and state guidelines governing the laboratory use of animals, and under approved protocols reviewed by the AAALAC-licensed Institutional Animal Care and Use Committee at Thomas Jefferson University. All animals were anesthetized by approved methods, and when required the animals were restrained using methods and devices specifically designed to provide a minimum of discomfort to the animal. Animals were euthanized in a halothane chamber, consistent with U.S. Department of Agriculture regulations and American Veterinary Medical Association recommendations.

In order to assess chimera distribution and imaging, 7.4–11.1 MBq (0.2–0.3 mCi) of the Tc-99m-chelator-PNA-peptides in 0.2 mL of sterile 0.1 M $Na_2HPO_4$, pH 7, were administered to each of five female immunocompromised mice (NIH) per group through a lateral tail vein using a sterile 27-gauge needle. For the 24 h distribution, 29.6–34.2 MBq (0.8–0.9 mCi) of probe was administered. At 4 and 24 h post-injection, mice were lightly anesthetized, then imaged using a Starcam (GE Medical, Milwaukee, WI) gamma camera equipped with a parallel hole collimator. For each image, 300,000 counts were collected. Digital scanning of region-of-interest intensities with the interfaced Entegra computer (GE Medical) across each scintigraphic image from the tumor-free left flank to the tumor-bearing right flank provided quantitation of tumor images.

To test our hypothesis that a complementary Tc-99m-AcGDAGGB-PNA-peptide probe specific for *MYC* mRNA and the IGF1 receptor could visualize a *MYC*-expressing tumor, we administered approximately 18.5 MBq (0.5 mCi) Tc-99m-AcGDAGGB-PNA-peptide *MYC* probes to cohorts of 5 female immunocompromised mice bearing approximately 0.5 cm MCF7:IGF1R xenografts to determine the specificity and sensitivity of scintigraphic imaging 4 and 24 h after administration (FIG. 15).[54] We previously tested whether the PNA-free chelator plus IGF1 analogue control probe would bind to tumor cells expressing high levels of IGF1 receptor, which it did not.[63] To test whether a probe containing four central PNA mismatches would bind to tumor cells expressing high levels of IGF1 receptor and *MYC* mRNA, we administered the PNA mismatch control, WT4235. We did not observe tumor

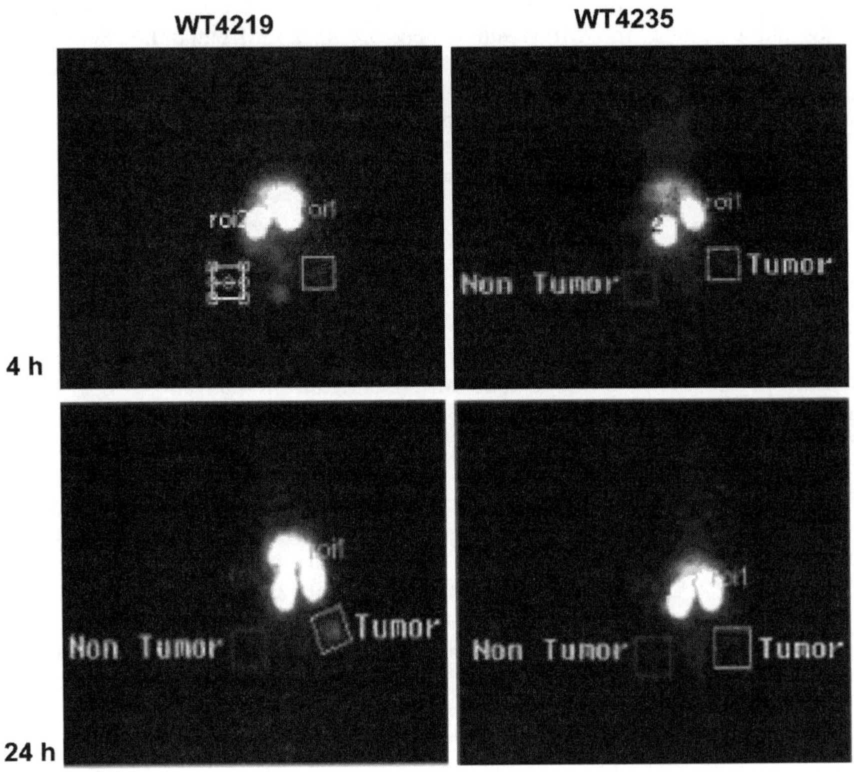


**FIGURE 15.** Scintigraphic images of γ–particles emitted by decaying Tc-99m in immunocompromised mice carrying human MCF7:IGF1R ER+ breast tumor cell xenografts at 4 hr. and 24 h after injection of Tc-99m-AcGDAGGB-PNA-peptides.[54] *Left*: Tc-99m-WT4219 *MYC* antisense probe; *right*: Tc-99m-WT4235 *MYC* mismatch control.

signals at 4 or 24 h post-injection (FIG. 15R). Finally, to test whether the complementary probe with correct IGF1 analogue would bind to tumor cells expressing high levels of IGF1 receptor and *MYC* mRNA, we administered the PNA antisense chimera, WT4219. In this case, we observed faint tumor signals at 4 h, and intermediate tumor signals at 24 h post-injection (FIG. 15L).

Digital scanning of the tumor site region-of-interest on the right flank vs. the mirror image tumor-free region-of-interest on the left flank enabled quantitation of tumor images. The ratios of tumor site:control site intensities are plotted in FIGURE 18 as a function of time.[16,17] One presumes that any ratio greater than 1 implies some preferential probe concentration. No tumor image was obvious in FIGURE 15 following administration of the PNA mismatch control, WT4235, which includes the IGF1 peptide analogue, but the digitized tumor site:control site ratio was $3.33 \pm 0.30$ at 4 h and $2.72 \pm 0.44$ at 24 h. A faint tumor image was apparent in FIGURE 15 four hours after administration of the antisense probe, WT4219, which correlated with the tu-

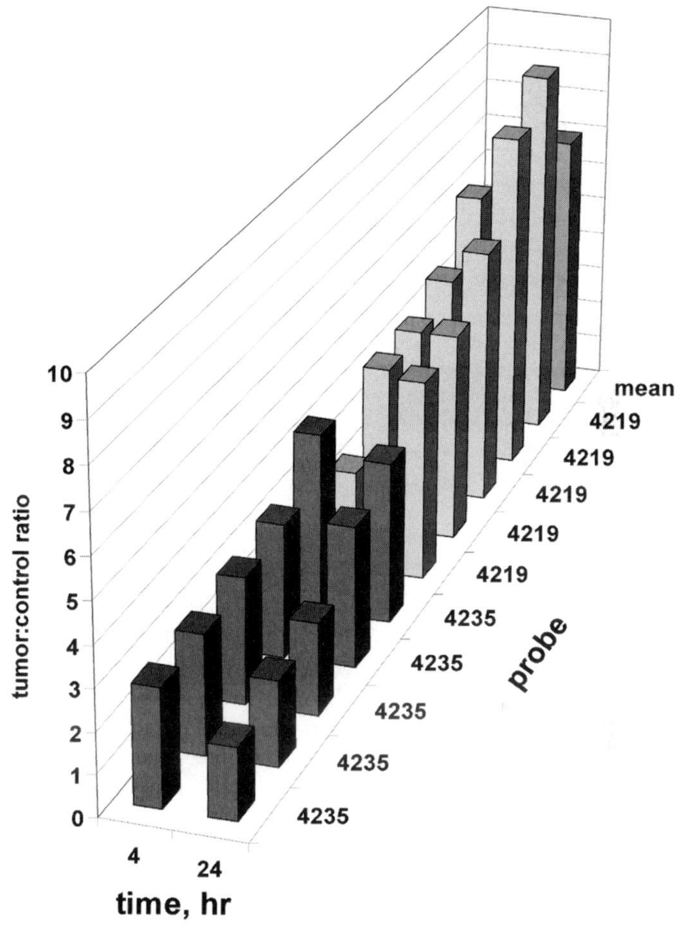


**FIGURE 16.** Tumor site:control site gamma intensity ratios after systemic administration of *MYC* Tc-99m-AcGDAGGB-PNA-peptide chimeras for all subjects in FIGURE 15.[1] Tc-99m-WT4235 *MYC* mismatch control (dark gray [red online]); Tc-99m-WT4219 *MYC* antisense probe (light gray [green online]).

mor site:control site ratio of 4.35 ± 0.58. At 24 h post-injection, the ratio increased to 7.01 ± 0.90.

Kruskal-Wallis one-way analysis of variance on ranks determined that the four groups were significantly different from each other ($P$ <0.001). When all four groups were compared by the Holm-Sidak method, the antisense group was not significantly different from the mismatch group at 4 h post-injection ($P = 0.244$). However, at 24 h post-injection, Holm-Sidak comparison revealed a statistically significant difference ($P$ <0.001) between the antisense group and the mismatch group. The test performed had a power of 0.985 with $\alpha = 0.050$.

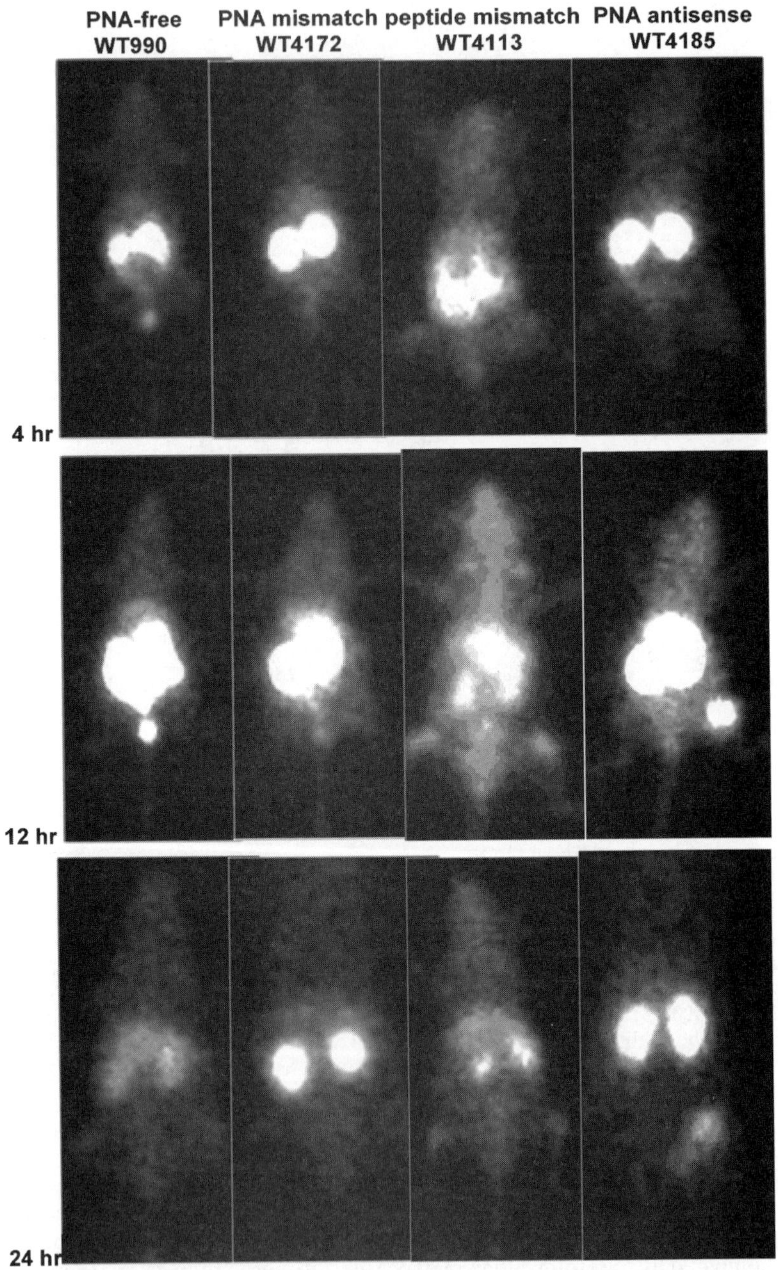


**FIGURE 17.** Scintigraphic images of γ–rays emitted by decaying Tc-99m in nude mice carrying human MCF7:IGF1R estrogen receptor-positive breast tumor cell xenografts at 4, 12, and 24 h after injection of PNA-free control, WT990, PNA *CCND1* mismatch control, WT4172, *CCND1* peptide mismatch control, WT4113, and PNA *CCND1* antisense probe, WT4185.[17]

To test our hypothesis that a complementary Tc-99m-AcGDAGGB-PNA-peptide probe specific for *CCND1* mRNA and the IGF1 receptor could visualize a *CCND1*-expressing tumor, we administered approximately 18.5 MBq (0.5 mCi) Tc-99m-AcGDAGGB-PNA-peptide *CCND1* probes to cohorts of 5 female immunocompromised mice bearing approximately 0.5 cm MCF7:IGF1R xenografts to determine the specificity and sensitivity of scintigraphic imaging 4, 12, and 24 h after administration (FIG. 17).[16,17]To test whether the probe would bind to tumor cells expressing high levels of IGF1 receptor, we administered the PNA-free chelator plus IGF1 analogue control, WT990, independent of internalization and mRNA binding. We did not observe tumor signals at 4, 12, or 24 h post-injection.

Similarly, to test whether a probe containing four central PNA mismatches would bind to tumor cells expressing high levels of IGF1 receptor and *CCND1* mRNA, we administered the PNA mismatch control, WT4172. We did not observe tumor signals at 4, 12, or 24 h post-injection. Next, to test whether the complementary probe with two central peptide mismatches would bind to tumor cells expressing high levels of IGF1 receptor and *CCND1* mRNA, we administered the peptide mismatch control, WT4113. We did not observe tumor signals at 4, 12, or 24 h post-injection.

Finally, to test whether the complementary probe with correct IGF1 analogue would bind to tumor cells expressing high levels of IGF1 receptor and *CCND1* mRNA, we administered the PNA antisense chimera, WT4185. In this case, we observed faint tumor signals at 4 h, strong tumor signals at 12 h, and intermediate tumor signals at 24 h post-injection.

Digital scanning of the tumor site region-of-interest on the right flank vs. the mirror image tumor-free region-of-interest on the left flank enabled quantitation of tumor images. The ratios of tumor site:control site intensities are plotted in FIGURE 18 as a function of time.[16,17] One presumes that any ratio greater than 1 implies some preferential probe concentration. Although no tumor image was obvious in FIGURE 17 following administration of the PNA-free control, WT990, the measured ratios of about 1.5 imply some weak binding. Similar ratios of about 1.5 were found for the PNA mismatch control, WT4172, which also includes the IGF1 peptide analogue. In the case of the peptide mismatch control, WT4113, some binding was apparent at 4 h post-administration, but not at 12 or 24 h. Only a faint tumor image was obvious in FIGURE 17 four hours after administration of the antisense probe, WT4185, which correlated with the average scanning ratio of $2.75 \pm 1.45$. At 12 h post-injection, the average ratio increased to $6.32 + 3.20$, and displayed a similar value of $6.65 \pm 1.31$ at 24 h. Kruskal-Wallis ANOVA determined that the 12 groups were significantly different from each other ($P < 0.001$).

When comparing each group against another at 4 h post-injection, Kruskal-Wallis ANOVA determined that there was not a statistically significant difference ($P = 0.182$) among them. However, at 12 h post-injection, Kruskal-Wallis ANOVA determined that there was a statistically significant difference ($P = 0.013$) among the four groups. Dunn's multiple comparison procedure determined that the PNA-free control, WT990, and the PNA mismatch, WT4172, groups were different ($P < 0.05$), and that the PNA mismatch, WT4172, and PNA antisense, WT4185, groups were different ($P < 0.05$), but that the peptide mismatch, WT4113, and PNA antisense, WT4185, groups were not different ($P > 0.05$). Similarly, at 24 h post-injection, Kruskal-Wallis ANOVA determined that there was a statistically significant difference ($P = 0.009$) among the four groups. Dunn's multiple comparison procedure again determined

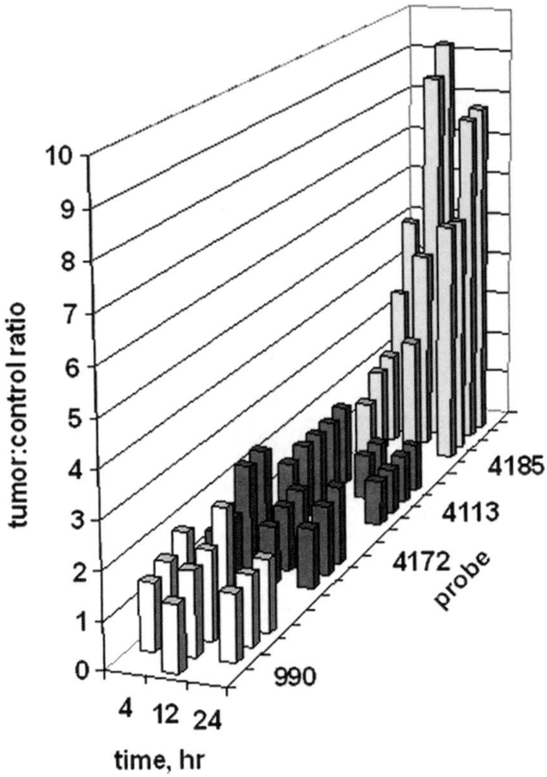


**FIGURE 18.** Tumor site:control site gamma intensity ratios after systemic administration of *CCND1* Tc-99m-AcGDAGGB-PNA-peptide chimeras for all subjects in FIGURE 17. PNA-free control, Tc-99m-WT990 (white [yellow online]); Tc-99m-WT4172 *CCND1* PNA mismatch control (dark gray [blue online]); Tc-99m-WT4113 *CCND1* peptide mismatch control (medium gray [red online]; Tc-99m-WT4185 *CCND1* antisense probe (light gray [green online]).[17]

that the PNA-free control, WT990, and the PNA mismatch, WT4172, groups were different ($P$ <0.05), and that the PNA mismatch, WT4172, and PNA antisense, WT4185, groups were different ($P$ <0.05), but that the peptide mismatch, WT4113, and PNA antisense, WT4185, groups were not different ($P$ >0.05).

For pancreatic cancer xenograft induction, $1 \times 10^7$ Panc-1 cells in 0.2 mL of culture medium were implanted intramuscularly through a sterile 27-gauge needle into the thighs of female Balb/c nu/nu mice (NIH). Panc-1 cells have the same *KRAS*-activating mutation as AsPC-1 cells and were maintained in the same medium. Tumors were allowed to grow to no more than 0.5 cm in diameter. Each injection included 10 mg of Matrigel (Becton Dickinson).

To test our hypothesis that a complementary Tc-99m-SBTG$_2$DAP-PNA-peptide probe specific for *KRAS* mRNA and the IGF1 receptor could visualize a *KRAS*-expressing tumor, we administered to cohorts of 5 tumor-bearing mice approximately 18.5 MBq (0.5 mCi) Tc-99m-WT4351 in 0.2 mL of sterile 0.1 M $Na_2HPO_4$, pH

7, through a lateral tail vein using a sterile 27-gauge needle. For the 24 h distribution, 29.6–34.2 MBq (0.8–0.9 mCi) of probe was administered. Scintigraphic imaging (FIG. 19) of Tc-99m-SBTG$_2$DAP-*KRAS* PNA-peptide in Panc-1 pancreatic xenografts showed tumor to contralateral muscle image intensity ratios of 5.4 at 4 h and 2.7 at 24 h after injection of probe into the tail vein.[55] Mismatch controls have not yet been carried out.

To test our hypothesis that the same SBTG$_2$DAP-PNA-peptide labeled with Cu-64 could image *KRAS* mRNA by PET, we administered to cohorts of 5 tumor-bearing

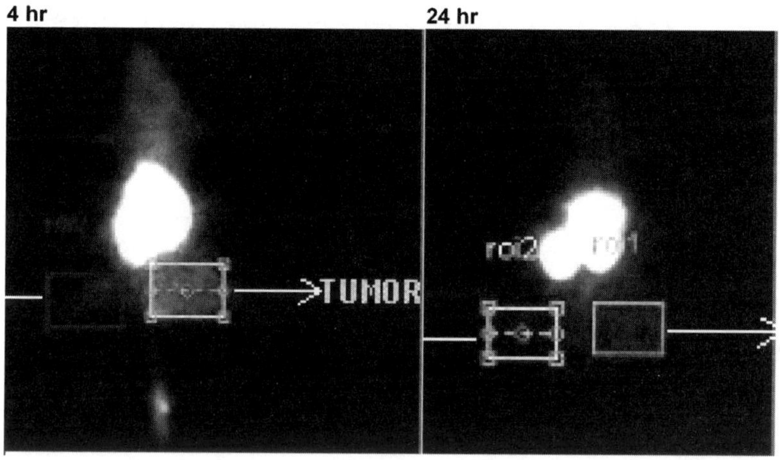


**FIGURE 19.** Scintigraphic imaging of Tc-99m-SBTG$_2$DAP-*KRAS* PNA-peptide in Panc-1 pancreatic xenografts 4 and 24 h after probe injection into the tail vein.[55]

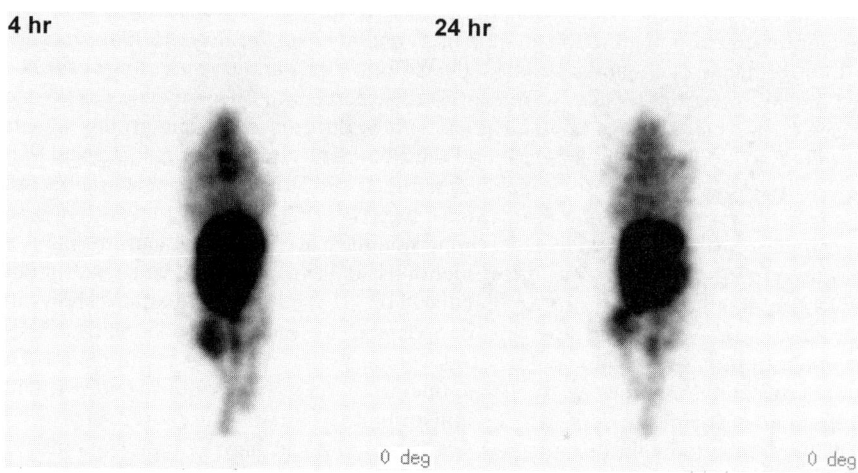


**FIGURE 20.** PET imaging of Cu-64-WT4351, SBTG$_2$DAP-*KRAS* PNA-peptide in AsPC1 pancreatic xenografts 4 and 24 h after injection of the probe into the tail vein.[55]

**TABLE 2. Tissue distribution (% injected dose/g) of the *MYC* antisense probe, Tc-99m-WT4219, and the *MYC* mismatch chimera, Tc-99m-WT4235, at 4 h after systemic administration ($n$ = 5)[54] 0}54**

| Tissue | Antisense | Mismatch | Null probability |
|---|---|---|---|
| Muscle | 0.08 ± 0.02 | 0.11 ± 0.03 | 0.11 |
| Intestine | 0.10 ± 0.03 | 0.11 ± 0.01 | 0.18 |
| Heart | 0.09 ± 0.02 | 0.68 ± 0.15 | 0.00003 |
| Lung | 0.52 ± 0.19 | 0.70 ± 0.27 | 0.25 |
| Blood | 0.18 ± 0.03 | 0.24 ± 0.03 | 0.01 |
| Spleen | 3.64 ± 1.71 | 4.44 ± 0.98 | 0.39 |
| Kidney | 31.54 ± 3.14 | 37.47 ± 3.42 | 0.02 |
| Liver | 5.55 ± 0.77 | 3.43 ± 0.51 | 0.00091 |
| Tumor | 0.20 ± 0.05 | 0.23 ± 0.05 | 0.47 |
| T/M ratio | 2.57 ± 0.96 | 2.26 ± 0.78 | 0.59 |
| T/B ratio | 1.14 ± 0.17 | 0.97 ± 0.29 | 0.30 |

mice approximately 7.4 MBq (0.2 mCi) Cu-64-WT4351 in 0.2 mL of sterile 0.1 M $Na_2HPO_4$, pH 7, through a lateral tail vein using a sterile 27-gauge needle. PET imaging (FIG. 20) of tumor-bearing mice showed tumor to contralateral muscle image intensity ratios of 2.0 at 4 h and 3.0 at 24 h.[55] Mismatch controls have not yet been carried out.

## TISSUE DISTRIBUTION

After imaging, mice were euthanized, and tissues were dissected. These were washed free of blood, blotted dry, weighed, and radioactivity associated with each tissue was counted in an automatic gamma counter (Packard Series 5000, Meridien, CT), together with a standard radioactive solution of a known quantity prepared at the time of injection. Results were expressed as percent of injected dose per gram of tissue (% injected dose/g). Statistical analysis of differences among groups was determined by applying the standard error of the mean, Student's $t$ test, Kruskal and Wallis' one-way analysis of variance on ranks, or the Holm-Sidak pairwise multiple comparison procedure, using SigmaStat 3.0 (SPSS, Chicago, IL).

Tissue distribution of each *MYC* probe was measured in all subjects at 4 and 24 h after administration.[54] TABLE 2 presents the data for the *MYC* antisense probe, WT4219, and the *MYC* mismatch probe, WT4235, at 4 h, while TABLE 3 shows the results at 24 h. As the time after injection elapsed, the radioactivity in all tissues decreased, including that in the tumors. However, the tumor to blood and tumor to muscle ratios increased for WT4219 as time went on. This is consistent with the scintigraphic images in FIGURE 15 and the tumor (right)-to-muscle (left) image intensity ratios provided in FIGURE 16, which were higher than the tumor/muscle distribution ratios from scintillation counting for WT4219. While the tumors were readily detectable by scintigraphy with WT4219, but not with WT4235, the tumor distribution counts of % injected dose/g for the antisense group and the mismatch

**TABLE 3. Tissue distribution (% injected dose/g) of the *MYC* antisense probe, Tc-99m-WT4219, and the *MYC* mismatch chimera, Tc-99m-WT4235, at 24 h after systemic administration ($n$ = 5)[54] 0}54**

| Tissue | Antisense | Mismatch | Null probability |
|---|---|---|---|
| Muscle | 0.04 ± 0.01 | 0.05 ± 0.01 | 0.45 |
| Intestine | 0.04 ± 0.00 | 0.05 ± 0.00 | 0.008 |
| Heart | 0.03 ± 0.00 | 0.24 ± 0.03 | 0.0000004 |
| Lung | 0.15 ± 0.04 | 0.25 ± 0.03 | 0.002 |
| Blood | 0.04 ± 0.01 | 0.05 ± 0.01 | 0.06 |
| Spleen | 3.47 ± 0.88 | 3.32 ± 1.41 | 0.84 |
| Kidney | 21.65 ± 6.50 | 20.06 ± 4.64 | 0.67 |
| Liver | 4.95 ± 0.58 | 2.93 ± 0.75 | 0.001 |
| Tumor | 0.10 ± 0.03 | 0.11 ± 0.03 | 0.63 |
| T/M ratio | 2.59 ± 0.88 | 2.19 ± 0.30 | 0.37 |
| T/B ratio | 2.48 ± 0.56 | 2.09 ± 0.55 | 0.30 |

**TABLE 4. Tissue distribution (% injected dose/g) of the PNA-free probe, WT990, at 4, 12, and 24 h after systemic administration ($n$ = 5)[16,17]1}17**

| Tissue | 4 h | 12 h | 24 h |
|---|---|---|---|
| Muscle | 0.14 ± 0.10 | 0.04 ± 0.01 | 0.08 ± 0.02 |
| Intestine | 0.09 ± 0.01 | 0.15 ± 0.19 | 0.06 ± 0.02 |
| Heart | 0.05 ± 0.01 | 0.05 ± 0.00 | 0.07 ± 0.01 |
| Lung | 0.16 ± 0.01 | 0.12 ± 0.02 | 0.14 ± 0.02 |
| Blood | 0.11 ± 0.01 | 0.07 ± 0.01 | 0.08 ± 0.00 |
| Spleen | 0.08 ± 0.01 | 0.13 ± 0.05 | 0.41 ± 0.16 |
| Kidney | 7.82 ± 1.21 | 4.78 ± 0.54 | 2.10 ± 0.28 |
| Liver | 0.36 ± 0.03 | 0.41 ± 0.09 | 0.77 ± 0.22 |
| Tumor | 0.16 ± 0.08 | 0.09 ± 0.03 | 0.09 ± 0.01 |
| T/M ratio | 1.31 ± 0.32 | 2.85 ± 1.48 | 1.06 ± 0.10 |
| T/B ratio | 1.43 ± 0.76 | 1.35 ± 0.42 | 1.10 ± 0.17 |

group were not remarkably different, except for the heart. The increased accumulation of the mismatch probe WT4235 in heart tissue invited a BLAST search with the WT4235 sequence for heart-specific or mitochondrial-specific murine mRNAs. Unfortunately, no complementary homologies were identified, so the concentration of mismatch probe in the heart remains unexplained. The tissue distribution data indicated that renal excretion was the primary route of elimination and renal uptake was highest among all tissues, but the extent differed from agent to agent.

Tissue distribution of each *CCND1* probe was measured in all subjects at 4, 12, and 24 h after administration. TABLE 4 presents the data for the PNA-free control, WT990; TABLE 5 for the PNA mismatch, WT4172; TABLE 6 for the peptide mismatch, WT4113; and TABLE 7 for the PNA antisense probe, WT4185. The tissue dis-

**TABLE 5. Tissue distribution (% injected dose/g) of the PNA mismatch probe, WT4172, at 4, 12, and 24 h after systemic administration ($n$ = 5)[16,17]1}17**

| Tissue | 4 h | 12 h | 24 h |
|---|---|---|---|
| Muscle | 0.15 ± 0.04 | 0.06 ± 0.01 | 0.06 ± 0.01 |
| Intestine | 0.17 ± 0.03 | 0.07 ± 0.01 | 0.05 ± 0.01 |
| Heart | 0.15 ± 0.01 | 0.08 ± 0.01 | 0.06 ± 0.01 |
| Lung | 0.39 ± 0.07 | 0.22 ± 0.03 | 0.14 ± 0.03 |
| Blood | 0.29 ± 0.02 | 0.12 ± 0.02 | 0.07 ± 0.01 |
| Spleen | 0.23 ± 0.02 | 0.19 ± 0.04 | 0.16 ± 0.02 |
| Kidney | 35.29 ± 8.41 | 23.07 ± 2.83 | 9.62 ± 2.61 |
| Liver | 0.89 ± 0.16 | 0.81 ± 0.10 | 0.47 ± 0.02 |
| Tumor | 0.23 ± 0.55 | 0.14 ± 0.03 | 0.07 ± 0.03 |
| T/M ratio | 1.63 ± 0.55 | 2.12 ± 0.23 | 1.26 ± 0.39 |
| T/B ratio | 0.80 ± 0.18 | 1.17 ± 0.16 | 1.05 ± 0.30 |

**TABLE 6. Tissue distribution (% injected dose/g) of the peptide mismatch probe, WT4113, at 4, 12, and 24 h after systemic administration ($n$ = 5)[16,17]1}17**

| Tissue | 4 h | 12 h | 24 h |
|---|---|---|---|
| Muscle | 0.33 ± 0.06 | 0.13 ± 0.02 | 0.13 ± 0.03 |
| Intestine | 0.39 ± 0.06 | 0.14 ± 0.00 | 0.16 ± 0.04 |
| Heart | 0.35 ± 0.02 | 0.29 ± 0.04 | 0.19 ± 0.05 |
| Lung | 0.63 ± 0.05 | 0.42 ± 0.08 | 0.31 ± 0.06 |
| Blood | 0.61 ± 0.04 | 0.40 ± 0.07 | 0.17 ± 0.03 |
| Spleen | 0.40 ± 0.04 | 0.53 ± 0.22 | 1.28 ± 0.53 |
| Kidney | 10.30 ± 1.07 | 4.22 ± 0.67 | 5.51 ± 1.15 |
| Liver | 2.00 ± 0.21 | 1.56 ± 0.25 | 2.74 ± 0.75 |
| Tumor | 0.53 ± 0.07 | 0.28 ± 0.04 | 0.20 ± 0.06 |
| T/M ratio | 1.64 ± 0.29 | 2.25 ± 0.69 | 1.74 ± 0.88 |
| T/B ratio | 0.88 ± 0.14 | 0.72 ± 0.22 | 1.23 ± 0.47 |

tribution data indicated that renal excretion was the primary route of elimination and renal uptake was highest among all tissues, but the extent of kidney accumulation differed from agent to agent. As the time after injection elapsed, the radioactivity in all tissues decreased, including that in the tumors. However, the tumor to blood and tumor to muscle ratios increased for WT4185 as time elapsed. This finding is consistent with the scintigraphic images in FIGURE 17 and the tumor (right)-to-muscle (left) image intensity ratios provided in FIGURE 18, which were higher than the tumor/muscle distribution ratios from scintillation counting for WT4185 in TABLE 7. While the tumors were readily detectable by scintigraphy with WT4185, but not with WT990, WT4172, or WT4113, the tumor distribution counts of % injected dose/g for WT990, WT4172, and WT4185 were not significantly different. This apparent contradiction is considered below in the DISCUSSION.

**TABLE 7. Tissue distribution (% injected dose/g) of the PNA antisense probe, WT4185, at 4, 12, and 24 h after systemic administration ($n$ = 5)[16,17]1}17**

| Tissue | 4 h | 12 h |
|---|---|---|
| Muscle | 0.12 ± 0.03 | 0.10 ± 0.05 |
| Intestine | 0.12 ± 0.01 | 0.09 ± 0.01 |
| Heart | 0.11 ± 0.01 | 0.07 ± 0.02 |
| Lung | 0.29 ± 0.03 | 0.19 ± 0.03 |
| Blood | 0.23 ± 0.02 | 0.11 ± 0.02 |
| Spleen | 0.17 ± 0.02 | 0.17 ± 0.02 |
| Kidney | 21.55 ± 2.90 | 19.10 ± 3.94 |
| Liver | 0.52 ± 0.04 | 0.81 ± 0.10 |
| Tumor | 0.20 ± 0.06 | 0.17 ± 0.06 |
| T/M ratio | 1.78 ± 0.53 | 1.85 ± 0.57 |
| T/B ratio | 0.88 ± 0.20 | 1.49 ± 0.34 |

**TABLE 8. Tissue distribution (% injected dose/g) of the PNA antisense probe, Tc-99m-WT4351, at 4 and 24 h after systemic administration**

| Tissue | **4 h** ($n$ = 4) | **24 h** ($n$ = 5) |
|---|---|---|
| Muscle | 0.19 ± 0.03 | 0.07 ± 0.03 |
| Intestine | 0.18 ± 0.09 | 0.07 ± 0.01 |
| Heart | 0.46 ±0.05 | 0.20 ± 0.08 |
| Lung | 0.49 ± 0.16 | 0.14 ± 0.03 |
| Blood | 0.27 ± 0.07 | 0.06 ± 0.01 |
| Spleen | 1.07 ± 0.26 | 1.00 ± 0.09 |
| Kidney | 90.18 ± 7.22 | 65.96 ± 5.76 |
| Liver | 5.19 ± 1.72 | 5.68 ± 0.46 |
| Tumor | 0.22 ± 0.03 | 0.14 ± 0.05 |
| T/M ratio | 1.14 ± 0.20 | 2.14 ± 0.74 |
| T/B ratio | 0.83 ± 0.19 | 2.37 ± 0.84 |

Tissue distribution of the *KRAS* antisense probe was measured in all subjects at 4 and 24 h after administration. TABLE 8 reveals rapid and extensive renal excretion of Tc-99m-WT4351, compared with the probes containing a GDAGGB chelator. TABLE 9, however, shows much less renal concentration, and significant buildup in the liver, although only one mouse has been analyzed so far. Cu-64 probe concentration in the tumor was 20-fold greater than the same probe labeled with Tc-99m, as was seen with $SBTG_2$-VIP.[51]

## *IN VIVO* STABILITY

Urine was collected up to 3 h post-injection from 5 mice injected with the *MYC* antisense probe, Tc-99m-WT4219, and the *MYC* mismatch chimera, Tc-99m-

**TABLE 9. Tissue distribution (% injected dose/g) of the PNA antisense probe, Cu-64-WT4351, at 24 h after systemic administration**

| Tissue | **24 h** ($n$ = 1) |
|---|---|
| Muscle | 1.72 |
| Intestine | 8.70 |
| Heart | 6.22 |
| Lung | 8.27 |
| Blood | 2.88 |
| Spleen | 5.98 |
| Kidney | 10.44 |
| Liver | 24.57 |
| Tumor | 4.00 |
| T/M ratio | 2.33 |
| T/B ratio | 1.39 |

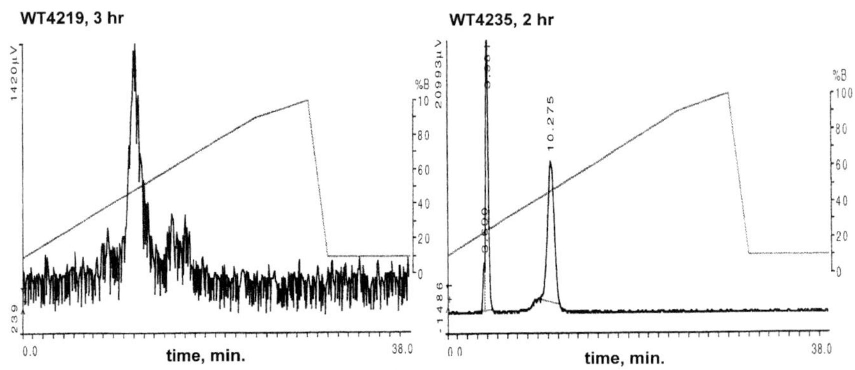


**FIGURE 21.** Analytical HPLC of Tc-99m-AcGDAGGB-PNA-peptide probes that were recovered from mouse urine 2–3 h after administration, chromatographed as in FIGURE 9 above.[54] *(Left) MYC* antisense probe, Tc-99m-WT4219, 3 h after administration; *(right) MYC* mismatch chimera, Tc-99m-WT4235, 2 h after administration.

WT4235, for assessment of probe stability.[54] Analytical HPLC of radioactivity in the combined deproteinized, lyophilized 3-h urine sample from mice injected with *MYC* antisense probe, Tc-99m-WT4219, showed no void volume peak of free Tc-99m, but only an intact probe peak at 10.7 min (FIG. 21, left). HPLC of radioactivity in the combined 2-h urine sample from mice injected with the *MYC* mismatch chimera, Tc-99m-WT4235, revealed a void volume peak of free Tc-99m, 44% of radioactivity, and a probe peak at 10.3 min with 56% of the radioactivity (FIG. 21, right). Breakdown fragments of the GDAGGB-PNA-peptide probes were not detected, consistent with the model that the PNA and the peptide moieties are resistant to proteases and nucleases.

## DISCUSSION

We set out to test the feasibility of using radiolabeled oncogene mRNA probes to visualize breast and pancreatic tumor xenografts from outside the body of murine hosts. To that end, we synthesized, purified, and characterized IGF1R-targeting agents with PNA hybridization probes to provide access to cancer cells overexpressing IGF1R, a receptor that is overexpressed in most malignant cells. Denaturing $NaDodSO_4$ gel electrophoresis of Tc-99m-GDAAGB-AEEA-CTGGTGTTCCAT-AEEA-D(CSKC), WT4185, showed a radioactive band that co-electrophoresed with the main radioactive band from the Tc-99m probe labeling mixture. We found by fluorescence microscopy that the chelator-PNA-peptide probes were taken up inside MCF7 breast cancer cells that overexpress IGF1R, if and only if the IGF1 peptide analogue sequence was correct. The measurements of fluorescent probe uptake, imaging of oncogene mRNAs in tumors, and intactness of probe recovered from urine demonstrate that the antisense chelator-PNA-peptide chimeras were stable *in vivo* for at least 24 h after administration.

We measured *CCND1* and *MYC* oncogene mRNA copy number in MCF7:IGF1R human breast cancer cells by qRT-PCR. Comparison of threshold cycle numbers for *CCND1* and *MYC* mRNA with those for TATA-box binding protein mRNA yielded estimates of 4,000–8,000/cell, permitting a theoretical estimate of maximum possible labeling. Assuming 6000 mRNAs per cell and $10^9$ cells per gram of tumor, there would be an estimated $6 \times 10^{12}$ mRNA copies available for binding in a one gram tumor. Our data suggest that 0.1% of the injected Tc-99m-WT4219 *MYC* probe, or 0.2% of the injected Tc-99m-WT4185 *CCND1* probe (specific activity 2 Ci/µmol) was associated with the tumors at 24 h. This suggests that approximately $3 \times 10^{11}$ molecules of Tc-99m-WT4219 *MYC* probe, or $6 \times 10^{11}$ molecules of Tc-99m-WT4185 *CCND1* were bound to the mRNA in a one-gram tumor, corresponding to about 5% of the *MYC* mRNAs, or about 10% of the *CCND1* mRNAs, despite nonuniform distribution of radioactivity in the tumor. Similar analyses yielded an estimate of about 2,000 *KRAS* mRNA/cell for AsPC1 pancreatic cancer cells. In a high specific activity or carrier-free preparation, this would be equivalent to about 500 µCi of $^{99m}$Tc, suggesting the possibility of up to 500 times greater sensitivity than we observed in this initial study.

To estimate the fraction of internalized PNA probes that could be hybridized to available *CCND1* or *MYC* mRNAs in live tumor cells, one must begin with the observed $T_m$ of approximately 80°C for 2.5 µM chelator-PNA-peptide 12-mers with 2.5 µM RNA.[52] A copy number of approximately 6000 *CCND1* or *MYC* mRNAs per 1 pL cell translates to 10 nM, or 3 nM for *KRAS* mRNA, while the tumor-localized Tc-99m-WT4219, Tc-99m-WT4185, or Tc-99m-WT4351 appeared to be about one-tenth of that, 1 nM, by 24 h. The $T_m$, the probe concentration, and the 10-fold excess mRNA concentration translate to a calculation[44] of virtually complete hybridization of available intracellular probe.

Interestingly, the concentration of label in tumors was very faint at 4 h after injection of the Tc-99m-WT4219 *MYC* probe or Tc-99m-WT4185 *CCND1* probe, although the digital scan revealed detectable concentrations of label. We interpret that observation to mean that uptake, intracellular trafficking, hybridization of label, and efflux of unbound label are all slow processes that do not reveal a strong tumor signal at 4 h. Because labeled antisense PNA in the tumors could be visualized at 24 h, we hypothesize that 24 h was sufficient for unbound probe to efflux from cells and to be excreted. With respect to the hybridized label, bound PNA probe dissociates negligibly from complementary RNA by 12–24 h.[44] In the end, we found that the MCF7:IGF1R xenografts that overexpress *CCND1* and *MYC* mRNA could be imaged reliably and specifically at 12–24 h post-injection. In contrast, Panc-1 and AsPC1 xenografts that overexpress *KRAS* mRNA could be imaged reliably and specifically by 4 h post-injection, with both Tc-99m and Cu-64. This faster response might reflect cellular differences between the indolent breast cancer cells and the aggressive pancreatic cancer cells.

The tissue distribution results are comparable to our previous observations with the antisense *MYC* PNA probe Tc-99m-GDAGGB-GCATCGTCGCGG, WT3613,[53] and to those of Stalteri and Mather,[64] as well as the tissue distribution of Tc-99m-GDAGGB-vasoactive intestinal peptide.[49,50,,65] Although there was no significant difference in tumor:muscle ratios between the *MYC* probe and its mismatch control, the MCF7:IGF1R xenografts were imaged clearly with WT4219, but not with WT4235. Similarly, the MCF7:IGF1R xenografts were imaged clearly with the *CCND1* probe WT4185, but not with WT990, WT4172, or WT4113. That is because the tissue distribution data report radioactivity in the entire excised masses, which include some surrounding normal tissue, the actively proliferating cells on the periphery of the tumors, and the necrotic cores, which exhibit poor uptake of macromolecules.[66]

By including the active and inactive portions of the tumors, as well as some surrounding normal tissue, the masses of actively proliferating tumors were overstated, and thereby the apparent % uptake of $^{99m}$Tc/g tumor and the ratios of tumor radioactivity to muscle radioactivity were decreased, reducing them to the range of the control agents. This same difference between clear scintigraphic images and modest % uptake of $^{99m}$Tc/g tumor was also observed earlier for Tc-99m-GDAGGB-vasoactive intestinal peptide, which revealed occult tumors in patients despite apparent tumor uptake of only 0.3% injected dose/g in xenografts in immunocompromised mice.[49,50,,65] Digital scanning, however, of scintigraphic intensities determined the radioactivity per pixel in the tumor region-of-interest, revealing *CCND1, MYC,* and *KRAS* mRNA expression in the actively proliferating cells of the tumors. In this case, the necrotic centers and the surrounding normal mouse tissue presumably did not contribute to the measurement, eliminating the possibility of label dilution. Thus, the tumor/contralateral scintifigraphic intensity ratios in FIGURES 15, 17, 19, and 20 probably provided more accurate results than the scintillation counting tissue distribution ratios in TABLES 2–9.

While the breast cancer xenografts were readily detectable by scintigraphy with the *MYC* probe Tc-99m-WT4219, but not with Tc-99m-WT4235, the tumor distribution counts of % injected dose/g for the antisense group and the mismatch group were not remarkably different, except for the heart. The increased accumulation of the mismatch probe Tc-99m-WT4235 in heart tissue invited a BLAST search with the WT4235 sequence for heart-specific or mitochondrial-specific murine mRNAs. Unfortunately, no complementary homologies were identified, so the concentration of mismatch probe in the heart remains unexplained. In the case of the *CCND1* probe Tc-99m-WT4113, with two D-Ala replacements in the peptide loop, the % tumor distribution values were higher than those for Tc-99m-WT4185; the kidney distribution values were lower and statistically significantly different ($P < 0.05$). Yet the tumors with Tc-99m-WT4113 were not detectable scintigraphically. Radioactivity uptake of Tc-99m-WT4113, for all time points, not only for the tumor, but for blood and muscle also, were three to four times greater ($P < 0.05$) than those for Tc-99m-WT4185. This greater uptake in blood and muscle may have contributed to the apparently greater uptake in the excised tumor due to the contribution of blood activity remaining in the tumor vasculature and by muscle, which could have contaminated the tumor during excision. The higher background radioactivity in the surrounding muscle rendered the tumors indistinguishable by scintigraphic scanning, even though the tissue counts showed higher Tc-99m-WT4113 radioactivity in muscle and tumors than Tc-99m-WT4185. This also resulted in lower intensity ratios, as determined by digital region-of-interest analyses shown in FIGURE 18. The two D-Ala replacements in the peptide loop of WT4113, in lieu of D-serine and D-lysine, precluded its binding to IGF1 receptor and reduced the net charge on WT4113. Both of those factors could have slowed its blood clearance. This was evidenced by a significantly lower renal uptake than that seen for Tc-99m-WT990, Tc-99m-WT4172, or Tc-99m-WT4185, all with the reversed, inverted IGF1 loop sequence, at each time point.

For most agents, renal clearance is predominantly determined by at least two parameters: first, the charge and second, the molecular size. In light of the neutrality of PNAs, the net charges on the PNA-free probe WT990, PNA mismatch probe WT4172, and PNA antisense probe WT4185 at pH 7.4 are probably the same: +1 from the N-terminal amine, and +1 from the D-lysine sidechain. The peptide mismatch probe, however, should only exhibit a charge of +1 from the N-terminal amine. The molecular masses of the chelator-PNA-peptide agents are not very different from one another, while the PNA-free chelator-peptide agent is much smaller. Hence, one would predict that the smaller PNA-free probe would clear most quickly, followed by the PNA mismatch and PNA antisense probes; then the peptide mismatch probe most slowly. *CCND1* expression has been reported to be high in renal cell carcinoma cells, but low in normal renal tissue.[67] Therefore, concentration of the PNA antisense probe WT4185 in the kidneys was probably not due to labeling of *CCND1* mRNA in kidney cells. Similarly, high-grade renal cell carcinomas exhibit elevated cytoplasmic Myc protein, but not in the nuclei and not in normal renal cells.[68] Therefore, concentration of the *MYC* probe Tc-99m-WT4219 in the kidneys was probably not due to labeling of *MYC* mRNA in kidney cells, but to nonspecific binding to negative charges on renal parenchyma. Consistent with that model, simultaneous L-lysine administration has been shown to reduce renal accumulation of In-111-DTPA-octreotide in rats.[69]

Urinalysis of the *MYC* antisense and mismatch Tc-99m-probes by reversed phase HPLC (FIG. 21) implied significant stability of the chelator-PNA-peptides *in vivo*, consistent with the hypothesis that a Tc-99m-D-peptide-PNA-D-peptide would be resistant to proteases and nucleases in blood and tissues. In the case of the mismatch probe, the free $^{99m}$Tc void volume peak probably resulted from re-oxidation of probe-bound $^{99m}$Tc(III) to free $^{99m}$Tc(VII) in the liver. The lack of a free $^{99m}$Tc void volume peak in the case of the antisense probe is remarkable. One may speculate that the antisense probe was only excreted upon the first pass through the kidney and that antisense probes that distributed to tissues did not re-enter the bloodstream to be metabolized by the liver, at least up to 3 h.

Our observation of scintigraphic imaging of *CCND1*, *MYC,* and *KRAS* mRNA expression in xenografts, and of positron imaging of *KRAS* mRNA expression in

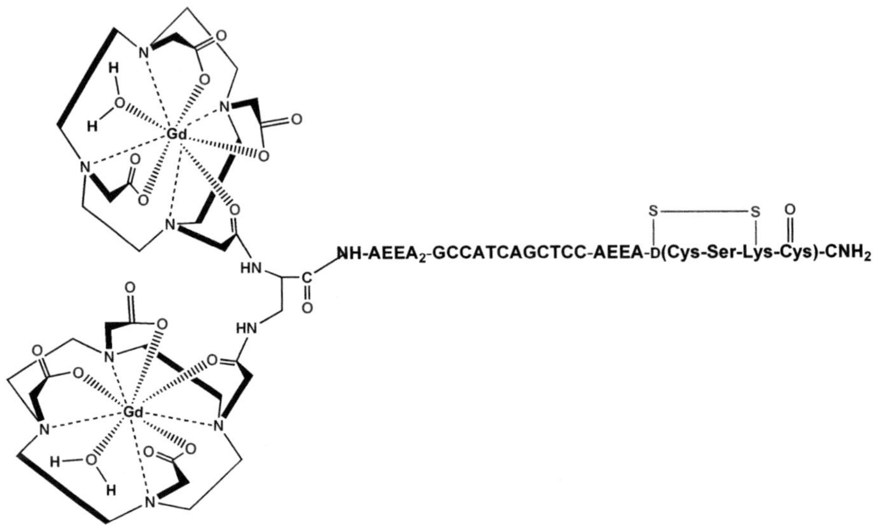


**FIGURE 22.** [Gd(III)-DOTA]$_2$DAP-PNA-peptide specific for *KRAS* mRNA and IGF1 receptor.

xenografts, could be applicable to patients at risk for new or recurrent cancer, including those with a strong family history of cancer, or when standard detection techniques provide ambiguous results. Imaging of mRNA expression with chelator-PNA-peptide chimeras labeled with Tc-99m, Cu-64, or other radionuclides, might also be applicable to other oncogenes or to other cell surface receptors. Other studies to image the breast, usually ultrasound or MRI, rely on morphologic changes between normal and abnormal breast tissue that may be present. Thus, not all malignant lesions are detected, and many invasive surgical procedures are performed to remove benign lesions. The latter problem results from the lack of specificity of current imaging techniques. We must confirm through histology the nature of masses detected by imaging studies. In this laboratory, we are also beginning to investigate MRI detection of mRNA overexpression via Gd(III) dendrimers (FIG. 22).[70]

## SUMMARY

Scintigraphic and positron imaging of cancer gene expression *in vivo* by noninvasive means could direct physicians to appropriate targets for intervention at the onset of disease and thereby significantly impact patient management. Until now, no method has been available to image specific overexpressed oncogene mRNAs *in vivo* by scintigraphic or positron imaging. We found that γ-emitting Tc-99m-chelator-PNA-peptides were taken up by human ER+ breast cancer xenografts, hybridized to complementary *CCND1* and *MYC* mRNA targets in the breast cancer cells, and concentrated sufficiently in tumor tissue to allow noninvasive imaging of oncogene overexpression. Similarly, a Tc-99m-chelator-PNA-peptide specific for *KRAS* mRNA could image pancreatic cancer xenografts by scintigraphic imaging, and the equivalent Cu-64-chelator-PNA-peptide could image pancreatic cancer xenografts by positron imaging.

In all cases, cellular uptake of the PNA probe by target cancer cells relied on the cyclized D(CSKC) analogue of IGF1 to enable binding and internalization by IGF1R overexpressed on the surface of the breast and pancratic cancer cells. The relatively low uptake in other normal tissues at both 4 and 24 h post-injection, except in the kidneys and liver, was also helpful in tumor delineation. These results suggest that Tc-99m-chelator-PNA-peptide probes and Cu-64-chelator-PNA-peptide probes could be applied for noninvasive imaging gene expression in tumors.

More sensitive and specific techniques are needed to detect disease as early as possible, minimizing diagnostic procedures and going directly to therapeutic intervention. While not sufficiently sensitive to be used alone, noninvasive measurement of mRNA expression by one or more oncogenes to confirm the presence or absence of cancer by gamma emission or by positron emission tomography when an imaging study is abnormal provides a mechanism for more accurate diagnosis of cancer.

## ACKNOWLEDGMENTS

We thank Dr. Eva Surmacz for her advice and the gift of MCF7 cells that constitutively overexpress IGF1R; Dr. Zhi-xian Lu for assistance in assembly of linear peptide-resin supports; and Dr. Richard Wassell for assistance in measuring mass spectra of peptide-PNA-peptides. This work was supported by Department of Energy/Biological Effects of Radiation grant ER63055, National Institutes of Health/National Cancer Institute (NIH/NCI) grant CA42960, NIH/NCI contract CO27175 to E.W., and by NIH grant HL59769 to M.L.T.

## REFERENCES

1. FONG, L.Y. *et al.* 2000. Muir-Torre-like syndrome in Fhit-deficient mice. Proc. Natl. Acad. Sci. USA **97:** 4742–4747.
2. BISHOP, J.M. 1991. Molecular themes in oncogenesis. Cell **64:** 235–248.
3. HILGERS, W. & S.E. KERN. 1999. Molecular genetic basis of pancreatic adenocarcinoma. Genes Chromosomes Cancer **26:** 1–12.
4. KNUDSON, A.G., JR. 1970. Genetics and cancer. Postgrad. Med. **48:** 70–74.
5. WOOSTER, R. 2000. Cancer classification with DNA microarrays. Is less more? Trends Genet. **16:** 327–329.
6. PEROU, C.M. *et al.* 1999. Distinctive gene expression patterns in human mammary epithelial cells and breast cancers. Proc. Natl. Acad. Sci. USA **96:** 9212–9217.
7. ALIZADEH, A., *et al.* 1998. Probing lymphocyte biology by genomic-scale gene expression analysis. J. Clin. Immunol. **18:** 373–379.
8. BARLUND, M. *et al.* 2000. Detecting activation of ribosomal protein S6 kinase by complementary DNA and tissue microarray analysis. J. Natl. Cancer Inst. **92:** 1252–1259.
9. CLARK, E.A. *et al.* 2000. Genomic analysis of metastasis reveals an essential role for RhoC. Nature **406:** 532–535.
10. PEROU, C.M. *et al.* 2000. Molecular portraits of human breast tumours. Nature **406:** 747–752.
11. AMERICAN CANCER SOCIETY. 2005. Cancer Facts and Figures. Atlanta, GA.

12. Rosenberg, R.D. *et al.* 1998. Effects of age, breast density, ethnicity, and estrogen replacement therapy on screening mammographic sensitivity and cancer stage at diagnosis: review of 183,134 screening mammograms in Albuquerque, New Mexico. Radiology **209:** 511–518.
13. Diekmann, F. *et al.* 2004. Evaluation of a wavelet-based computer-assisted detection system for identifying microcalcifications in digital full-field mammography. Acta Radiol. **45:** 136–141.
14. Fahy, B.N. *et al.* 2001. Cost-benefit analysis of biopsy methods for suspicious mammographic lesions. Arch. Surg. **136:** 990–994; discussion 994–995.
15. Evans, D.B., J.L. Abbruzzese & C.G. Willett. 2001. Cancer of the pancreas. *In* Cancer: Principles and Practice of Oncology. V.T. DeVita, S. Hellman & S.A. Rosenberg, Eds.: 1126–1161. Lippincott, Williams & Wilkins. Philadelphia.
16. Sauter, E.R. *et al.* 2000. Prolonged response to antisense cyclin D1 in a human squamous cancer xenograft model. Clin. Cancer Res. **6:** 654–660.
17. Tian, X. *et al.* 2004. External imaging of *CCND1* cancer gene activity in experimental human breast cancer xenografts with Tc-99m-peptide-PNA-peptide chimeras. J. Nucl. Med. **45:** 2070–2082.
18. Vaughn, J.P. *et al.* 1995. Antisense DNA downregulation of the ERBB2 oncogene measured by a flow cytometric assay. Proc. Natl. Acad. Sci. USA **92:** 8338–8342.
19. Wickstrom, E. & F.L. Tyson. 1997. Differential oligonucleotide activity in cell culture versus mouse models. Oligonucleotides as therapeutic agents. Ciba Found. Symp. **209:** 124–137; discussion 137–141.
20. Andrews, D.W. *et al.* 2001. Results of a pilot study involving the use of an antisense oligodeoxynucleotide directed against the insulin-like growth factor type I receptor in malignant astrocytomas. J. Clin. Oncol. **19:** 2189–2200.
21. Wickstrom, E.L. *et al.* 1988. Human promyelocytic leukemia HL-60 cell proliferation and c-Myc protein expression are inhibited by an antisense pentadecadeoxynucleotide targeted against c-*MYC* mRNA. Proc. Natl. Acad. Sci. USA **85:** 1028–1032.
22. Wickstrom, E., T.A. Bacon & E.L. Wickstrom. 1992. Down-regulation of c-Myc antigen expression in lymphocytes of Eμ-c-*myc* transgenic mice treated with anti-c-*myc* DNA methylphosphonates. Cancer Res. **52:** 6741–6745.
23. Huang, Y. *et al.* 1995. Prevention of tumor formation in a mouse model of Burkitt's lymphoma by 6 weeks of treatment with anti-c-*myc* DNA phosphorothioate. Mol. Med. **1:** 647–658.
24. Smith, J.B. & E. Wickstrom. 1998. Antisense c-*myc* and immunostimulatory oligonucleotide inhibition of tumorigenesis in a murine B-cell lymphoma transplant model. J. Natl. Cancer Inst. **90:** 1146–1154.
25. Aoki, K. *et al.* 1995. Liposome-mediated in vivo gene transfer of antisense K-ras construct inhibits pancreatic tumor dissemination in the murine peritoneal cavity. Cancer Res. **55:** 3810–3816.
26. Kawada, M. *et al.* 1997. Inhibition of anchorage-independent growth of ras-transformed cells on polyHEMA surface by antisense oligodeoxynucleotides directed against K-ras. Biochem. Biophys. Res. Commun. **231:** 735–737.
27. Okada, F. *et al.* 1998. Impact of oncogenes in tumor angiogenesis: mutant K-ras upregulation of vascular endothelial growth factor/vascular permeability factor is necessary, but not sufficient for tumorigenicity of human colorectal carcinoma cells. Proc. Natl. Acad. Sci. USA **95:** 3609–3614.
28. Kita, K. *et al.* 1999. Growth inhibition of human pancreatic cancer cell lines by antisense oligonucleotides specific to mutated K-ras genes. Int. J. Cancer **80:** 553–558.
29. Cogoi, S. *et al.* 2004. Antiproliferative activity of a triplex-forming oligonucleotide recognizing a Ki-ras polypurine/polypyrimidine motif correlates with protein binding. Cancer Gene Ther. **11:** 465–476.
30. Bishop, M.R. *et al.* 1997. Ex vivo treatment of bone marrow with phosphorothioate oligonucleotide OL(1)p53 for autologous transplantation in acute myelogenous leukemia and myelodysplastic syndrome. J. Hematother. **6:** 441–446.
31. Bayever, E. *et al.* 1994. Selective cytotoxicity to human leukemic myeloblasts produced by oligodeoxyribonucleotide phosphorothioates complementary to p53 nucleotide sequences. Leukemia & Lymphoma **12:** 223–231.

32. BRADLEY, J.D. *et al.* 2004. Implementing biologic target volumes in radiation treatment planning for non-small cell lung cancer. J. Nucl. Med. **45:** 96S–101S.
33. NAMAVARI, M. *et al.* 2000. Synthesis of 8-[(18)F]fluoroguanine derivatives: in vivo probes for imaging gene expression with positron emission tomography. Nucl. Med. Biol. **27:** 157–162.
34. PONOMAREV, V. *et al.* 2000. PET imaging of p53 gene expression in tumors. J. Nucl. Med. **41:** 263P–264P.
35. LEYTON, J. *et al.* 2005. Early detection of tumor response to chemotherapy by 3′-deoxy-3′-[18F]fluorothymidine positron emission tomography: the effect of cisplatin on a fibrosarcoma tumor model in vivo. Cancer Res. **65:** 4202–4210.
36. EISENHUT, M. & U. HABERKORN. 2000. [123I]VIP receptor scintigraphy in patients with pancreatic adenocarcinomas. Eur. J. Nucl. Med. **27:** 1589–1590.
37. GOLD, D.V. *et al.* 2001. Localization of pancreatic cancer with radiolabeled monoclonal antibody PAM4. Crit. Rev. Oncol. Hematol. **39:** 147–154.
38. WICKSTROM, E. 1992. Strategies for administering targeted therapeutic oligodeoxynucleotides. Trends Biotechnol. **10:** 281–287.
39. GRAY, G.D., S. BASU & E. WICKSTROM. 1997. Transformed and immortalized cellular uptake of oligodeoxynucleoside phosphorothioates, 3′-alkylamino oligodeoxynucleotides, 2′-O-methyl oligoribonucleotides, oligodeoxynucleoside methylphosphonates, and peptide nucleic acids. Biochem. Pharmacol. **53:** 1465–1476.
40. WALDER, R.Y. & J.A. WALDER. 1988. Role of RNase H in hybrid-arrested translation by antisense oligonucleotides. Proc. Natl. Acad. Sci. USA **85:** 5011–5015.
41. AGRAWAL, S. 1996. Antisense oligonucleotides: towards clinical trials. Trends Biotechnol. **14:** 376–387.
42. BUCHARDT, O. *et al.* 1993. Peptide nucleic acids and their potential applications in biotechnology. Trends Biotechnol. **11:** 384–386.
43. GOOD, L. & P.E. NIELSEN. 1997. Progress in developing PNA as a gene-targeted drug. Antisense Nucleic Acid Drug Dev. **7:** 431–437.
44. EGHOLM, M. *et al.* 1993. PNA hybridizes to complementary oligonucleotides obeying the Watson-Crick hydrogen-bonding rules. Nature **365:** 566–568.
45. BONHAM, M.A. *et al.* 1995. An assessment of the antisense properties of RNase H-competent and steric-blocking oligomers. Nucleic Acids Res. **23:** 1197–1203.
46. ARMENGOL, G. *et al.* 2000. DNA copy number changes and evaluation of MYC, IGF1R, and FES amplification in xenografts of pancreatic adenocarcinoma. Cancer Genet. Cytogenet. **116:** 133–141.
47. PIETRZKOWSKI, Z. *et al.* 1992. Inhibition of cellular proliferation by peptide analogues of insulin- like growth factor 1. Cancer Res. **52:** 6447–6451.
48. BASU, S. & E. WICKSTROM. 1997. Synthesis and characterization of a peptide nucleic acid conjugated to a D-peptide analog of insulin-like growth factor 1 for increased cellular uptake. Bioconjugate Chem. **8:** 481–488.
49. THAKUR, M.L. *et al.* 2000. Imaging vascular thrombosis with 99mTc-labeled fibrin alpha-chain peptide. J. Nucl. Med. **41:** 161–168.
50. THAKUR, M.L. *et al.* 2000. 99mTc-labeled vasoactive intestinal peptide analog for rapid localization of tumors in humans. J. Nucl. Med. **41:** 107–110.
51. THAKUR, M.L. *et al.* 2004. PET imaging of oncogene overexpression using $^{64}$Cu-vasoactive intestinal peptide (VIP) analog: comparison with $^{99m}$Tc-VIP analog. J. Nucl. Med. **45:** 1381–1389.
52. TIAN, X. & E. WICKSTROM. 2002. Continuous solid-phase synthesis and disulfide cyclization of peptide-PNA-peptide chimeras. Organic Lett. **4:** 4013–4016.
53. RAO, P.S. *et al.* 2003. $^{99m}$Tc-peptide-peptide nucleic acid probes for imaging oncogene mRNAs in tumours. Nucl. Med. Commun. **24:** 857–863.
54. TIAN, X. *et al.* 2005. Noninvasive molecular imaging of *MYC* mRNA expression in human breast cancer xenografts with a [$^{99m}$Tc]peptide-peptide nucleic acid-peptide chimera. Bioconjugate Chem. **16:** 70–79.
55. CHAKRABARTI, A. *et al.* 2005. Synthesis of novel PNA-peptide chimera for non-invasive imaging of cancer. Nucleosides, Nucleotides & Nucleic Acids **24:** 409–415.
56. SCHNEIDER, R.F. *et al.* 1984. N,N′-bis(S-benzoylmercaptoacetamido) ethylenediamine and propylenediamine ligands as renal function imaging agents. I. Alternate synthetic methods. J. Nucl. Med. **25:** 223–229.

57. GARIEPY, J. *et al.* 2002. A simple two-step approach for introducing a protected diaminedithiol chelator during solid-phase assembly of peptides. Bioconjug. Chem. **13:** 679–684.
58. BARTUCCI, M. *et al.* 2001. Differential insulin-like growth factor I receptor signaling and function in estrogen receptor (ER)-positive MCF-7 and ER-negative MDA-MB-231 breast cancer cells. Cancer Res. **61:** 6747–6754.
59. BIÈCHE, I. *et al.* 2002. Prognostic value of CCND1 gene status in sporadic breast tumours, as determined by real-time quantitative PCR assays. Br. J. Cancer **86:** 580–586.
60. BIÈCHE, I. *et al.* 1999. Quantitation of MYC gene expression in sporadic breast tumors with a real-time reverse transcription-PCR assay. Cancer Res. **59:** 2759–2765.
61. TAN, M.H. & T.M. CHU. 1985. Characterization of the tumorigenic and metastatic properties of a human pancreatic tumor cell line (AsPC-1) implanted orthotopically into nude mice. Tumour Biol. **6:** 89–98.
62. YASUDA, D., *et al.* 1993. Possible association of nm23 gene expression and Ki-ras point mutations with metastatic potential in human pancreatic cancer-derived cell lines. Int. J. Oncol. **3:** 641–644.
63. TIAN, X. *et al.* 2003. Imaging oncogene expression. *In* Therapeutic Oligonucleotides: Antisense, RNAi, Triple Helix, DNA Decoys, and DNA Chips. N.Y. Acad. Sci. **1002:** 1083–1099.
64. STALTERI, M.A. & S.J. MATHER. 2000. In-vitro studies on 99m-Tc-labeled HYNIC-conjugated oligonucleotides. Nucl. Med. Commun. **21:** 374.
65. PALLELA, V.R. *et al.* 1999. 99mTc-labeled vasoactive intestinal peptide receptor agonist: functional studies. J. Nucl. Med. **40:** 352–360.
66. JAIN, R.K. 1998. The next frontier of molecular medicine: delivery of therapeutics. Nat. Med. **4:** 655–657.
67. HEDBERG, Y. *et al.* 1999. Cyclin-D1 expression in human renal-cell carcinoma. Int. J. Cancer **84:** 268–272.
68. LIPPONEN, P., M. ESKELINEN & K. SYRJANEN. 1995. Expression of tumour-suppressor gene Rb, apoptosis-suppressing protein Bcl-2 and c-Myc have no independent prognostic value in renal adenocarcinoma. Br. J. Cancer **71:** 863–867.
69. DE JONG, M. *et al.* 1996. Inhibition of renal uptake of indium-111-DTPA-octreotide in vivo. J. Nucl. Med. **37:** 1388–1392.
70. AMIRKHANOV, N.V. & E. WICKSTROM. 2005. Synthesis of novel polydiamidopropanoate dendrimer PNA-peptide chimeras for non-invasive magnetic resonance imaging of cancer. Nucleosides, Nucleotides & Nucleic Acids **24:** 423–426.

# Functional Validation of Genes Implicated in Lymphomagenesis

## An *in Vivo* Selection Assay Using a Myc-Induced B-Cell Tumor

DUONAN YU, DIANA COZMA, ANDREA PARK, AND ANDREI THOMAS-TIKHONENKO

*Department of Pathobiology, University of Pennsylvania, Philadelphia, Pennsylvania 19104, USA*

**ABSTRACT: The involvement of the c-Myc transcription factor in neoplastic transformation is well documented. However, which of its numerous target genes are crucial for tumorigenesis remains a frequently contested issue. We have recently established a non-transgenic murine model for B-cell lymphoma based on neoplastic conversion of p53-null bone marrow cells by conditionally active Myc. Using this model, we have identified a number of genes whose expression levels are affected by Myc during B-lymphomagenesis. Here we discuss their possible roles in neoplastic processes and describe an experimental approach allowing *in vivo* validation of these roles. We demonstrate that lymphoma cells overexpressing one of the Myc targets, the interleukin-10 receptor gene, have a very strong selective advantage over low IL10R expressors. Furthermore, Mcl1, a presumptive IL10R effector, also confers selective advantages when overexpressed in Myc-transformed hematopoietic cells. Thus, both IL10R and Mcl1 might be amenable to therapeutic interventions, and new targets can be identified and validated using the selection approach.**

**KEYWORDS: c-Myc; B-cell lymphoma; target genes; Mcl1; IL10**

## INTRODUCTION

c-Myc, an oncogenic transcription factor, is a crucial regulator of cell expansion. It was realized early on that activation of Myc forces quiescent fibroblasts to re-enter the cell cycle[1] and that rodent fibroblasts with targeted disruption of Myc are severely deficient in cell proliferation.[2] Thus, in mice (but curiously not in Drosophila[3]), decreased expression of Myc results in hypoplasia.[4] Predictably, some of the best-recognized Myc targets are crucial regulators of cell homeostasis: cdk4[5] and telomerase[6] (upregulation) and cdk inhibitors[7–11] and gadd45[12] (downregulation). In addition, Myc regulates, at the transcriptional level, a dazzling array of genes per-

Address for correspondence: Andrei Thomas-Tikhonenko, Department of Pathobiology, University of Pennsylvania, M/C 6051, 3800 Spruce Street, Philadelphia, PA 19104-6051. Voice: 215-573-5138; fax: 215-746-0380.
andreit@mail.vet.upenn.edu

**Ann. N.Y. Acad. Sci. 1059: 145–159 (2005). © 2005 New York Academy of Sciences.
doi: 10.1196/annals.1339.047**

taining to numerous physiological and pathological processes, such as cell growth and cell death.[13,14] In all, the database of Myc-regulated genes currently contains 1,697 entries (http://www.myccancergene.org/). It is often pointed out that many of these genes are indirect targets and that only a fraction of them might contain *bona fide* Myc-binding sites. Yet recent research using chromatin immunoprecipitation and other approaches has revealed that Myc binds to and regulates up to 15% of all genes (reviewed in Ref. 15). The abundance of Myc target genes raises the question of how crucial mediators of Myc-induced tumorigenesis could be identified.

Below we describe a simple approach that has allowed us to assign functional significance to Myc-induced variations in interleukin-10 receptor levels in transformed bone marrow cells. According to our data, the *il10ra* gene is downregulated by Myc,[16] and its expression levels become rate-limiting for B-lymphomagenesis. However, in the absence of active Myc, IL10R protein levels rapidly recover. This boosts cell expansion and ultimately correlates with Myc-independent tumor relapse. We envision that the same approach could be used to functionally validate various Myc targets as well as other genes tentatively implicated in B-lymphomagenesis.

## MATERIALS AND METHODS

### *Tumor Production and Analysis*

Generation of Myc- and MycER-induced murine B-lymphomas has been described earlier.[16–18] Syngeneic C57BL6/J mice (NCI, Frederick, MD) were used as hosts for tumor production. Lymphoma cells ($5–10 \times 10^6$) were injected subcutaneously into the flanks, and tumor growth was monitored over the course of several weeks. For 4-OHT treatment, the hormone powder (H6278, Sigma, St. Louis, MO) was dispersed in corn oil (Sigma) at the concentration of 10 mg/mL. The administration of 4-OHT was performed daily via intraperitoneal injections (1 mg per mouse). For the selection assay, tumors were harvested and dissected approximately 3 weeks after implantation. Neoplastic cells were used for flow cytometric analyses or subsequent passages *in vivo*.

### *Microarray Analysis*

Total RNAs from MycER tumors were used for cDNA synthesis. Labeled probes were hybridized to the U74v2 gene chip (Affymetrix, Inc. Santa Clara, CA) using the PENN Microarray Facility's standard protocol (http://www.med.upenn.edu/microarr/Data%20Analysis/Affymetrix/methods.htm). Affymetrix MAS 5 probeset signals and presence/absence flags were calculated. The LPE (Local Pooled Error) test for differential expression as implemented in S+ArrayAnalyzer v 1.1 (Insightful Corporation, Seattle, WA) was applied with 1% Bonferonni multiple testing correction to median IQR normalized MAS 5 signal values. The resulting list of 686 genes was imported into GeneSpring v 6.1 (Silicon Genetics, San Carlos, CA), filtered for presence (per Affymetrix MAS5 analysis) in 2 of 2 samples in one or more conditions ($Myc^{ON}$ or $Myc^{OFF}$), and then filtered for fold change.

### *Generation of Recombinant Retroviruses*

The murine IL10Rα-encoding retrovirus has been described earlier.[16] To generate an IL10Rα mutant lacking the intracellular domain, the PCRII-mIL10Rα plasmid[16] was cut with BamH I and Xma I, and the truncated IL10R insert was subcloned into the pSL1180 phagemid vector (Amersham Pharmacia, Piscataway, NJ). In this vector, the polylinker segment between Xma I and Sal I site was replaced with the double-stranded oligonucleotide (CCGGGTTA**G**AATTACCTCAG) containing a single T-to-G substitution shown in bold. This substitution resulted in a stop-codon (underlined) positioned in-frame with the IL10R coding sequence. The IL10RSTOP sequence was cut out with Bgl II and Sal I and inserted into the bicistronic GFP-expressing retroviral vector pMIGRI[19] linearized with Bgl II and Xho I. The full length murine mcl-1 cDNA was purchased from the American Type Culture Collection (Manassas, VA, catalog # MGC-13884, IMAGE ID: 4190996). The cDNA was released from the pCMV-SPORT6 vector using Not I and EcoR V restriction enzymes, cloned into pSL1180, and then recloned, using Bgl II and Hpa I restriction sites, into MIGR1.

### *Cell Propagation, Transfection, and Infection*

Myc3 B-lymphoma cells were cultured on monolayers of gamma-irradiated S17 cells as described previously.[18] BOSC and GP293 packaging cells were cultured in DMEM with 10% FBS. For *in vitro* infections, either of these cell lines was transfected with retroviral clones using Lipofectamine 2000 (Invitrogen, Carlsbad, CA). Conditioned media were harvested and added to Myc3 cells for 2 to12 h. Three days post infection, the percentages of GFP-positive cells in infected cultures were determined using flow cytometry.

### *Flow Cytometric Analyses*

To detect expression of mIL10Rα and the mIL10RSTOP truncated protein, transiently transfected packaging cells were stained on ice for 45 min with a biotin-conjugated anti-mouse IL10R antibody (559913, Pharmingen, San Diego, CA), followed by staining with APC-conjugated streptavidin (SA1005, Caltag Laboratories, Burlingame, CA). All samples were analyzed using a FACScalibur flow cytometer (Becton Dickinson, Mountain View, CA) with the CELLQuest software (Becton Dickinson).

## RESULTS AND DISCUSSION

### *Improved Survival of Neoplastic Cells following Myc Inactivation*

We have recently established a new mouse model for B-cell lymphoma based on infection of p53-null bone marrow cells with retroviruses encoding either constitutively active Myc[17] or a fusion between Myc and the mutant form of the estrogen receptor (MycER),[20] requiring the presence of the synthetic estrogen 4-hydroxy-tamoxifen (4-OHT) for activity.[16] The use of conditionally active Myc allowed us to address the role of Myc in tumor maintenance (FIG. 1). To this end, cells obtained from primary tumors were injected subcutaneously into flanks of syngeneic mice, and administration of the estrogen was maintained until palpable neoplasms have formed. Animals were then randomized into three groups. Mice in the first group continued to receive 4-OHT and rapidly developed large tumors (FIG. 2, tumors 1 and 2). In the second group, 4-OHT treatment was permanently discontinued (tumors 3 and 4). In the third group, 4-OHT treatment was suspended for two weeks and resumed on day 21 (tumors 5 and 6). We observed that in animals deprived of 4-OHT, tumor growth decreased dramatically, but the neoplasms did not undergo overt regression. Instead tumors remained stable for approximately two weeks. If 4-OHT was re-administered, extremely rapid neoplastic growth ensued (tumors 5 and 6), attesting to the viability of cells with inactivated Myc. Moreover, even without estrogen re-administration, MycER tumors began to slowly regrow after only two weeks of dormancy (FIG. 2 and Ref. 16).

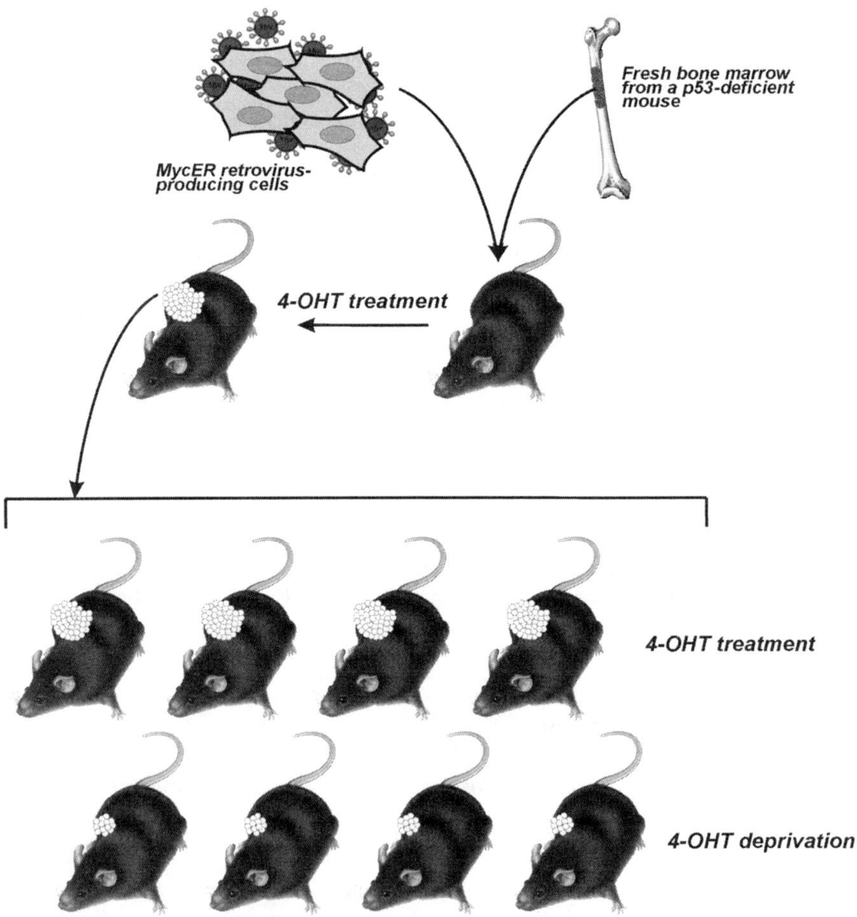


**FIGURE 1.** The non-transgenic mouse model of B-cell lymphoma based on the expression of conditionally active Myc in p53-null bone marrow cells. The use of 4-OHT deprivation allows the analysis of the role of Myc in tumor maintenance.

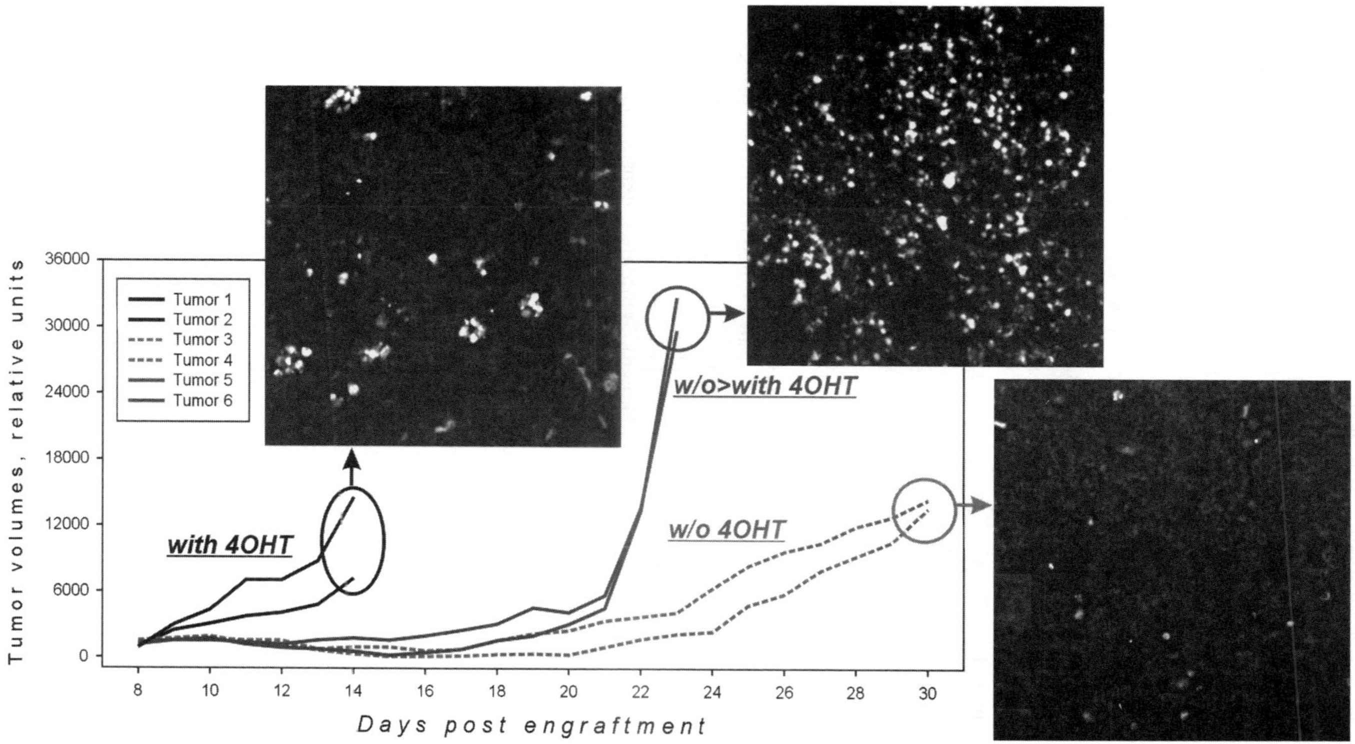


**FIGURE 2.** MycER activity correlates with rapid tumor growth and high rates of apoptosis. Plots refer to tumor sizes in animals continuously treated with the estrogen (with 4OHT), deprived of the estrogen (w/o 4OHT), and retreated with the estrogen after a 2-week hiatus (w/o > with 4OHT). The insets depict TUNEL staining performed on representative tumor samples from each group.

To correlate tumor dormancy with neoplastic cell survival, hematoxylin/eosin and TUNEL stainings of formalin-fixed tumor sections were performed. We observed that while the rate of cell proliferation decreased upon inactivation of Myc (data not shown), so did the rate of cell death. Interestingly, tumors with reactivated Myc exhibited yet higher rates of apoptosis, as judged by the percentage of TUNEL-positive cells (FIG. 2). Conversely, relapsing tumors with inactivated MycER had modest rates of cell proliferation but almost no apoptosis.

### *Transcriptional Signatures of Myc$^{ON}$ and Myc$^{OFF}$ Tumors*

In order to correlate Myc-induced changes in cell proliferation and survival to alterations in gene expression, we performed a series of microarray experiments. In these experiments transcriptional signatures of tumors with active and inactive MycER were compared. Differentially expressed genes were identified as described in MATERIALS AND METHODS. Forty-four genes were upregulated more than fourfold in Myc$^{ON}$ cells and 68 genes in Myc$^{OFF}$ cells (TABLES 1 and 2).

The functions of many Myc-upregulated and Myc-downregulated genes were consistent with the biological findings. Several genes implicated in cell proliferation maintained high transcription levels only in the *presence* of functional MycER, for example, cyclins B1 and B2, cdc2A, and DP1 (TABLE 1). On the other hand, many of the genes upregulated in the *absence* of Myc were known to contribute to B-cell survival and expansion, in particular, in response to antigen or cytokine stimulation. This list included components of B-cell receptor signaling pathways (receptor type protein tyrosine phosphatase C and B-lymphoid kinase),[21] NF-κB–activators (lymphotoxin B),[22] direct apoptosis inhibitors (Mcl1),[23] and cytokine receptors (interleukin 10 receptor)[24] (TABLE 2 and data not shown). While their expression correlated with neoplastic B-cell survival and eventual relapse, some of them were incompletely characterized or even reported to suppress tumorigenesis. For example, while IL10 has been known to stimulate proliferation of normal B cells *in vitro,*[25] its *in vivo* effects on both normal and neoplastic B cells are not well understood. In addition, anti-angiogenic, and thus anti-neoplastic, effects of IL10 have been reported.[26–28] Thus, we were interested in developing an unbiased approach capable of revealing both tumor-promoting and tumor-inhibiting properties of IL10R and other Myc target proteins.

### *An* in Vivo *Selection Assay for Cells Overexpressing Myc Target Genes*

The following approach was devised in order to assign functional significance to genes implicated in B-lymphomagenesis, such as IL10R. Its full-length cDNA was inserted into a retroviral vector MIGR1, co-expressing through the IRES element green fluorescent protein (GFP).[19] Retroviral constructs were transfected into packaging cells, and viral supernatants were harvested 48 h later. Then Myc-overexpressing B-lymphoma cells (Myc3[18]) were infected *in vitro* with either MIGR1/IL10R or just MIGR1 (empty vector). By varying the amount of viral supernatants, the infection rate of approximately 10% was achieved, as judged by flow cytometry for GFP. Partially but stably infected cultures were used for tumor production in syngeneic animals. The resulting tumors were analyzed using flow cytometry and percentages of GFP-positive cells were determined again. By enumerating GFP-positive cells be-

**TABLE 1. Myc-activated genes**

| Fold Induction | Affy ID | Common name | Description |
|---|---|---|---|
| 38.2 | 97473_at | Tm4sf7 | transmembrane 4 superfamily member 7 |
| 24.4 | 102632_at | Calmbp1 | calmodulin binding protein 1 |
| 14.3 | 96293_at | 2410015N17Rik | RIKEN cDNA 2410015N17 gene |
| 13.7 | 94971_at | Cdkn3 | cyclin-dependent kinase inhibitor 3 |
| 12.9 | 104423_at | 2810047L02Rik | RIKEN cDNA 2810047L02 gene |
| 7.4 | 96269_at | Idi1 | isopentenyl-diphosphate delta isomerase |
| 6.5 | 97124_at | Fin15 | fibroblast growth factor inducible 15 |
| 6.5 | 103525_at | Hnrpll | heterogeneous nuclear ribonucleoprotein L-like |
| 6.4 | 97411_at | Ect2 | ect2 oncogene |
| 6.1 | 103203_f_at | 4432406C08Rik | RIKEN cDNA 4432406C08 gene |
| 6.1 | 160159_at | Ccnb1 | cyclin B1 |
| 5.6 | 160501_at | Kif20a | kinesin family member 20A |
| 5.4 | 92840_at | Nup54 | nucleoporin 54 |
| 5.3 | 95755_at | Csda | cold-shock domain protein A |
| 5.3 | 160906_i_at | E430003D02Rik | RIKEN cDNA E430003D02 gene |
| 5.3 | 99578_at | Top2a | topoisomerase (DNA) II alpha |
| 5 | 93099_f_at | Plk | polo-like kinase homolog (Drosophila) |
| 5 | 160395_at | D11Ertd603e | DNA segment, Chr 11, ERATO Doi 603, expressed |
| 5 | 93250_r_at | Hmgb2 | high-mobility group box 2 |
| 5 | 101065_at | Pcna | proliferating cell nuclear antigen |
| 4.9 | 160069_at | Gmnn | geminin |
| 4.9 | 94292_at | Strap | serine/threonine kinase receptor–associated protein |
| 4.7 | 97527_at | Cks2 | CDC28 protein kinase regulatory subunit 2 |
| 4.7 | 101589_at | Hmgn2 | high-mobility group nucleosomal binding domain 2 |
| 4.7 | 100612_at | Rrm1 | ribonucleotide reductase M1 |

**TABLE 1. (*continued*) Myc-activated genes**

| Fold Induction | Affy ID | Common name | Description |
|---|---|---|---|
| 4.6 | 99457_at | Mki67 | antigen identified by monoclonal antibody Ki 67 |
| 4.5 | 92807_at | Txn1 | thioredoxin 1 |
| 4.5 | 100128_at | Cdc2a | cell division cycle 2 homologue A (S. pombe) |
| 4.5 | 94255_g_at | Clic4 | chloride intracellular channel 4 (mitochondrial) |
| 4.4 | 102911_at | Brca2 | breast cancer 2 |
| 4.4 | 97468_at | Cks1 | CDC28 protein kinase 1 |
| 4.3 | 100116_at | 2810417H13Rik | RIKEN cDNA 2810417H13 gene |
| 4.3 | 94274_at | Ube2s | ubiquitin-conjugating enzyme E2S |
| 4.3 | 96784_at | Anln | anillin, actin-binding protein (scraps homolog, Drosophila) |
| 4.3 | 94953_at | Racgap1 | Rac GTPase-activating protein 1 |
| 4.2 | 100512_at | Uchl5 | ubiquitin carboxyl-terminal esterase L5 |
| 4.2 | 160955_at | 2010309E21Rik | RIKEN cDNA 2010309E21 gene |
| 4.2 | 101521_at | Birc5 | baculoviral IAP repeat-containing 5 (survivin) |
| 4.2 | 92790_at | Kpna2 | karyopherin (importin) alpha 2 |
| 4.2 | 104097_at | Bub1 | budding uninhibited by benzimidazoles 1 homologue (S. cerevisiae) |
| 4.1 | 94294_at | Ccnb2 | cyclin B2 |
| 4.1 | 101959_r_at | Tfdp1 | transcription factor Dp 1 |
| 4 | 92639_at | Stk6 | serine/threonine kinase 6 |
| 4 | 99098_at | Fdps | farnesyl diphosphate synthetase |

**TABLE 2. Myc-repressed genes**

| Fold repression | Affy ID | Common name | Description |
|---|---|---|---|
| −21.8 | 99446_at | CD20 (a.k.a. Ms4a1) | membrane-spanning 4 domains, subfamily A, member 1 |
| −21.7 | 96109_at | Klf2 | Kruppel-like factor 2 (lung) |
| −21 | 103061_at | Gad1 | glutamic acid decarboxylase 1 |
| −20.5 | 96515_at | Il4i1 | interleukin-4 induced 1 |
| −20.4 | 98034_at | H2-DMb1 | histocompatibility 2, class II, locus Mb1 |
| −18.9 | 96525_at | Il10ra | interleukin-10 receptor, alpha |
| −17.1 | 96207_at | Rbms1 | RNA binding motif, single stranded interacting protein 1 |
| −16.7 | 160667_at | Evl | Ena-vasodilator stimulated phosphoprotein |
| −16.5 | 103985_at | Map4k2 | mitogen-activated protein kinase kinase kinase kinase 2 |
| −16.1 | 101845_s_at | Csprs | component of Sp100-rs |
| −13.6 | 102940_at | Ltb | lymphotoxin B |
| −13.4 | 103299_at | AI132321 | expressed sequence AI132321 |
| −10.8 | 102378_at | Sspn | Sarcospan |
| −10.2 | 94354_at | Abca1 | ATP-binding cassette, sub-family A (ABC1), member 1 |
| −9.7 | 103422_at | Cd1d1 | CD1d1 antigen |
| −9 | 98859_at | Acp5; TRAP | acid phosphatase 5, tartrate resistant |
| −8.8 | 98974_at | Igh-4 | similar to immunoglobulin delta-chain |
| −8.7 | 93714_f_at | LOC436489 | similar to MHC class I–alpha |
| −8.4 | 100011_at | Klf3 | Kruppel-like factor 3 (basic) |
| −7.8 | 92471_i_at | Slfn2 | schlafen 2 |
| −7.8 | 95373_at | Cd2 | CD2 antigen |
| −7.7 | 101792_at | | Mouse-gene fragment for delta-immunoglobulin (exon 8) |
| −7.6 | 92866_at | H2-Aa | histocompatibility 2, class II antigen A, alpha |

**TABLE 2.** *(continued)* **Myc-repressed genes**

| Fold repression | Affy ID | Common name | Description |
|---|---|---|---|
| –7.3 | 103596_at | Dgka | diacylglycerol kinase, alpha |
| –7.3 | 98402_at | Macf1 | microtubule-actin crosslinking factor 1 |
| –7.2 | 103202_at | Gbp3 | guanylate nucleotide binding protein 3 |
| –6.8 | 94224_s_at | Ifi205 | interferon-activated gene 205 |
| –6.6 | 92740_at | Iga | mouse Ig germline D-J-C region alpha gene and secreted tail. |
| –6.6 | 103697_at | A230075M04Rik | RIKEN cDNA A230075M04 gene |
| –6.1 | 99511_at | Prkcb | protein kinase C, beta |
| –6.1 | 160754_at | Pygm | muscle glycogen phosphorylase |
| –5.9 | 100998_at | H2-Ab1 | histocompatibility 2, class II antigen A, beta 1 |
| –5.7 | 101912_at | 1100001G20Rik | RIKEN cDNA 1100001G20 gene |
| –5.5 | 101054_at | Ii | Ia-associated invariant chain |
| –5.5 | 93683_at | Rag1 | recombination activating gene 1 |
| –5.4 | 94834_at | Ctsh | cathepsin H |
| –5.3 | 98035_g_at | H2-DMb1 | histocompatibility 2, class II, locus Mb1 |
| –5.2 | 94713_at | Myo7a | myosin VIIa |
| –5.1 | 104429_at | H2-Ob | histocompatibility 2, O region beta locus |
| –5 | 93026_at | Mgst1 | microsomal glutathione S-transferase 1 |
| –5 | 103531_f_at | 1300013B24Rik | RIKEN cDNA 1300013B24 gene |
| –5 | 93657_at | Spib | Spi-B transcription factor (Spi-1/PU.1 related) |
| –4.9 | 97313_at | Gdi1 | guanosine diphosphate (GDP) dissociation inhibitor 1 |
| –4.8 | 99623_s_at | Olfm1 | olfactomedin 1 |
| –4.8 | 93104_at | Btg1 | B-cell translocation gene 1, anti-proliferative |
| –4.8 | 101048_at | Ptprc | protein tyrosine phosphatase, receptor type, C |

**TABLE 2. (*continued*) Myc-repressed genes**

| Fold repression | Affy ID | Common name | Description |
|---|---|---|---|
| –4.8 | 93688_at | Cmah | cytidine monophospho-N-acetylneuraminic acid hydroxylase |
| –4.7 | 98001_at | Arhgef1 | Rho guanine nucleotide exchange factor (GEF) 1 |
| –4.5 | 92436_at | Stk23 | serine/threonine kinase 23 |
| –4.5 | 160781_r_at | Unc93b1 | unc-93 homologue B1 (C. elegans) |
| –4.4 | 100295_at | Lgl | mouse Ig germline lambda-chain gene Vx-J2-C2-region, clone 30X2. |
| –4.4 | 161819_f_at | Laptm5 | lysosomal-associated protein transmembrane 5 |
| –4.4 | 99953_at | Rgl2 | ral guanine nucleotide dissociation stimulator-like 2 |
| –4.3 | 161005_at | 5730420B22Rik | RIKEN cDNA 5730420B22 gene |
| –4.3 | 94285_at | H2-Eb1 | histocompatibility 2, class II antigen E beta |
| –4.2 | 93321_at | Ifi203 | interferon activated gene 203 |
| –4.2 | 95119_at | 1110038D17Rik | RIKEN cDNA 1110038D17 gene |
| –4.2 | 160812_at | Gga2 | Golgi-associated, gamma adaptin ear containing, ARF-binding protein 2 |
| –4.2 | 98980_at | Cd37 | CD37 antigen |
| –4.1 | 97963_at | Sipa1 | signal-induced proliferation associated gene 1 |
| –4.1 | 160773_at | Zcchc7 | zinc finger, CCHC domain containing 7 |
| –4.1 | 97173_f_at | H2-K2; H-2K2 | similar to MHC class I–alpha |
| –4.1 | 95893_at | Blk | B lymphoid kinase |
| –4.1 | 98931_at | Gns | glucosamine (N-acetyl)-6-sulfatase |
| –4.1 | 101331_f_at | Igk-V8 | immunoglobulin kappa chain variable 8 (V8) |
| –4.1 | 93092_at | H2-DMa | histocompatibility 2, class II, locus DMa |
| –4.1 | 100511_at | 6330406L22Rik | RIKEN cDNA 6330406L22 gene |
| –4 | 103970_at | Dri2 | dead ringer homologue 2 (Drosophila) |

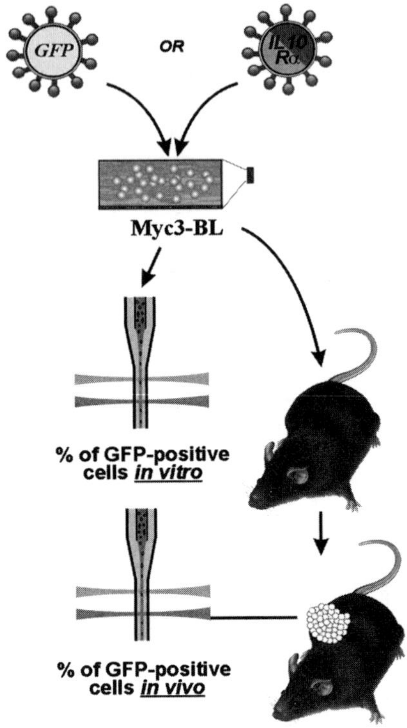


**FIGURE 3.** An *in vivo* selection assay for cells overexpressing Myc target genes. See text for more explanations.

fore and after passaging *in vivo*, both positive and negative effects of the gene of interest on B-lymphomagenesis could be revealed (FIG. 3).

### *Cells Overexpressing Interleukin 10 Receptor or Its Presumptive Downstream Target Mcl1 Are Selected during B-Lymphomagenesis*

The approach described above was applied to determine whether levels of IL10R are rate-limiting during B-lymphomagenesis. IL10Rα full-length cDNA is described in MATERIALS AND METHODS. As a negative control, we also generated and utilized its truncated version (IL10RSTOP) retaining the extracellular and transmembrane domains but lacking the cytoplasmic tail (see MATERIALS AND METHODS). Transfection of both constructs into the packaging cells resulted in expression of polypeptides of expected lengths (immunoblotting data not shown) located on the cell surface (flow cytometry data in FIG. 4A). The IL10R and IL10RSTOP retroviruses were used to infect Myc3 cultures as described in the previous section.

When transduced cells were used for tumor production *in vivo*, a steady increase in the percentages of IL10R-overexpressing, GFP-positive cells was apparent: after only three passages *in vivo* such cells accounted for over 90% of total neoplastic cells, up from 10% observed after infection *in vitro* (FIG. 4B). No increase was ob-

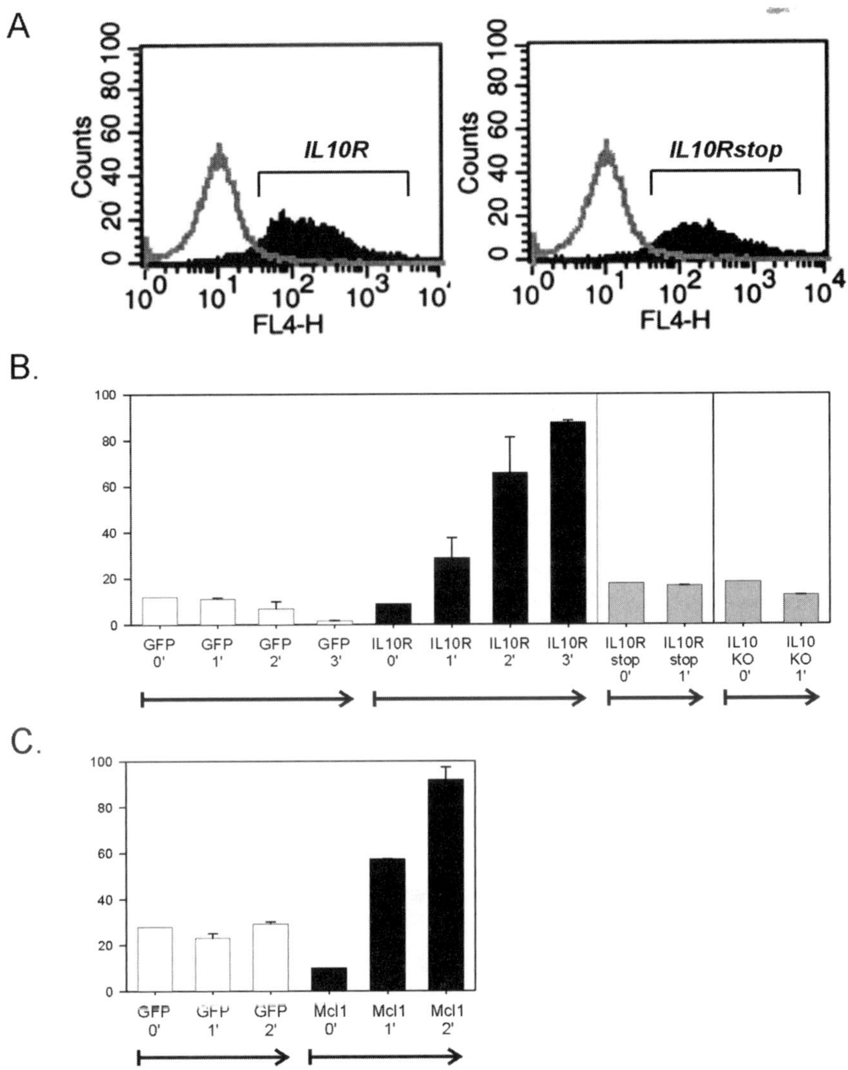


**FIGURE 4.** (**A**) Retrovirus-driven expression of IL10R and IL10Rstop on the surface of transfected BOSC23 cells. Live cells were stained with an anti-IL10R antibody as described in Materials and Methods and analyzed using flow cytometry (APC fluorophor). (**B**) Positive selection for cells overexpressing IL10R. Percentages of GFP-positive cells in Myc3 B-cell lymphoma cells transduced with either empty vector (GFP) or IL10R/GFP and IL10Rstop/GFP-expressing retroviruses. 0′ refers to cells passaged *in vitro*. 1′, 2′, and 3′ refer to tumors propagated *in vivo* for the indicated number of passages. The last panel depicts the IL10R selection experiment performed in IL10-null hosts. (**C**) Positive selection for cells overexpressing Mcl1. All designations are the same as in **B**.

served with GFP- or IL10RSTOP-overproducing cells. Additionally, no increase was observed when the experiment was performed in IL10-deficient mice,[29] suggesting that the positive selection for IL10R-overexpressing cells depends on the availability of its cognate ligand.

IL-10 is known to signal predominantly through the STAT3 pathway (reviewed in Ref. 30), which activates expression of several anti-apoptotic genes including Bcl-2, Bcl-xl, survivin, and Mcl1.[31] Consistent with this, Mcl1 was upregulated in Myc$^{OFF}$ tumors, albeit slightly less than fourfold (data not included in TABLE 2). We thus asked whether positive selection for Mcl1-overexpressing cells would also be in place. We generated a murine Mcl1/GFP-encoding retrovirus and repeated the basic experiment. As evidenced by data in FIGURE 4C, after only two passages *in vivo,* Mcl1-transduced cells accounted for almost 100% of the total cell population. Thus, it is possible that the contribution of the IL10 pathway to B-lymphomagenesis is based on its ability to inhibit apoptosis and improve tumor-cell survival. Consequently, targeting of the IL10 pathway using soluble IL10R$\alpha$[32] or a dominant-negative STAT3[33] could block expansion of lymphoma cells. Finally, functional validation of other Myc-regulated genes, which is under way in our laboratory, might yield new therapeutic targets.

## ACKNOWLEDGMENTS

We thank Drs. Emma Wilson and Christopher Hunter (University of Pennsylvania) for providing us with IL10-null mice and Dr. Michael Dews for stimulating discussions and helpful comments on the manuscript. This work was supported by National Institutes of Health Grants CA 097932 and CA 102709 and the Commonwealth of Pennsylvania Health Research Formula Fund #4100020574 to A.T.-T.

## REFERENCES


1. EILERS, M., D. PICARD, K.R. YAMAMOTO & J.M. BISHOP. 1989. Chimaeras of Myc oncoprotein and steroid receptors cause hormone-dependent transformation of cells. Nature **340:** 66–68.
2. MATEYAK, M.K., A.J. OBAYA, S. ADACHI & J.M. SEDIVY. 1997. Phenotypes of c-Myc-deficient rat fibroblasts isolated by targeted homologous recombination. Cell Growth & Differentiation **8:** 1039–1048.
3. JOHNSTON, L.A., D.A. PROBER, B.A EDGAR, *et al.* 1999. Drosophila myc regulates cellular growth during development. Cell **98:** 779–790.
4. TRUMPP, A., Y. REFAELI, T. OSKARSSON, *et al.* 2001. c-Myc regulates mammalian body size by controlling cell number but not cell size. Nature **414:** 768–773.
5. HERMEKING, H., C. RAGO, M. SCHUHMACHER, *et al.* 2000. Identification of CDK4 as a target of c-MYC. Proc. Natl. Acad. Sci. USA **97:** 2229–2234.
6. WANG, J., L.Y. XIE, S. ALLAN, *et al.* 1998. Myc activates telomerase. Genes Dev. **12:** 1769–1774.
7. MITCHELL, K.O. & W.S. EL-DEIRY. 1999. Overexpression of c-Myc inhibits p21WAF1/CIP1 expression and induces S-phase entry in 12-O-tetradecanoylphorbol-13-acetate (TPA)-sensitive human cancer cells. Cell Growth Differ .**10:** 223–230.
8. CLAASSEN, G.F. & S.R.HANN. 2000. A role for transcriptional repression of p21CIP1 by c-Myc in overcoming transforming growth factor beta -induced cell-cycle arrest. Proc. Natl. Acad. Sci. USA **97:** 9498–9503.
9. GARTEL, A.L., X. YE, E. GOUFMAN, *et al.* 2001. Myc represses the p21(WAF1/CIP1) promoter and interacts with Sp1/Sp3. Proc. Natl. Acad. Sci. USA **98:** 4510–4515.

10. SEOANE, J., C. POUPONNOT, P. STALLER, *et al.* 2001. TGFβ influences Myc, Miz-1 and Smad to control the CDK inhibitor p15INK4b. Nature Cell. Biol. **3:** 400–408.
11. STALLER, P., K. PEUKERT, A. KIERMAIER, *et al.* 2001. Repression of p15INK4b expression by Myc through association with Miz-1. Nature Cell. Biol. **3:** 392–399.
12. MARHIN, W.W., S. CHEN, L.M. FACCHINI, *et al.* 1997. Myc represses the growth arrest gene gadd45. Oncogene **14:** 2825–2834.
13. OSTER, S.K., C.S. HO, E.L. SOUCIE & L.Z. PENN. 2002. The myc oncogene: marvelously complex. Adv. Cancer Res. **84:** 81–154.
14. O'CONNELL, B.C., A.F. CHEUNG, C.P. SIMKEVICH, *et al.* 2003. A large scale genetic analysis of c-Myc-regulated gene expression patterns. J. Biol. Chem. **278:** 12563–12573.
15. PATEL, J.H., A.P. LOBODA, M.K. SHOWE, *et al.* 2004. Analysis of genomic targets reveals complex functions of MYC. Nat. Rev. Cancer **4:** 562–568.
16. YU, D., M. DEWS, A. PARK, *et al.* 2005. Inactivation of Myc in two-hit B-lymphomas causes dormancy with elevated levels of interleukin-10 receptor and CD20: implications for adjuvant therapies. Cancer Res. **65:** 5454–5461.
17. YU, D. & A. THOMAS-TIKHONENKO. 2002. A non-transgenic mouse model for B-cell lymphoma: in vivo infection of p53-null bone marrow progenitors by a Myc retrovirus is sufficient for tumorigenesis. Oncogene **21:** 1922–1927.
18. YU, D., D. ALLMAN, M. GOLDSCMIDT, *et al.* 2003. Oscillation between B-lymphoid and myeloid lineages in Myc-induced hematopoietic tumors following spontaneous silencing/reactivation of the EBF/Pax5 pathway. Blood **101:** 1950–1955.
19. PEAR, W.S., J.P. MILLER, L. XU, *et al.* 1998. Efficient and rapid induction of a chronic myelogenous leukemia-like myeloproliferative disease in mice receiving P210 bcr/abl-transduced bone marrow. Blood **92:** 3780–3792.
20. LITTLEWOOD, T.D., D.C. HANCOCK, P.S. DANIELIAN, *et al.* 1995. A modified oestrogen receptor ligand-binding domain as an improved switch for the regulation of heterologous proteins. Nucleic Acids Res. **23:** 1686–1690.
21. KUPPERS, R. 2005. Mechanisms of B-cell lymphoma pathogenesis. Nat. Rev. Cancer **5:** 251–262.
22. WEIH, F. & J. CAAMANO. 2003. Regulation of secondary lymphoid organ development by the nuclear factor-κB signal transduction pathway. Immunol. Rev. **195:** 91–105.
23. PACKHAM, G. & F.K. STEVENSON. 2005. Bodyguards and assassins: Bcl-2 family proteins and apoptosis control in chronic lymphocytic leukaemia. Immunology **114:** 441–449.
24. MOORE, K.W., M.R. DE WAAL, R.L. COFFMAN & A. O'GARRA. 2001. Interleukin-10 and the interleukin-10 receptor. Annu. Rev. Immunol. **19:** 683–765.
25. ROUSSET, F., E. GARCIA, T. DEFRANCE, *et al.* 1992. Interleukin 10 is a potent growth and differentiation factor for activated human B lymphocytes. Proc. Natl. Acad. Sci. USA **89:** 1890–1893.
26. HUANG, S., K. XIE, C.D. BUCANA, *et al.* 1996. Interleukin 10 suppresses tumor growth and metastasis of human melanoma cells: potential inhibition of angiogenesis. Clin. Cancer Res. **2:** 1969–1979.
27. SILVESTRE, J.S., Z. MALLAT, M. DURIEZ, *et al.* 2000. Antiangiogenic effect of interleukin-10 in ischemia-induced angiogenesis in mice hindlimb. Circ. Res. **87:** 448–452.
28. CERVENAK, L., L. MORBIDELLI, D. DONATI, *et al.* 2000. Abolished angiogenicity and tumorigenicity of Burkitt lymphoma by interleukin-10. Blood **96:** 2568.
29. KUHN, R., J. LOHLER, D. RENNICK, *et al.* 1993. Interleukin-10-deficient mice develop chronic enterocolitis. Cell **75:** 263–274.
30. GAMERO, A.M., H.A. YOUNG & R.H. WILTROUT. 2004. Inactivation of Stat3 in tumor cells: releasing a brake on immune responses against cancer? Cancer Cell **5:** 111–112.
31. BUETTNER, R., L.B. MORA & R. JOVE. 2002. Activated STAT signaling in human tumors provides novel molecular targets for therapeutic intervention. Clin. Cancer Res. **8:** 945–954.
32. HO, A.S., Y. LIU, T.A. KHAN, *et al.* 1993. A receptor for interleukin 10 is related to interferon receptors. Proc. Natl. Acad. Sci. USA **90:** 11267–11271.
33. NIU, G., R. HELLER, R. CATLETT-FALCONE, *et al.* 1999. Gene therapy with dominant-negative Stat3 suppresses growth of the murine melanoma B16 tumor in vivo. Cancer Res. **59:** 5059–5063.

# The Proteasome Inhibitor Bortezomib (Velcade) Sensitizes Some Human Tumor Cells to Apo2L/TRAIL-Mediated Apoptosis

ALAN D. BROOKS,[a] TERESA RAMIREZ,[b] UHI TOH,[c] JENNIFER ONKSEN,[b] PETER J. ELLIOTT,[d] WILLIAM J. MURPHY,[e] AND THOMAS J. SAYERS[a]

[a]*Basic Research Program, SAIC-Frederick Inc. and*
[b]*Laboratory of Experimental Immunology, National Cancer Institute Frederick, Frederick, Maryland, USA*

[c]*Department of Surgery, Kurume University, Kurume, Japan*

[d]*Combinatorex, Boston, Massachusetts, USA*

[e]*University of Nevada, Reno, Nevada, USA*

ABSTRACT: **On testing a panel of different human cancer cell lines, we observed that the proteasome inhibitor bortezomib could dramatically sensitize some lines to the apoptotic effects of Apo2L/TRAIL. Certain renal, colon, or breast tumor cell lines were dramatically sensitized, whereas other tumor lines from the same tissue of origin remained resistant. This sensitization did not correlate with either the p53 status of the individual tumor cell lines or their intrinsic sensitivity to Apo2L/TRAIL. Colon cancer cell lines lacking p53 or Bax were sensitized by bortezomib, suggesting that neither p53 nor Bax levels were crucial for sensitization. Although the molecular basis of bortezomib sensitization of tumor cells to Apo2L/TRAIL remains to be determined, this combination can have an enhanced apoptotic effect over either agent alone for certain human cancer cells.**

KEYWORDS: **apoptosis; bortezomib; velcade; Apo2L/TRAIL**

## INTRODUCTION

The proteasome inhibitor bortezomib (Velcade, formerly PS-341) was recently approved for the treatment of multiple myeloma[1] and has also entered clinical trials (alone and in combination with other agents) for other types of cancer. Bortezomib can promote apoptosis in some tumor cells, yet its molecular mechanism of action remains unclear.[2] Tumor necrosis factor (TNF)-related apoptosis-inducing ligand (Apo2L/TRAIL) is a member of the TNF family that preferentially induces apoptosis in tumor cells as opposed to normal cells.[3] Apo2L/TRAIL and agonist antibodies to its death-inducing receptors (DR4 and DR5) have also recently entered clinical

Address for correspondence: Thomas J. Sayers, Basic Research Program, SAIC-Frederick, NCI Frederick, Frederick, MD 21702-1201. Voice: 301-846-5729; fax: 301-846-1673. sayers@mail.ncifcrf.gov

**Ann. N.Y. Acad. Sci. 1059: 160–167 (2005).** 
**doi: 10.1196/annals.1339.042**

trials as single agents. A number of recent studies have indicated that proteasome inhibition can sensitize certain tumor cells to the apoptotic effects of Apo2L/TRAIL. The molecular mechanisms underlying this sensitization by bortezomib to Apo2L/TRAIL apoptosis also remain unclear. Bortezomib can inhibit activation of NF-κB in many cells, but the importance of this inhibition for apoptosis sensitization has been questioned.[4] Bortezomib has also been reported to increase the levels of p53,[5,6] as well as the Apo2L/TRAIL death receptor DR5,[7] and to decrease amounts of the antiapoptotic protein c-FLIP.[4] All of these molecular changes could contribute to an increased sensitivity to Apo2L/TRAIL. In particular, increases in DR5 and decreases in c-FLIP could result in an increased activation of caspase 8 which may amplify any apoptotic signal. Two signaling pathways are reported to be involved in death receptor–mediated apoptosis, depending on the individual cell type.[8,9] In type I cells, caspase 8 activation can directly induce apoptosis in the absence of mitochondrial involvement, the so-called extrinsic apoptotic pathway. In type II cells, caspase 8 activation induces cleavage of the proapoptotic protein Bid, resulting in mitochondrial damage. This mitochondrial damage acts as a crucial amplifying signal linking the extrinsic to intrinsic apoptotic pathways, and in type II cells mitochondria play a major role in the death signaling. To date, a limited number of human cancer cells have been analyzed for their sensitization to Apo2L/TRAIL-mediated apoptosis by bortezomib. We have examined the effects of this combination on the National Cancer Institute panel of 60 cancer cell lines *in vitro* and report some of these findings here. In addition, to further assess potential molecular mechanisms underlying this apoptotic sensitization by bortezomib, we have utilized the HCT116 colon carcinoma cell line together with its isogenic variants that lack either Bax or p53.

## METHODS

The renal cell cancer cells lines A498, ACHN, CAKI-1, SN12C, TK-10, UO-31, and 786-0; colon carcinoma cells COLO 205, HCT-15, KM12, and SW-620; and breast cancer cells BT-549, HS 578T, MCF7, MDA-MB-231, MDA-MB-435, and T-47D were all obtained from the DTP Molecular Targets Program at the National Cancer Institute Frederick. The HCT116 cells and the isogenic variants $p53^{-/-}$ or $Bax^{-/-}$ were kindly provided by Dr. Bert Vogelstein (Johns Hopkins University, Baltimore, MD). Cells at 5 or $10 \times 10^3$ per well were added to flat-bottomed microtiter plates for overnight incubation at 37°C, 5% $CO_2$. Bortezomib, kindly provided by Millennium Pharmaceuticals, Cambridge, MA, was then added at a various concentrations. After a 3-h incubation, recombinant human Apo2L/TRAIL (zinc-trimerized preparation provided by Genentech/Amgen) was added at various concentrations for a final volume of 100 μL, and plates were incubated for a further 18 h. For a quantification of viable cells, 20 μL of 3-[4,5-dimethyiazol-2-yl-5]-[3-carboxymeethyloxyphenyl]-2-[4-sulfophenyl]-2H tetrazolium (MTS) was added to each well and plates were incubated for another four hours. Absorbance at 490 nm was then measured on a microtiter plate reader and percent growth inhibition or cell survival was calculated for experimental groups as compared to appropriate controls. In some experiments, tumor cells incubated overnight with bortezomib, then were labeled with $^{111}$[In] Ox prior to Apo2L/TRAIL addition. After a further 18-h incu-

**TABLE 1. Effect of bortezomib plus Apo2L/TRAIL on the survival of human renal cancer cells**

| Renal cells[a] | Bortezomib (20 nM) | Apo2L/TRAIL (50 ng/mL) | Bortezomib + Apo2L/TRAIL | p53 Status |
|---|---|---|---|---|
| A498 | 82 ± 10[b] | 84 ± 3 | 2 ± 2 | wt |
| ACHN | 75 ± 7 | 91 ± 3 | 6 ± 9 | wt |
| **CAKI-1** | **82 ± 9** | **100 ± 1** | **83 ± 2** | **wt** |
| **SN12C** | **88 ± 2** | **100 ± 1** | **81 ± 3** | **mut** |
| TK-10 | 73 ± 6 | 92 ± 3 | 38 ± 5 | mut |
| UO-31 | 75 ± 8 | 80 ± 2 | 12 ± 6 | wt |
| **786-0** | **76 ± 7** | **100 ± 1** | **73 ± 1** | **mut** |

[a]Renal cancer cell lines in bold type are not sensitized to Apo2L/TRAIL by bortezomib.
[b]Percent cell survival as determined by MTS staining.
wt, wild type; mut, mutation.

bation at 37°C, supernatants were harvested as previously described[10] and counted on a gamma counter.

Cytotoxicity was calculated based on the formula:

$$\%\text{ cytotoxicity} = \frac{\text{experimental sample(cpm)} - \text{spontaneous release(cpm)}}{\text{total release(cpm)} - \text{spontaneous release(cpm)}} \times 100$$

In certain experiments the pan-caspase inhibitor zVAD-FMK, the caspase 8 inhibitor zIETD-FMK, and the caspase 9 inhibitor zLEHD-FMK were added at concentrations of 20 μM at two hours prior to the addition of Apo2L/TRAIL.

## RESULTS AND DISCUSSION

As seen from TABLE 1, bortezomib could effectively sensitize some tumor cells to Apo2L/TRAIL. Therefore, the renal cancer cells A498 and ACHN were very effectively sensitized to the apoptotic effects of Apo2L/TRAIL, whereas CAKI-1, 786-0, and SN12C were not. TK-10 and UO-31 were moderately sensitized by bortezomib treatment. The reduction in cell number observed was due to apoptosis because cells exhibited all the morphological characteristics of apoptotic cell death, and the effects could be blocked by caspase inhibition (data not shown). In a similar manner, breast cancer cells HS 578T and MDA-MB-435 were dramatically sensitized to Apo2L/TRAIL; BT-549 and MDA-MB-231 cells were only very weakly sensitized; whereas MCF7 and T-47D were very resistant to sensitization by bortezomib (FIG. 1). For colon carcinoma cells KM-12 and SW-620, cells were sensitized to Apo2L/TRAIL, whereas COLO 205 and HCT-15 were not (FIG. 2). The pattern observed for renal, colon, and breast cancer cells was also noted for other tumors in the 60-cell panel—that is, about 20–30% of the tumor cells were dramatically sensitized to Apo2L/TRAIL by bortezomib treatment. Some were only weakly sensitized and others were completely resistant to the effects of bortezomib on Apo2L/TRAIL-mediated apoptosis. Therefore, the original tissue of origin of the tumor did not give

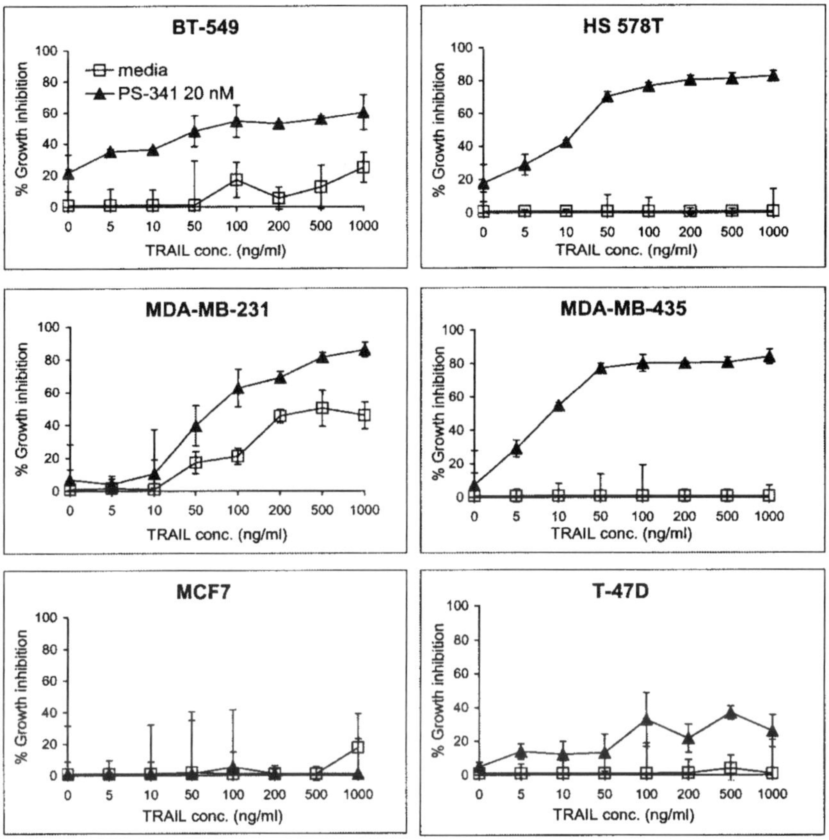


**FIGURE 1.** Various breast cancer cells lines were tested for the effects of bortezomib combined with Apo2L/TRAIL on growth inhibition.

a clear indication as to whether it would be sensitized to Apo2L/TRAIL by bortezomib treatment. Furthermore, the p53 status of these cancer cells is known, and there was no direct correlation between p53 status and sensitization by bortezomib. Although both of the renal cancer cell lines (A498 and ACHN) dramatically sensitized to Apo2L/TRAIL by bortezomib are p53 wild type (TABLE 1), one of the resistant lines CAKI-1 also has wild-type p53. In addition, the bortezomib-sensitized colon cancer (KM-12, SW-640) and breast cancer cell lines (HS 578T, MDA-MB-435) all exhibit p53 mutations. The intrinsic sensitivity of tumor cell lines to Apo2L/TRAIL as a single agent also did not correlate with the sensitization following bortezomib treatment. This is particularly noticeable in the breast cancer cell lines (FIG. 1) where the Apo2L/TRAIL killing of the sensitive MDA-MB-231 cells is only weakly augmented by bortezomib treatment, in contrast to the Apo2L/TRAIL resistant HS 578T and MDA-MB-435 cells that were dramatically sensitized. Regarding the renal cancer cell lines, we recently reported that all seven of these lines are sensitized to

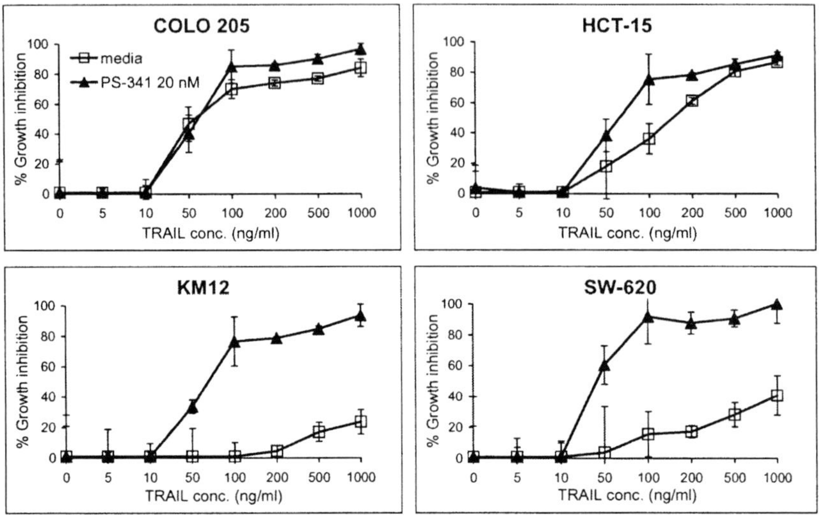


**FIGURE 2.** The colon carcinoma cell lines were tested for the effects of bortezomib and Apo2L/TRAIL on growth inhibition.

Apo2L/TRAIL by treatment with cycloheximide.[11] This suggests that the Apo2L/TRAIL apoptotic pathway is intact in all of these cells, and the mechanism(s) of Apo2L/TRAIL sensitization by cycloheximide and bortezomib may be quite different. Cycloheximide treatment of the renal cancer cells did not affect surface expression of any of the Apo2L/TRAIL receptors, but did cause a dramatic decrease in levels of c-FLIP in all cases. Preliminary findings with renal cancer cells following bortezomib treatment suggest that some changes in death receptors and c-FLIP can occur following bortezomib treatments. However, further studies are required to confirm whether these changes are crucial events in the sensitization of renal cancer cells to Apo2L/TRAIL.

In an attempt to further study the mechanism underlying bortezomib sensitization of cells to the proapoptotic effect of Apo2L/TRAIL, we performed further studies with the HCT116 colon carcinoma cell line and its well-defined isogenic variants that lack Bax or p53. The HCT116 variants were confirmed to lack Bax or p53 by Western blotting (data not shown). In contrast to some of the other colon carcinoma cells tested, bortezomib sensitization of HCT116 cells was only moderate. However, as seen in FIGURE 3A, low concentrations of bortezomib (20 nM) can sensitize these cells to Apo2L/TRAIL. Interestingly, this process did not involve p53 because both $p53^{+/+}$ and $p53^{-/-}$ cells were sensitized to an equal degree. This finding, in combination with the previous findings where no correlation existed between p53 status and bortezomib sensitization, suggests that the p53 status of cells does not influence bortezomib sensitization to Apo2L/TRAIL. Since many cancer cells have mutations in p53, it would be anticipated that at least some of these tumor cells could still be sensitized to Apo2L/TRAIL apoptosis by bortezomib. $Bax^{-/-}$ HCT116 cells were more resistant than $Bax^{+/+}$ HCT116 to Apo2L/TRAIL as a single agent as previously

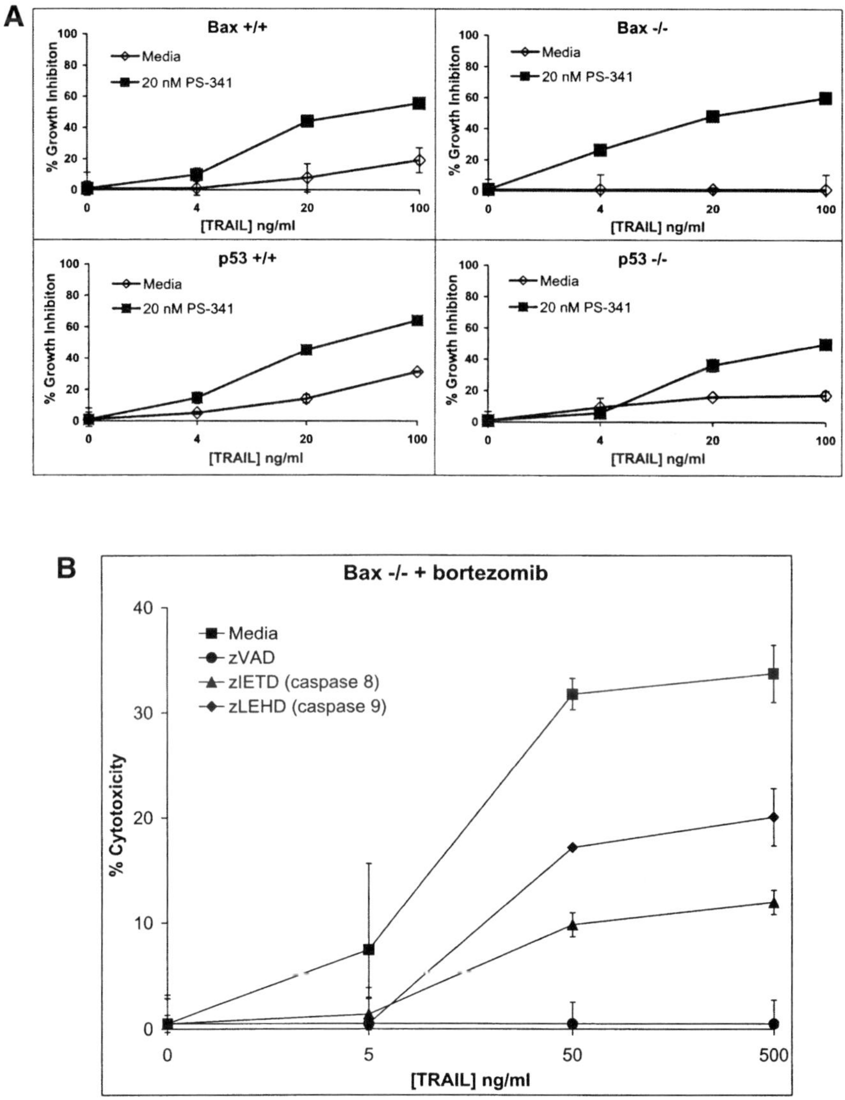


**FIGURE 3.** (**A**) The effects of bortezomib treatment on Apo2L/TRAIL sensitivity of HCT116 cells lacking either Bax or p53 were assessed using the MTS assay. (**B**) The cytotoxic effects of Apo2L/TRAIL on HCT116 $Bax^{-/-}$ cells that had been pretreated with 10 nM bortezomib were determined by indium release in the presence or absence of zVAD-FMK (pan caspase inhibitor), zIETD-FMK (caspase 8 inhibitor), and zLEHD-FMK (caspase 9 inhibitor).

reported;[12] however, following bortezomib treatment both $Bax^{+/+}$ and $Bax^{-/-}$ cells were sensitized. Therefore, Bax does not seem to be necessary for sensitization of cells to Apo2L/TRAIL, at least in HCT116 cells. Bax is regarded as an important mediator of the mitochondrial damage that occurs following signaling through the intrinsic apoptotic pathway. The lack of an effect of Bax on bortezomib sensitization to Apo2L/TRAIL can be interpreted in at least two ways. First, as suggested by others, there may be some redundancy in molecules required for the intrinsic apoptotic pathway, and other proteins such as Bak may functionally substitute for a lack of Bax.[7] Second, an alternative explanation could be that bortezomib may amplify the extrinsic apoptotic signaling pathway, such that the mitochondrial amplification loop was no longer crucially required for apoptosis to occur. In this case, HCT116 cells that have previously been designated as type II cells could be converted to a type I phenotype following bortezomib treatment. Bortezomib treatment substantially increased caspase 8 activation following Apo2L/TRAIL exposure in some cells,[7] suggesting that it can amplify apoptotic signaling. However, both caspase-8 and -9 inhibitors significantly inhibit Apo2L/TRAIL killing of $Bax^{-/-}$ HCT116 cells following bortezomib treatment (FIG. 3B), consistent with an involvement of the mitochondrial pathway.[13] Nonetheless, the importance of the mitochondrial component of the apoptotic pathway is perhaps best approached by the overexpression of the anti-apopototic proteins Bcl-2 or Bcl-xL to block the mitochondrial contribution to the intrinsic apoptotic pathway. Following Bcl-2 overpression in a murine acute myeloid leukemia, we did not see any decreased sensitivity to bortezomib plus Apo2L/TRAIL (data not shown). Further, human prostate cancer cells overexpressing Bcl-xL were still quite sensitive to bortezomib combined with Apo2L/TRAIL.[7] Therefore, the importance of mitochondrial changes for bortezomib sensitization to Apo2L/TRAIL apoptosis remains to be determined, and indeed may be cell type–dependent.

In conclusion, bortezomib can sensitize a variety of human tumor cells from different tissues to the apoptotic affects of Apo2L/TRAIL. The exact molecular mechanism(s) underlying this sensitization remains unclear. Since not all tumor cells are sensitized, it is likely that this process involves specific molecular events that differ in sensitized and resistant cells following proteasome inhibition. Identification of these molecular changes may allow for an advance prediction as to whether a particular cell could be sensitized to Apo2L/TRAIL apoptosis by bortezomib. Furthermore, this may allow for the identification of new molecular targets that could be modified by agents more specific than bortezomib to enhance the sensitivity of tumor cells to death ligand–mediated apoptosis.

## ACKNOWLEDGMENTS

This project has been funded with federal funds from the National Cancer Institute, National Institutes of Health, under contract number N01-C0-12400.

The content of this publication does not necessarily reflect the views or policies of the Department of Health and Human Services, nor does the mention of trade names, commercial products, or organizations imply endorsement by the U.S. Government.

## REFERENCES

1. Kane, R.C., P.F. Bross, A.T. Farrell, *et al.* 2003. Velcade: U.S. FDA approval for the treatment of multiple myeloma progressing on prior therapy. Oncologist **8:** 508–513.
2. Adams, J., V.J. Palombella, E.A. Sausville, *et al.* 1999. Proteasome inhibitors: a novel class of potent and effective antitumor agents. Cancer Res. **59:** 2615–2622.
3. LeBlanc, H.N. & A. Ashkenazi. 2003. Apo2L/TRAIL and its death and decoy receptors. Cell Death Differ. **10:** 66–75.
4. Sayers, T.J., A.D. Brooks, C.Y. Koh, *et al.* 2003. The proteasome inhibitor PS-341 sensitizes neoplastic cells to TRAIL-mediated apoptosis by reducing levels of c-FLIP. Blood **102:** 303–310.
5. An, W.G., S.G. Hwang, J.B. Trepel, *et al.* 2000. Protease inhibitor-induced apoptosis: accumulation of wt p53, p21WAF1/CIP1, and induction of apoptosis are independent markers of proteasome inhibition. Leukemia **14:** 1276–1283.
6. Williams, S.A. & D.J. McConkey. 2003. The proteasome inhibitor bortezomib stabilizes a novel active form of p53 in human LNCaP-Pro5 prostate cancer cells. Cancer Res. **63:** 7338–7344.
7. Johnson, T.R., K. Stone, M. Nikrad, *et al.* 2003. The proteasome inhibitor PS-341 overcomes TRAIL resistance in Bax and caspase 9-negative or Bcl-xL overexpressing cells. Oncogene **22:** 4953–4963.
8. Scaffidi, C., S. Fulda, A. Srinivasan, *et al.* 1998. Two CD95 (APO-1/Fas) signaling pathways. EMBO J. **17:** 1675–1687.
9. Ozoren, N. & W.S. el Deiry. 2002. Defining characteristics of Types I and II apoptotic cells in response to TRAIL. Neoplasia **4:** 551–557.
10. Sayers, T.J., A.D. Brooks, N. Seki, *et al.* 2000. T cell lysis of murine renal cancer: multiple signaling pathways for cell death via Fas. J. Leukoc. Biol. **68:** 81–86.
11. Brooks, A.D. & T.J. Sayers. 2005. Reduction of the antiapoptotic protein cFLIP enhances the susceptibility of human renal cancer cells to TRAIL apoptosis. Cancer Immunol. Immunother. **54:** 499–505.
12. LeBlanc, H., D. Lawrence, E. Varfolomeev, *et al.* 2002. Tumor-cell resistance to death receptor—induced apoptosis through mutational inactivation of the proapoptotic Bcl-2 homolog Bax. Nat. Med. **8:** 274–281.
13. Kim, S.H., K. Kim, J.G. Kwagh, *et al.* 2004. Death induction by recombinant native TRAIL and its prevention by a caspase 9 inhibitor in primary human esophageal epithelial cells. J. Biol. Chem. **279:** 40044–40052.

# The Role of Tuberin in Cellular Differentiation

## Are B-Raf and MAPK Involved?

MAGDALENA KARBOWNICZEK AND ELIZABETH PETRI HENSKE

*Fox Chase Cancer Center, Philadelphia, Pennsylvania, USA*

**ABSTRACT: Tuberous sclerosis complex (TSC) is a tumor suppressor gene syndrome whose manifestations can include seizures, mental retardation, autism, and tumors in the brain, retina, kidney, heart, and skin. The products of the *TSC1* and *TSC2* genes, hamartin and tuberin, respectively, heterodimerize and inhibit the mammalian target of rapamycin (mTOR). This review focuses on the genetic and biochemical basis of the renal and pulmonary manifestations of TSC, angiomyolipomas, and lymphangiomyomatosis, respectively. Genetic analyses of sporadic angiomyolipomas revealed that all three components (smooth muscle, vessels, and fat) derive from a common progenitor cell, indicating the ability of cells lacking tuberin to differentiate into multiple lineages. Other genetic studies showed that the benign smooth muscle cells of pulmonary lymphangiomyomatosis have the ability to migrate to other organs. These findings suggest that tuberin and hamartin play a role in the regulation of cellular migration and differentiation. We have found that tuberin activates B-Raf kinase and p42/44 MAPK and that cells lacking tuberin have low levels of B-Raf activity. We hypothesize that aberrant B-Raf activity in angiomyolipomas leads to abnormal cellular differentiation and migration.**

**KEYWORDS: TSC; tuberous sclerosis complex; mTOR; LAM; lymphangiomyomatosis; TSC2; tuberin; TSC1; hamartin; Rheb; MAPK; B-Raf; C-Raf**

## INTRODUCTION

Tuberous sclerosis complex (TSC) is a tumor suppressor gene syndrome whose clinical features include seizures, mental retardation, autism, and tumors in the brain, retina, kidney, heart, and skin. Mutations in either of two genes, *TSC1* on chromosome 9q34[1] and *TSC2* on chromosome 16p13,[2] cause TSC. Tuberin, the *TSC2* gene product, interacts with the product of the *TSC1* gene, hamartin,[3,4] and functions in multiple cellular pathways, including vesicular trafficking,[5] regulation of the G1 phase of the cell cycle,[6–10] steroid hormone regulation,[11] and Rho activation.[12,13] Hyperphosphorylation of p70 S6 kinase (S6K) and/or its substrate, ribosomal protein S6, occurs in cells lacking hamartin or tuberin.[14–18] Regulation of S6K by the tuberin-hamartin complex is mediated by the mammalian target of rapamycin (mTOR).[9,10,19–21] Tuberin possesses a highly conserved domain near the carboxy-terminus with homology to rap1 GTPase–activating protein (GAP),[5,22] and Rheb (Ras

Address for correspondence: Magdalena Karbowniczek, Fox Chase Cancer Center, 333 Cottman Avenue, Philadelphia, PA 19111. Voice: 215-728-2955; fax: 215-214-1623.
Magdalena.Karbowniczek@fccc.edu

**Ann. N.Y. Acad. Sci. 1059: 168–173 (2005). © 2005 New York Academy of Sciences.**
**doi: 10.1196/annals.1339.045**

homologue-enriched in brain), a member of the Ras/Rap/Ral subfamily of Ras proteins,[23] was shown to be a direct downstream target of tuberin's GAP domain.[24–30] Rheb has also been shown to negatively regulate an upstream activator of p42/44 mitogen-activated protein kinase (MAPK), B-Raf kinase.[31,32]

The clinical manifestations of TSC include lymphangiomyomatosis (LAM), which is characterized by widespread pulmonary proliferation of abnormal smooth muscle cells and cystic changes within the lung parenchyma. For reasons that are not yet understood, LAM affects predominantly young women. LAM can also occur sporadically in women who do not have TSC. Renal angiomyolipomas, which occur in most TSC patients, also occur in approximately 50% of patients with sporadic LAM.[33] Angiomyolipomas are distinctive tumors with three components: dysplastic vessels, abnormal smooth muscle cells, and fat. We and others have found that all three components of angiomyolipomas are derived from a common precursor cell lacking TSC1 or TSC2[17,34] and that the pathogenesis of LAM involves the metastasis of histologically benign smooth muscle cells lacking TSC1 or TSC2.[35]

The Ras/Raf/MEK/MAP kinase signaling cascade is essential to the integration of signals from the extracellular membrane to cellular effectors and transcription factors in the nucleus. MAPK influences cell fate by regulating cellular differentiation, apoptosis, and migration.[36,37] This drew our attention to p42/44 MAPK signaling as a potential link to the phenotypes observed in angiomyolipomas and LAM. Three mammalian Raf homologues (Raf-1, B-Raf, and A-Raf) have been shown to bind to MEK1/2 and lead to the sequential activation of MEK and p42/44 MAPK *in vitro*.[38–40] Recent evidence suggests that B-Raf may be the most important physiological MEK/MAPK activator.[39]

## DIFFERENTIATION PLACTICITY IN RENAL ANGIOMYOLIPOMAS

The presence of mesenchymal tumors in the kidneys of patients with TSC suggests that the TSC proteins (tuberin and hamartin) could regulate differentiation of an early renal precursor cell. To better understand cellular differentiation in cells lacking tuberin, we analyzed separately the three components of angiomyolipoma: fat, smooth muscle, and vessels. Genetic examination of angiomyolipomas from patients with sporadic LAM revealed that the smooth muscle component, the fat component, and four of the five types of vessels have TSC2 loss of heterozygosity. This confirmed that angiomyolipoma vessel walls are derived from the same progenitor cell as the fat and smooth muscle.[17] Loss of heterozygosity was not present in endothelial cells covering the vessels indicating that normal endothelial cells are recruited in the process of forming vascular structures. This is possibly related to the expression of vascular endothelial growth factor by cells lacking tuberin.[41] Taken together, these data demonstrate that loss of both alleles of TSC2 contribute to vessel formation in angiomyolipomas, and implicate tuberin and hamartin as regulators of cellular differentiation.

Interestingly, angiomyolipomas seem to be the first and thus far the only vascular tumor in which the vascular component is neoplastic.[42] Data obtained from hemangioblastomas and retinal angiomas associated with von Hippel-Lindau disease indicate that the stromal, not the vascular component, contains the second-hit mutation.[43–45] This suggests that tuberin and hamartin may play a role in the regulation of a novel mechanism of blood vessel formation.

## PULMONARY LYMPHANGIOLEIOMYOMATOSIS: THE BENIGN METASTASIS MODEL

The occurrence of angiomyolipomas in both sporadic LAM and tuberous sclerosis complex suggested a common genetic basis.[46,47] Genetic analysis of LAM cells and angiomyolipomas from the same patients with the sporadic form of LAM revealed the same TSC2 mutation in both tissues.[48] These findings led to the hypothesis that pulmonary LAM results from the metastatic spread of angiomyolipoma smooth muscle cells. This was surprising because angiomyolipomas are histologically benign tumors. Additional data supporting a metastatic model of LAM were obtained from a patient with sporadic LAM, who underwent lung transplantion and subsequently had a recurrence of LAM. Genetic analysis revealed that the recurrent LAM cells from the transplanted donor's lung had the same one base-pair frameshifting deletion in exon 18 as the native pulmonary LAM. This mutation was not present in normal bronchial epithelial cells derived from either the patient's or donor's lung. Four separate mediastinal lymph nodes from this patient contained LAM cells with this exon 18 mutation.[35] The presence of the same TSC2 mutation in the original pulmonary LAM, the recurrent LAM, and lymph node LAM strongly support a migratory or metastatic character of LAM cells *in vivo*. However, the model in which LAM cells migrate from angiomyolipoma to the lung is challenged by the fact that about 50% of patients with LAM, including the patient we studied with recurrent LAM, do not have angiomyolipomas.[35]

## THE MAPK SIGNALING PATHWAY: IS THERE A LINK BETWEEN TUBERIN, RHEB, RAF, AND ABNORMAL DIFFERENTIATION?

We found that tuberin expression increases B-Raf kinase activity and the phosphorylation of p42/44 MAPK, and siRNA downregulation of tuberin decreases B-Raf kinase activity.[32] In addition, expression of Rheb, a small GTP-ase which activates mTOR and is inhibited by the tuberin's GAP domain,[24–30] decreased B-Raf kinase activity and inhibited B-Raf–induced phosphorylation of p42/44 MAPK.

We also found that Rheb's inhibition of B-Raf and p42/44 MAPK is resistant to 24 hours of rapamycin treatment, indicating that it is not mediated by mTOR complex 1.[49] This has potential clinical relevance because rapamycin is currently in clinical trials for patients with TSC and/or LAM. Binding of B-Raf to Rheb has been shown by our group and by Im *et al.*[31,32] We also found that interaction between endogenous Rheb and B-Raf was enhanced twofold with serum stimulation or Ras expression in HEK293 cells, suggesting that the Rheb/B–Raf interaction is regulated by growth factors.[32] We propose that Rheb's inhibition of B-Raf kinase is a direct, mTOR-independent function of Rheb (FIG. 1).

Animal models have provided insights into the involvement of Raf kinase in embryonal development and organogenesis. B-Raf knockout mice die *in utero* from massive hemorrhage into body cavities as a consequence of endothelial cells defects.

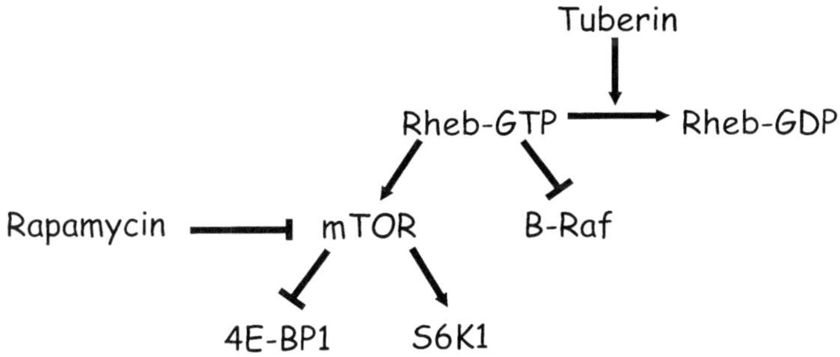


**FIGURE 1.** Model of Rheb, which directly inhibits B-Raf kinase in an mTOR-independent manner.

The mice show enlarged blood vessels and disturbed growth and differentiation of neuroepithelium, resulting in anatomical abnormalities in neuronal tissue.[50] These abnormalities are reminiscent of the enlarged and dysplastic blood vessels in renal angiomyolipomas, which can also result in massive hemorrhages, and suggest a link between B-Raf signaling and the clinical manifestations of TSC.

## REFERENCES

1. van Slegtenhorst, M. *et al.* 1997. Identification of the tuberous sclerosis gene TSC1 on chromosome 9q34. Science **277:** 805–808.
2. The European Chromosome 16 Tuberous Sclerosis Consortium. 1993. Cell **75:** 1305–1315.
3. Plank, T.L., R.S. Yeung & E.P. Henske. 1998. Hamartin, the product of the tuberous sclerosis 1 (TSC1) gene, interacts with tuberin and appears to be localized to cytoplasmic vesicles. Cancer Res. **58:** 4766–4770.
4. van Slegtenhorst, M. *et al.* 1998. Interaction between hamartin and tuberin, the TSC1 and TSC2 gene products. Hum. Mol. Genet. **7:** 1053–1057.
5. Xiao, G.H. *et al.* 1997. The tuberous sclerosis 2 gene product, tuberin, functions as a Rab5 GTPase activating protein (GAP) in modulating endocytosis. J. Biol. Chem. **272:** 6097–6100.
6. Ito, N. & G.M. Rubin. 1999. Gigas, a Drosophila homolog of tuberous sclerosis gene product-2, regulates the cell cycle. Cell **96:** 529–539.
7. Soucek, T. *et al.* 1997. Role of the tuberous sclerosis gene-2 product in cell cycle control. Loss of the tuberous sclerosis gene-2 induces quiescent cells to enter S phase. J. Biol. Chem. **272:** 29301–29308.
8. Miloloza, A. *et al.* 2000. The TSC1 gene product, hamartin, negatively regulates cell proliferation. Hum. Mol. Genet. **9:** 1721–1727.
9. Potter, C.J., H. Huang & T. Xu. 2001. Drosophila Tsc1 functions with Tsc2 to antagonize insulin signaling in regulating cell growth, cell proliferation, and organ size. Cell **105:** 357–368.
10. Tapon, N. *et al.* 2001. The Drosophila tuberous sclerosis complex gene homologs restrict cell growth and cell proliferation. Cell **105:** 345–355.
11. Henry, K.W. *et al.* 1998. J. Biol. Chem. **273:** 20535–20539.
12. Lamb, R.F. *et al.* 2000. The TSC1 tumour suppressor hamartin regulates cell adhesion through ERM proteins and the GTPase Rho. Nat. Cell. Biol. **2:** 281–287.
13. Astrinidis, A. *et al.* 2002. Tuberin, the tuberous sclerosis complex 2 tumor suppressor gene product, regulates Rho activation, cell adhesion and migration. Oncogene **21:** 8470–8476.

14. KWIATKOWSKI, D.J. *et al.* 2002. A mouse model of TSC1 reveals sex-dependent lethality from liver hemangiomas, and up-regulation of p70S6 kinase activity in Tsc1 null cells. Hum. Mol. Genet. **11:** 525–534.
15. GONCHAROVA, E.A. *et al.* 2002. Tuberin regulates p70 S6 kinase activation and ribosomal protein S6 phosphorylation. A role for the TSC2 tumor suppressor gene in pulmonary lymphangioleiomyomatosis (LAM). J. Biol. Chem. **277:** 30958–30967.
16. KENERSON, H.L. *et al.* 2002. Activated mammalian target of rapamycin pathway in the pathogenesis of tuberous sclerosis complex renal tumors. Cancer Res. **62:** 5645–5650.
17. KARBOWNICZEK, M., J. YU & E.P. HENSKE. 2003. Renal angiomyolipomas from patients with sporadic lymphangiomyomatosis contain both neoplastic and non-neoplastic vascular structures. Am. J. Pathol. **162:** 491–500.
18. EL-HASHEMITE, N. *et al.* 2003. Mutation in TSC2 and activation of mammalian target of rapamycin signalling pathway in renal angiomyolipoma. Lancet **361:** 1348–1349.
19. RADIMERSKI, T. *et al.* 2002. Lethality of Drosophila lacking TSC tumor suppressor function rescued by reducing dS6K signaling. Genes Dev. **16:** 2627–2632.
20. INOKI, K. *et al.* 2002. TSC2 is phosphorylated and inhibited by Akt and suppresses mTOR signalling. Nat. Cell Biol. **4:** 648–657.
21. GAO, X. *et al.* 2002. Tsc tumour suppressor proteins antagonize amino-acid-TOR signalling. Nat. Cell Biol. **4:** 699–704.
22. WIENECKE, R., A. KONIG & J.E. DECLUE. 1995. Identification of tuberin, the tuberous sclerosis-2 product. Tuberin possesses specific Rap1GAP activity. J. Biol. Chem. **270:** 16409–16414.
23. YAMAGATA, K. *et al.* 1994. Rheb, a growth factor- and synaptic activity-regulated gene, encodes a novel Ras-related protein. J. Biol. Chem. **269:** 16333–16339.
24. STOCKER, H. *et al.* 2003. Rheb is an essential regulator of S6K in controlling cell growth in Drosophila. Nat. Cell. Biol. **5:** 559–566.
25. SAUCEDO, L.J. *et al.* 2003. Rheb promotes cell growth as a component of the insulin/TOR signalling network. Nat. Cell Biol. **5:** 566–571.
26. ZHANG, Y. *et al.* 2003. Rheb is a direct target of the tuberous sclerosis tumour suppressor proteins. Nat. Cell Biol. **5:** 578–581.
27. TEE, A.R. *et al.* 2003. Tuberous sclerosis complex gene products, Tuberin and Hamartin, control mTOR signaling by acting as a GTPase-activating protein complex toward Rheb. Curr . Biol. **13:** 1259–1268.
28. INOKI, K. *et al.* 2003. Rheb GTPase is a direct target of TSC2 GAP activity and regulates mTOR signaling. Genes Dev. **17:** 1829–1834.
29. GARAMI, A. *et al.* 2003. Insulin activation of Rheb, a mediator of mTOR/S6K/4E-BP signaling, is inhibited by TSC1 and 2. Mol. Cell **11:** 1457–1466.
30. CASTRO, A.F. *et al.* 2003. Rheb binds tuberous sclerosis complex 2 (TSC2) and promotes S6 kinase activation in a rapamycin- and farnesylation-dependent manner. J. Biol. Chem. **278:** 32493–32496.
31. IM, E. *et a*l. 2002. Rheb is in a high activation state and inhibits B-Raf kinase in mammalian cells. Oncogene **21:** 6356–6365.
32. KARBOWNICZEK, M. *et al.* 2004. Regulation of B-Raf kinase activity by tuberin and Rheb is mammalian target of rapamycin (mTOR)-independent. J. Biol. Chem. **279:** 29930–29937.
33. AVILA, N.A. *et al.* 2000. Lymphangioleiomyomatosis:Abdominopelvic CT and US findings. Radiology **216:** 147–153.
34. NIIDA, Y. *et al.* 2001. Survey of somatic mutations in tuberous sclerosis complex (TSC) hamartomas suggests different genetic mechanism for pathogenesis of TSC lesions. Am. J. Hum. Genet. **69:** 493–503.
35. KARBOWNICZEK, M. *et al.* 2003. Recurrent lymphangiomyomatosis after transplantation: genetic analyses reveal a metastatic mechanism. Am. J. Respir. Crit. Care Med. **167:** 976–982.
36. DICKSON, B. & E. HAFEN. 1994. Genetics of signal transduction in vertebres. Curr. Opin. Genet. Dev. **4:** 64–70.
37. MARAIS, R. & C.J. MARSHALL. 1996. Control of the ERK MAP kinase cascade by Ras and Raf. Cancer Surv. **27:** 101–125.

38. HAGEMANN, C. & U.R. RAPP. 1999. Isotype-specific functions of Raf kinases. Exp. Cell Res. **253:** 34–46.
39. MARAIAS, R. *et al.* 1997. Differential regulation of Raf-1, A-Raf and B-Raf by oncogenic ras and tyrosine kinases. J. Biol. Chem. **272:** 4378–4383.
40. PRITCHARD, C.A. *et al.* 1995. Conditionally oncogenic forms of the A-Raf and B-Raf protein kinases display different biological and biochemical properties in NIH 3T3 cells. Mol. Cell. Biol. **15:** 6430–6442.
41. ARBISER, J.L. *et al.* 2002. Tuberous sclerosis-associated lesions of the kidney, brain, and skin are angiogenic neoplasms. J. Am. Acad. Dermatol. **46:** 376–380.
42. MARCHUK, D.A. 2001. Pathogenesis of hemangioma. J. Clin. Invest. **107:** 665–666.
43. VORTMEYER, A.O. *et al.* 1997. von Hippel-Lindau gene deletion detected in the stromal cell component of cerebellar hemangioblastoma associated with von Hippel-Lindau disease. Hum. Pathol. **28:** 540–543.
44. LEE, J.Y. *et al.* 1998. Loss of heterozygosity and somatic mutations of the *VHL* tumor suppressor gene in sporadic cerebellar hemangioblastomas. Cancer Res. **58:** 504–508.
45. CHAN, C.C. *et al.* 1999. *VHL* gene deletion and enhanced VEGF gene expression detected in the stromal cells of retinal angioma. Arch. Ophthalmol. **117:** 625–630.
46. SMOLAREK, T.A. *et al.* 1998. Evidence that lymphangiomyomatosis is caused by *TSC2* mutations: chromosome 16p13 loss of heterozygosity in angiomyolipomas and lymph nodes from women with lmphangiomyomatosis. Am. J. Hum. Genet. **62:** 810–815.
47. CARSILLO, T., A. ASTRINIDIS & E.P. HENSKE. 2000. Mutations in the tuberous sclerosis complex gene *TSC2* are a cause of sporadic pulmonary lymphangioleiomyomatosis. Proc. Natl. Acad. Sci. USA **97:** 6085–6090.
48. YU, J., A. ASTRINIDIS & E.P. HENSKE. 2001. Chromosome 16 loss of heterozygosity in tuberous sclerosis and sporadic lymphangiomyomatosis. Am. J. Respir. Crit. Care Med. **164:** 1537–1540.
49. JACINTO, E. *et al.* 2004. Mammalian TOR complex 2 controls the actin cytoskeleton and is rapamycin insensitive. Nat. Cell Biol. **6:** 1122–1128.
50. WOJNOWSKI, L. *et al.* 1998. Craf-1 protein kinase is essential for mouse development. Mech. Dev. **76:** 141–149.

# A Role for Hath1, a bHLH Transcription Factor, in Colon Adenocarcinoma

CHING CHING LEOW,[a] PAUL POLAKIS,[b] AND WEI-QIANG GAO[a]

*Departments of Molecular Oncology[a] and of Cancer Pathways and Targets,[b] Genentech, Inc., South San Francisco, California 94080, USA*

**ABSTRACT: A significant reduction or loss of goblet cells is often observed in clinical samples of colon adenocarcinomas, which is the predominant form of colon carcinoma. Mice lacking Math1, a bHLH transcription factor downstream of the Notch signaling pathway, demonstrates that Math1 is necessary for cell fate determination of the intestinal secretory cells, including goblet cells. Examination of *Hath1*, the human orthologue of *Math1*, expression in multiple colon tumor samples and colon cancer cell lines reveals a dramatic decrease in Hath1 expression in colon tumor samples and colon cancer cell lines. Hath1 expression in the HT29 colon cancer cell line can significantly inhibit its proliferation and anchorage-independent growth both *in vitro* and *in vivo*. At the molecular level, Hath1 may regulate the expression of MUC2, a mucin secreted by goblet cells, and Hath1 may also be a novel factor normally repressed as a consequence of activation of the Wnt signaling pathway, which has been clearly implicated in colon tumorigenesis.**

**KEYWORDS: Hath1; Math1; colorectal cancer; colon adenocarcinoma; goblet cells; mucin**

## INTRODUCTION

Colorectal cancer is one of the major cancer types to afflict both men and women in the United States.[1,2] One of the earliest signs of cancer involves expansion of the proliferative crypt compartment in the colon accompanied by a delay or inhibition in cellular differentiation and apoptosis.[3] Although goblet cells constitute the major secretory population in the colon, only a few mucin-secreting goblet cells are present in moderately well-differentiated colon carcinoma.[4–7] This suggests that homeostasis of the mucin-secreting, goblet cell population might have a critical effect on colon cancer progression. Incidentally, mice lacking the *mucin 2* (*MUC2*) gene reportedly developed intestinal adenomas.[8]

Hath1 is a basic helix-loop-helix (bHLH) transcription factor homologous to the Drosophila *atonal* and mouse *Math1*.[9] Math1, which is downstream of the Notch signaling pathway, regulates terminal cell differentiation in the developing brain and

Address for correspondence: Ching Ching Leow, Department of Molecular Biology, MS #72, Genentech, Inc., 1 DNA Way, South San Francisco, CA 94080. Voice: 650-225-6908; fax: 650-225-6240.
ching2@gene.com

**Ann. N.Y. Acad. Sci. 1059: 174–183 (2005).** 
**doi: 10.1196/annals.1339.048**

inner ear hair cells.[10–15] Intestines of *Math1* null mice fail to develop all three secretory cell lineages, including the goblet cells.[16] Hes1, a major target of the Notch pathway, likely represses Math1 because Jensen *et al.*[17] showed elevated Math1 expression upon removal of Hes1. Mice that are null for Hes1 produced excessive goblet cells in the intestine.[17] In addition, co-electroporation of Hes1 and Math1 into the inner ear tissue can block hair cell differentiation induced by Math1.[18]

Constitutive activation of the canonical Wnt signaling pathway is often implicated in a majority of colon cancers.[19,20–24] Other factors shown to contribute to the multistage process of colon cancer progression include *K-ras*, *p53*, *Cox-2, EGFR,* and *TGF*β.[25] In addition, deregulated expression of genes involved in cell cycle regulation such as *cyclin D1, p21,* and *p27* have also been implicated in colon cancer.[26–29] Both *in vitro* and *in vivo* studies place Hath1 within the preceding list of molecular targets that are deregulated during the malignant transformation of normal colonic mucosa.[30]

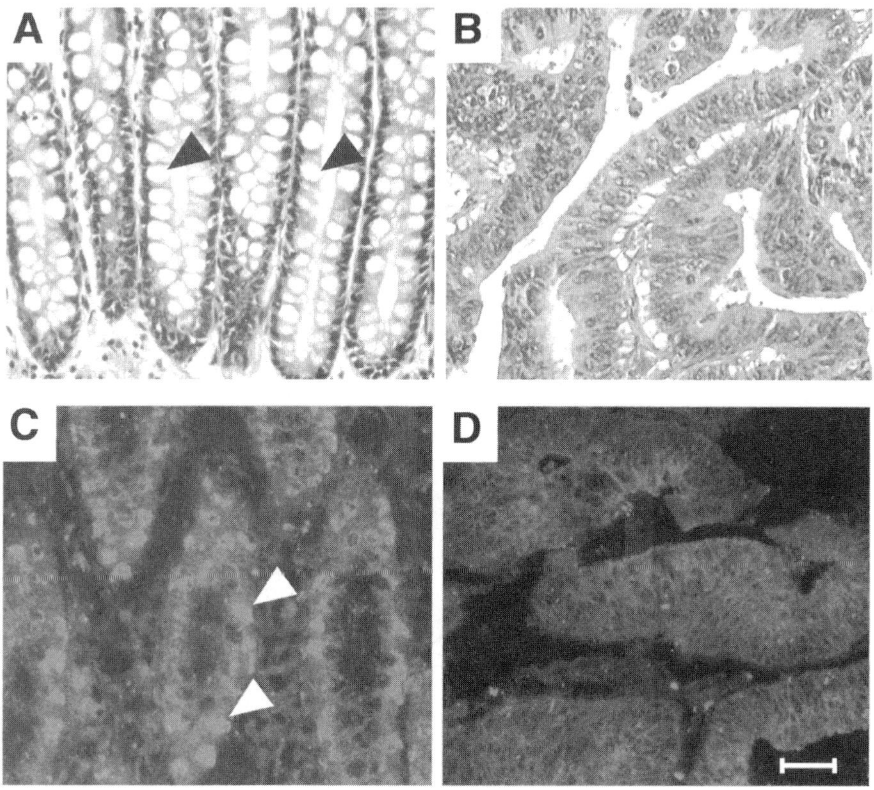


**FIGURE 1.** Fewer goblet cells are detected in colon carcinoma. Paraffin sections of paraffin-embedded tissues from normal colon (**A, C**) and colon adenocarcinomas (**B, D**) are stained with H& E (**A, B**), and MUC2 protein expression is detected by immunofluorescence (**C, D**). While goblet cells are abundant in the normal colon (*black and white arrowheads*), there are very few goblet cells in colon adenocarcinomas. *Bar* in **D** is 50 μm. (From Leow *et al.*[30] Reprinted by permission from *Cancer Research.*)

## HATH1 AND GOBLET CELLS ARE DRAMATICALLY REDUCED IN COLON ADENOCARCINOMAS

Several histological and molecular markers for goblet cells were used to confirm the abundance of these cells in normal colon versus colon adenocarcinoma. Goblet cells in normal colonic mucosa have a distinct goblet-like morphology identifiable by hematoxylin and eosin (H&E) staining (black arrowhead, FIG. 1A). Mucin2 (MUC2) is uniquely produced by goblet cells and can be detected using anti-MUC2

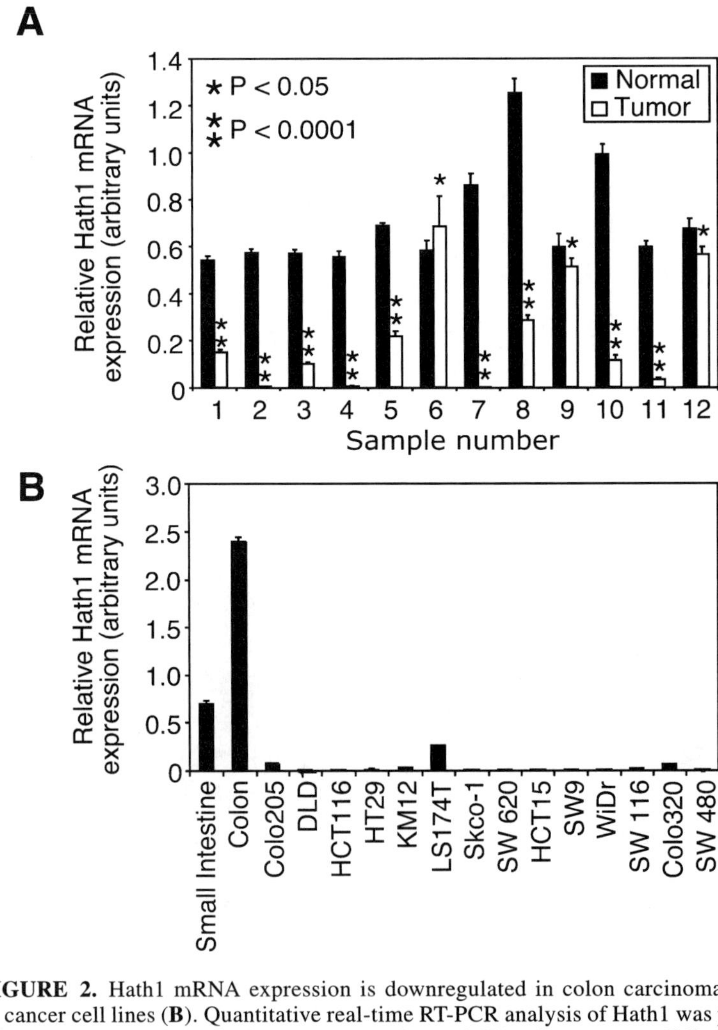


**FIGURE 2.** Hath1 mRNA expression is downregulated in colon carcinomas (**A**) and colon cancer cell lines (**B**). Quantitative real-time RT-PCR analysis of Hath1 was performed on (**A**) paired normal versus colon tumor samples and (**B**) colon cancer cell lines. All RT-PCR were performed in triplicate. Data were plotted as relative Hath1 mRNA expression following RPL19 normalization, and Student's *t* test was used for statistical analyses. (From Leow *et al.*[30] Reprinted by permission from *Cancer Research.*)

immunofluorescent staining (white arrowhead, FIG. 1C).[31] Goblet cells also produce acidic mucins detectable by Alcian blue staining.[30,32] Colon sections from 18 colon adenocarcinoma cases, which included normal colon and colon adenocarcinoma sections from each case, were scrutinized for goblet cells using the techniques described above. It is striking to note that while there are numerous goblet cells lining the normal colonic mucosa, H&E staining (FIG. 1B), MUC2 immunofluorescent staining (FIG. 1D), and Alcian blue staining (not shown) reveal few goblet cells in colon adenocarcinoma.[30]

A correlation between Hath1 and colon cancer can be demonstrated using quantitative real-time RT–PCR analysis of *Hath1* mRNA expression in clinical colon tumor samples and colorectal cancer cell lines. *Hath1* mRNA expression was significantly downregulated in 11 of 12 clinical samples of invasive colon adenocarinoma, with the exception of a mucinous adenocarcinoma sample, which is a rare

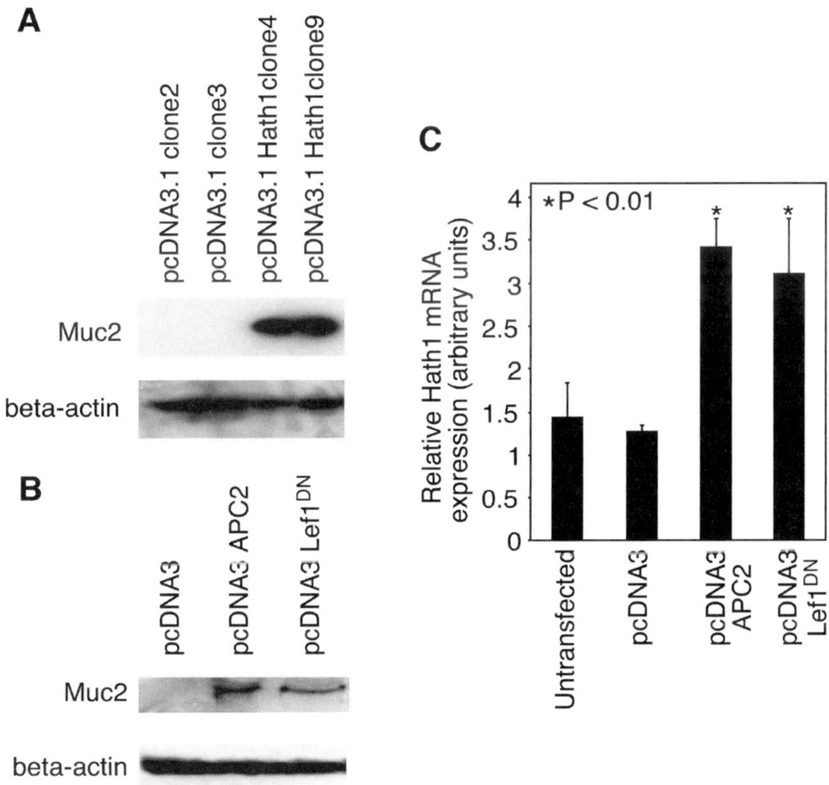


**FIGURE 3.** Expression of Hath1 in HT29 colon cancer cells upregulates MUC2 protein (**A**) whereas HT29 cells stably expressing pcDNA3.1 (clone 2 and clone 3) do not induce MUC2 expression. Wnt inhibition through expression of APC2 and Lef1$^{DN}$ results in elevated MUC2 protein expression (**B**) and enhanced Hath1 expression. (From Leow *et al.*[30] Reprinted by permission from *Cancer Research*.)

form of colorectal carcinoma with goblet cells making up more than 50% of cells (FIG. 2A). Similarly, Hath1 mRNA was also downregulated in various colon cancer cell lines examined except for LS174T (FIG. 2B). It is interesting to note that Hath1 expression is slightly elevated in the one case of mucinous adenocarcinoma and LS174T, a cell line reported to express higher levels of MUC2.

Consistent with a previous finding that demonstrated a role for Math 1 in inducing differentiation of intestinal epithelial cells, we also demonstrated evidence of Hath1 driving progenitor cells into terminal differentiation in colon cancer cells. *In vitro*, only HT29 cells overexpressing Hath1 upregulated MUC2, a marker of goblet cell differentiation, by Western blot analysis (clone 4 and clone 9) (FIG. 3A). Our finding has recently been confirmed in the $Apc^{Min}$ mouse model of intestinal neoplasia whereby inactivation of the Notch signaling pathway, which resulted in enhanced Math1 expression, can induce differentiation of adenoma cells into goblet cells.[33]

Finally, a survey of the subscription-based Gene Logic database, which consists of expression data for normal and tumor tissues determined by Affymetrix microarray analyses, reveals that *Hath1* expression in normal tissues is highest in colon and small intestine but relatively low in other types of normal tissue.[30] Consistent with the finding from the clinical colon adenocarcinoma samples and colon cancer cell lines, Gene Logic data indicated that *Hath1* expression was also downregulated in neoplastic tissues originating from colon and small intestine.[30]

## HATH1 INHIBITS GROWTH OF HT29 COLORECTAL CANCER CELL LINE BOTH *IN VITRO* AND *IN VIVO*

Introduction of Hath1 inhibited proliferation of HT29 colon cancer cells. HT29 clones stably overexpressing Hath1 incorporated less tritiated-thymidine ([$^3$H]-thymidine) and thymidine analogue, 5-bromo-2-deoxyuridine (BrdUrd) in comparison to clones transfected with pcDNA3.1 (Student's $t$ test, $P < 0.001$).[30] It should be noted that Hath1 overexpression was not toxic because no apoptosis was detected either by caspase 3 staining and DAPI-stained nuclei.[30] Since cell cycle checkpoint regulators are often deregulated during cancer progression,[34–36] we examined the effect of Hath1 expression on p27 and cyclin D1 expression. Our results showed that Hath1 positively regulates p27 but negatively regulates cyclin D1.[30]

Cancer cells often display anchorage-independent growth. In fact, we show that Hath1 expression in HT29 colon cancer cells can have a negative effect on anchorage-independent growth of HT29 colon cancer cells in soft agar. After 10 days in culture, HT29 cell lines stably expressing pcDNA3.1 Hath1 (clone 4 and clone 9) formed 10-fold fewer colonies ($n = 3$, ANOVA, $P < 0.001$), and the colonies that did form on the soft agar were much smaller in size in comparison to HT29 pcDNA3.1 cell lines (clone 2 and clone 3) (FIG. 4A and B). When HT29 stably transfected cells were injected subcutaneously (s.c.) into athymic nude mice and monitored for tumor growth, tumor formation by HT29 cells expressing Hath1 (clone 4 and 9) was significantly inhibited (ANOVA, $P < 0.01$) 20 days after xenograft implantation, whereas untransfected and pcDNA 3.1–transfected (clone 3) HT29 cells continued to grow robustly (clone 4, ANOVA, $P < 0.01$; clone 9, ANOVA, $P < 0.05$) (FIG. 4C).

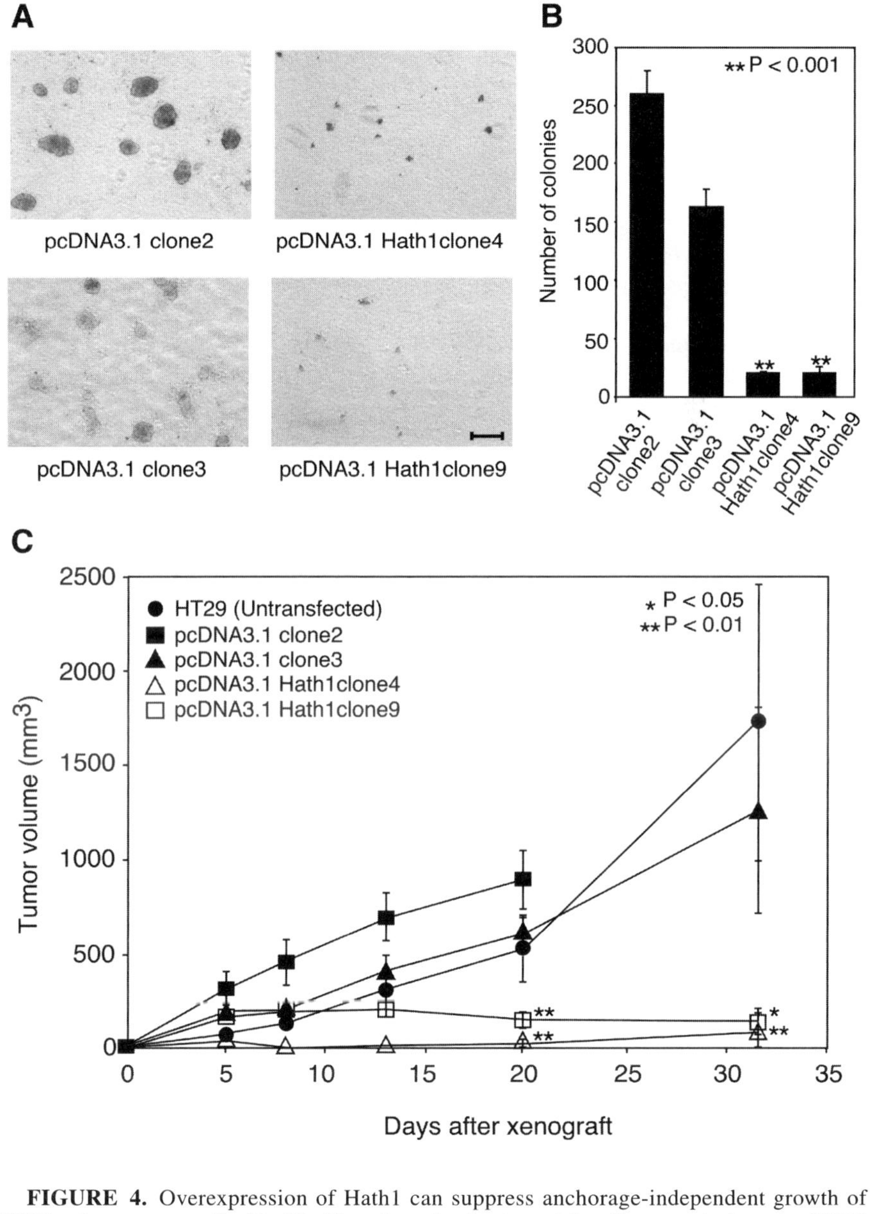


**FIGURE 4.** Overexpression of Hath1 can suppress anchorage-independent growth of HT29 colon cancer cells (**A, B**). The size of colonies arising from control vector HT29 clones is markedly bigger than stable clones overexpressing Hath1 (**A**). *Bar* in **A** is 400 μm. Xenograft of HT29 stably expressing pcDNA3.1 (clone 2 and clone 3) and pcDNA3.1 Hath1 (clone 4 and clone 9) measured over a period of 32 days reveals that tumor growth in untransfected and pcDNA3.1-expressing HT29 cells were robust in comparison to those expressing pcDNA3.1 Hath1 (**C**). Data were plotted as mean ± SEM, and ANOVA was used for statistical analyses. (From Leow *et al.*[30] Reprinted by permission from *Cancer Research*.)

## RELATIONSHIP BETWEEN HATH1 AND WNT SIGNALING IN COLON ADENOCARCINOMA

HT29 colorectal cells are known to possess APC mutations,[37] and transient expression of wild-type APC (pcDNA3 APC2) and dominant negative lymphocyte enhancer factor ( pcDNA3 Lef1$^{DN}$) can inhibit Wnt signaling.[38–40] Recently, it has been shown that inhibition of Wnt pathway in LS174T colon cancer cells can upregulate MUC2 expression.[40] Inhibition of Wnt signaling in HT29 colon cancer cells also upregulated MUC2 expression (FIG. 3B). Since Hath1 can induce MUC2 expression as well (FIG. 3A), we examined Wnt regulation of Hath1 in HT29 colon cancer cells. Taqman RT-PCR analysis revealed that inhibition of Wnt signaling with either wild-type APC or dominant negative Lef1 increased *Hath1* expression approximately twofold in HT29 cells (ANOVA, $P < 0.01$) (FIG. 3C); this suggests that Hath1 is negatively regulated upon Wnt activation. The level of MUC2 induction by Hath1 (FIG. 3A) was greater than the level of induction by Wnt activation (FIG. 3C). This could be the result of more than a twofold upregulation of Hath1 expression in the stable clones whereas activation of the Wnt pathway only resulted in a twofold increase in Hath1 expression (FIG. 3C). Although direct interaction between TCF/Lef transcription factors and Hath1 promoter has not been reported, there exists a core TCF/Lef-binding site (5′ A/T A/T CAAAG 3′) in the Hath1 promoter.[30] Consistent with our findings, a recent microarray study examining the gene expression profile of Wnt signaling inhibition in LS174T colon cancer cells revealed an increase in MUC2 expression.[40] Interestingly, Pretlow and Pretlow[41] show that goblet cells are already absent from aberrant crypt foci (ACF), which are precursors to adenoma and colon adenocarcinoma. Since APC mutation is also involved in the initiation of ACF,[41] it is possible that the loss of Hath1 expression in aberrant crypt foci may represent an early event in colon tumorigenesis.

Consistent with our observation of enhanced MUC2 expression upon inhibition of Wnt signaling, van de Wetering *et al.*[40] also demonstrated that inhibition of Wnt signaling by dominant negative Tcf4 in LS174T colon cancer cells resulted in elevated MUC2 expression. In future studies, it would be interesting to determine whether Hath1 expression could also be enhanced in LS174T cells expressing dominant negative Tcf4. Also in agreement with our findings that Hath1 is negatively regulated by Wnt, Pinto *et al.*[42] reported that Math1 expression and goblet cells were maintained in Tcf4-deficient mice. In addition, Van Es *et al.*[33] reported that adenomas from Apc$^{Min}$ mice contained less than 1% Math1-positive goblet cells, which once again suggests that active Wnt signaling may repress Hath1 and that upon Notch inhibition the number of Math1-positive goblet cells was increased. This may represent another level of Hath1 regulation because inactivation of the Notch pathway is sufficient to induce Math1 expression and differentiate adenoma cells in Apc$^{Min}$ mice. It should be noted that, contrary to our findings, Pinto *et al.*[42] reported intestines of transgenic mice ectopically expressing Dickkopf1 (Dkk1) lacked goblet cells and Math1 expression. The primary function of Dkk1 is to inhibit the low-density receptor-related protein (LRP), which is a Wnt coreceptor.[43] A recent publication suggests that LRP competes for gamma secretase,[44] whose enzymatic activity is required for Notch activation.[23] This reconciles our findings[30] with those of Pinto *et al.*[42] because the presence of Dkk1 could sequester LRP from competing for gamma secretase. This would in turn lead to enhanced Hes1 expression, which suppresses Math1 and subsequently leads to a reduction of goblet cells in the Dkk1 transgenic mice. Ultimately, our understanding of the interaction between Notch signaling and Wnt signaling in the context of normal colon versus colon adenocarcinoma is still in its infancy, and more work will have to be done to decipher the intricate relationship between the two pathways.

## CONCLUSION

Our study suggests a role for Hath1 in colon cancer progression. Hath1 can inhibit cell proliferation, induce a goblet-cell differentiation marker, MUC2, in a colon cancer cell line, suppress anchorage-independent growth of colon cancer cells in a soft agar colony formation assay and, more significantly, inhibit growth of HT29 colon cancer cells in xenograft experiments. The orthologue of Hath1 is not only required for differentiation of goblet cells in mice[16] but can also induce differentiation of colon cancer cells.[30] Few, if any, Hath1-positive cells are detected in colon adenocarcinoma samples, which suggests a potential role for loss of Hath1 in colon tumorigenesis.[30] Our results demonstrate that Hath1 may be negatively regulated by Wnt signaling, a pathway critical in colon tumor progression.

## REFERENCES

1. JEMAL, A., T. MURRAY, A. SAMUELS, *et al.* 2003. Cancer statistics, 2003. CA Cancer J. Clin. **53:** 5–26.
2. JEMAL, A., A. THOMAS, T. MURRAY, *et al.* 2002. Cancer statistics, 2002. CA Cancer J. Clin. **52:** 23–47.
3. AUGENLICHT, L., A. VELCICH, J. MARIADASON, *et al.* 1999. Colonic cell proliferation, differentiation, and apoptosis. Adv. Exp. Med. Biol. **470:** 15–22.
4. HANSKI, C., E. RIEDE, A. GRATCHEV, *et al.* 1997. MUC2 gene suppression in human colorectal carcinomas and their metastases: in vitro evidence of the modulatory role of DNA methylation. Lab. Invest. **77:** 685–695.
5. HO, S.B., G.A. NIEHANS, C. LYFTOGT, *et al.* 1993. Heterogeneity of mucin gene expression in normal and neoplastic tissues. Cancer Res. **53:** 641–651.
6. AUDIE, J.P., A. JANIN, N. PORCHET, *et al.* 1993. Expression of human mucin genes in respiratory, digestive, and reproductive tracts ascertained by in situ hybridization. J. Histochem. Cytochem. **41:** 1479–1485.
7. SYLVESTER, P.A., N. MYERSCOUGH, B.F. WARREN, *et al.* 2001. Differential expression of the chromosome 11 mucin genes in colorectal cancer. J. Pathol. **195:** 327–335.
8. VELCICH, A., W. YANG, J. HEYER, *et al.* 2002. Colorectal cancer in mice genetically deficient in the mucin Muc2. Science **295:** 1726–1729.
9. AKAZAWA, C., M. ISHIBASHI, C. SHIMIZU, *et al.* 1995. A mammalian helix-loop-helix factor structurally related to the product of Drosophila proneural gene atonal is a positive transcriptional regulator expressed in the developing nervous system. J. Biol. Chem. **270:** 8730–8738.
10. BEN-ARIE, N., H.J. BELLEN, D.L. ARMSTRONG, *et al.* 1997. Math1 is essential for genesis of cerebellar granule neurons. Nature **390:** 169–172.
11. HELMS, A.W. & J.E. JOHNSON. 1998. Progenitors of dorsal commissural interneurons are defined by MATH1 expression. Development **125:** 919–928.
12. BERMINGHAM, N.A., B.A. HASSAN, S.D. PRICE, *et al.* 1999. Math1: an essential gene for the generation of inner ear hair cells. Science **284:** 1837–1841.
13. ISAKA, F., M. ISHIBASHI, W. TAKI, *et al.* 1999. Ectopic expression of the bHLH gene Math1 disturbs neural development. Eur. J. Neurosci. **11:** 2582–2588.

14. BEN-ARIE, N., B.A. HASSAN, N.A. BERMINGHAM, *et al.* 2000. Functional conservation of atonal and Math1 in the CNS and PNS. Development **127:** 1039–1048.
15. KAGEYAMA, R., T. OHTSUKA, J. HATAKEYAMA, *et al.* 2005. Roles of bHLH genes in neural stem cell differentiation. Exp. Cell. Res. **306:** 343–348.
16. YANG, Q., N.A. BERMINHAM, M.J. FINEGOLD, *et al.* 2001. Requirement of Math1 for secretory cell lineage commitment in the mouse intestine. Science **294:** 2155–2158.
17. JENSEN, J., E.E. PEDERSEN, P. GALANTE, *et al.* 2000. Control of endodermal endocrine development by Hes-1. Nat. Genet. **24:** 36–44.
18. ZHENG, J.L. & W.Q. GAO. 2000. Overexpression of Math1 induces robust production of extra hair cells in postnatal rat inner ears. Nat. Neurosci. **3:** 580–586.
19. BIENZ, M. & H. CLEVERS. 2000. Linking colorectal cancer to Wnt signaling. Cell **103:** 311–320.
20. OVING, I.M. & H.C. CLEVERS. 2002. Molecular causes of colon cancer. Eur. J. Clin. Invest. **32:** 448–457.
21. POLAKIS, P. 2000. Wnt signaling and cancer. Genes Dev. **14:** 1837–1851.
22. PINTO, D. & H. CLEVERS. 2005. Wnt, stem cells and cancer in the intestine. Biol. Cell. **97:** 185–196.
23. RADTKE, F. & H. CLEVERS. 2005. Self-renewal and cancer of the gut: two sides of a coin. Science **307:** 1904–1909.
24. GREGORIEFF, A. & H. CLEVERS. 2005. Wnt signaling in the intestinal epithelium: from endoderm to cancer. Genes Dev. **19:** 877–890.
25. MARKOWITZ, S.D., D.M. DAWSON, J. WILLIS, *et al.* 2002. Focus on colon cancer. Cancer Cell **1:** 233–236.
26. MCKAY, J.A., J.J. DOUGLAS, V.G. ROSS, *et al.* 2002. Analysis of key cell-cycle checkpoint proteins in colorectal tumours. J. Pathol. **196:** 386–393.
27. YANG, W., L. BANCROFT, C. NICHOLAS, *et al.* 2003. Targeted inactivation of p27kip1 is sufficient for large and small intestinal tumorigenesis in the mouse, which can be augmented by a Western-style high-risk diet. Cancer Res. **63:** 4990–4996.
28. YANG, W., A. VELCICH, J. MARIADASON, *et al.* 2001. p21(WAF1/cip1) is an important determinant of intestinal cell response to sulindac in vitro and in vivo. Cancer Res. **61:** 6297–6302.
29. SUTTER, T., S. DOI, K.A. CARNEVALE, *et al.* 1997. Expression of cyclins D1 and E in human colon adenocarcinomas. J. Med. **28:** 285–309.
30. LEOW, C.C., M.S. ROMERO, S. ROSS, *et al.* 2004. Hath1, down-regulated in colon adenocarcinomas, inhibits proliferation and tumorigenesis of colon cancer cells. Cancer Res. **64:** 6050–6057.
31. LEE, H.W., D.H. AHN, S.C. CRAWLEY, *et al.* 2002. Phorbol 12-myristate 13-acetate upregulates the transcription of MUC2 intestinal mucin via Ras, ERK, and NF-kappa B. J. Biol. Chem. **277:** 32624–32631.
32. GAFFNEY, E. 1994. Laboratory Methods in Histotechnology. American Registry of Pathology. Washington, D.C.
33. VAN ES, J.H., M.E. VAN GUN, O. RICCIO, *et al.* 2005. Notch/gamma-secretase inhibition turns proliferative cells in intestinal crypts and adenomas into goblet cells. Nature **435:** 959–963.
34. HANAHAN, D. & R.A. WEINBERG. 2000. The hallmarks of cancer. Cell **100:** 57–70.
35. SHERR, C.J. 1996. Cancer cell cycles. Science **274:** 1672–1677.
36. SHERR, C.J. 2000. The Pezcoller lecture: cancer cell cycles revisited. Cancer Res. **60:** 3689–3695.
37. ILYAS, M., I.P. TOMLINSON, A. ROWAN, *et al.* 1997. Beta-catenin mutations in cell lines established from human colorectal cancers. Proc. Natl. Acad. Sci. USA **94:** 10330–10334.
38. RUBINFELD, B., B. SOUZA, I. ALBERT, *et al.* 1995. The APC protein and E-cadherin form similar but independent complexes with alpha-catenin, beta-catenin, and plakoglobin. J. Biol. Chem. **270:** 5549–5555.
39. MUNEMITSU, S., I. ALBERT, B. SOUZA, *et al.* 1995. Regulation of intracellular beta-catenin levels by the adenomatous polyposis coli (APC) tumor-suppressor protein. Proc. Natl. Acad. Sci. USA **92:** 3046–3050.

40. VAN DE WETERING, M., E. SANCHO, C. VERWEIJ, *et al.* 2002. The beta-catenin/TCF-4 complex imposes a crypt progenitor phenotype on colorectal cancer cells. Cell **111:** 241–250.
41. PRETLOW, T.P. & T.G. PRETLOW. 1998. Putative preneoplastic changes identified by enzyme histochemical and immunohistochemical techniques. J. Histochem. Cytochem. **46:** 577–583.
42. PINTO, D., A. GREGORIEFF, H. BEGTHEL, *et al.* 2003. Canonical Wnt signals are essential for homeostasis of the intestinal epithelium. Genes Dev. **17:** 1709–1713.
43. ZORN, A.M. 2001. Wnt signalling: antagonistic Dickkopfs. Curr. Biol. **11:** R592–595.
44. LLEO, A., E. WALDRON, C.A. VON ARNIM, *et al.* 2005. Low density lipoprotein receptor-related protein (LRP) interacts with presenilin 1 and is a competitive substrate of the amyloid precursor protein (APP) for gamma-secretase. J. Biol. Chem. **280:** 27303–27309.

# Alterations in DNA Repair Gene Expression under Hypoxia

## Elucidating the Mechanisms of Hypoxia-Induced Genetic Instability

RANJIT S. BINDRA,[a,b] PAUL J. SCHAFFER,[c] ALICE MENG,[d] JENNIFER WOO,[d] KÅRSTEIN MÅSEIDE,[d] MATT E. ROTH,[c] PAUL LIZARDI,[b,c] DAVID W. HEDLEY,[d] ROBERT G. BRISTOW,[d] AND PETER M. GLAZER[a,e]

[a]*Department of Therapeutic Radiology, Yale University School of Medicine, New Haven, Connecticut 06520, USA*

[b]*Department of Experimental Pathology, Yale University School of Medicine, New Haven, Connecticut 06520, USA*

[c]*Agilix Corporation, New Haven, Connecticut 06519, USA*

[d]*Ontario Cancer Institute/Princess Margaret Hospital (University Health Network) and Department of Medical Biophysics, University of Toronto, Toronto, Ontario M5G2M9, Canada*

[e]*Department of Genetics, Yale University School of Medicine, New Haven, Connecticut 06520, USA*

**ABSTRACT: Hypoxia is a common feature of solid tumors and is associated with genetic instability and tumor progression. It has been shown previously that alterations in the expression of DNA repair genes in response to hypoxic stress may account for a proportion of such genetic instability. Here, we demonstrate that the expression of *RAD51*, a critical mediator of homologous recombination (HR), is repressed by hypoxia in numerous cell lines derived from a wide range of tissues. Repression of this gene by hypoxia occurs in a cell cycle– and hypoxia-inducible factor (HIF)–independent manner, and decreased *RAD51* expression was observed to persist during the post-hypoxic period. In addition, decreases in Rad51 expression were correlated with functional impairments in HR repair in hypoxic and post-hypoxic cells. Based on these data, we propose a novel mechanism of hypoxia-induced genetic instability via suppression of the HR pathway in cancer cells within the tumor microenvironment.**

**KEYWORDS: tumor microenvironment; hypoxia; DNA repair; genetic instability**

Address for correspondence: Peter M. Glazer, Department of Therapeutic Radiology, Yale University School of Medicine, P.O. Box 208040, New Haven, CT 06520-8040. Voice: 203-737-2788; fax: 203-737-2630.
peter.glazer@yale.edu

**Ann. N.Y. Acad. Sci. 1059: 184–195 (2005). © 2005 New York Academy of Sciences.
doi: 10.1196/annals.1339.049**

## INTRODUCTION

We and others have shown that aspects of the tumor microenvironment such as hypoxia can contribute to genetic instability and tumor progression.[1–5] Given the profound and complex gene expression changes observed under low-oxygen tensions,[6,7] we have been studying whether altered expression of DNA repair genes might account for a proportion of hypoxia-induced genetic instability. We recently found that severe hypoxia (0.01% $O_2$) downregulates the expression of the DNA mismatch repair (MMR) gene, *MLH1*, at the level of transcription, resulting in increased mutagenesis under these conditions.[1] Along these lines, it has also been shown recently that hypoxia can induce the transcriptional repression of another MMR gene, *MSH2*, in a p53- and HIF-1α–dependent manner in numerous cell lines that also leads to genetic instability.[8] Here we report that the expression of *RAD51*, a critical mediator of homologous recombination (HR) in cells, is specifically repressed by hypoxia. Repression of *RAD51* gene expression is not dependent on hypoxia-inducible factor (HIF) expression or cell cycle profile, and decreased expression persists during the post-hypoxic phase following reoxygenation. In addition, decreased Rad51 protein expression is associated with functional impairments in the ability to carry out HR in hypoxic and post-hypoxic cells. Based on these data, we propose a novel mechanism of genetic instability in the tumor microenvironment mediated by hypoxia-induced suppression of the HR pathway in cancer cells.

## MATERIALS AND METHODS

### *Cells*

MCF-7, A549, RKO, SW-480, HeLa, SiHa, PC3, and A431 cells were obtained from the American Type Culture Collection (Manassas, VA) and were grown as per supplier instructions. Cell lines (786-0) were from Dr. W.G. Kaelin and have been described previously.[9]

### *Plasmids and Transfections*

The HIF-1α expression vector, pCEP$_4$/HIF-1α, was obtained from Dr. G. Semenza, and the 5X-HRE luciferase reporter plasmid was obtained from Dr. Zhong Yun.[10] Transfections were performed using the Fugene 6 reagent (Roche Diagnostics Corporation, Indianapolis, IN) according to the manufacturer's recommendations.

### *Hypoxia Exposure*

Severe hypoxia (0.01% $O_2$) was established as described previously,[2] using a continuous flow of a humidified mixture of 95% $N_2$ and 5% $CO_2$ gas certified to contain less than 10 ppm $O_2$ (Airgas Northeast, Cheshire, CT). Treatment with desferrioxamine mesylate (DFX) (Sigma, St. Louis, MO) was carried out by supplementation of culture medium at a concentration of 250 μM under normoxic conditions for 24 h.

### *Western Blot Analysis*

RIPA protein lysates were prepared and Western blot analyses were performed as described previously.[1,11] The following antibodies were used for these analyses: Rad51 (BD Pharmingen, Franklin Lakes, NJ), tubulin (clone B-512; Sigma), β-actin (Research Diagnostics, Flanders, NJ), HIF-1α (Clone 54; BD Transduction Laboratories, Franklin Lakes, NJ), and Glut1 (Alpha Diagnostic International, San Antonio, TX).

### *Semiquantitative Real-Time (RT) Polymerase Chain Reaction (PCR) Analysis*

Semiquantitative RT-PCR analyses were performed using the SuperScript One-step RT-PCR kit (Life Technologies, Carlsbad, CA) according to the manufacturer's instructions.

### *Northern Blot Analysis*

Total RNA was isolated using the TRIzol RNA isolation system (Life Technologies), according to the manufacturer's recommendations. Northern blot analyses were performed as described previously,[1] and primer sequences for all probes are available upon request. Blots were visualized via autoradiography and quantified either by phosphoimager analysis or NIH-Image software.

### *Protein and mRNA Stability Analyses*

To assess protein and mRNA stability, cells were grown in the presence or absence of DFX (250 μm) for 24 h, followed by the addition of either cycloheximide (CHX; 10 μg/mL; Sigma) to inhibit new protein synthesis, or actinomycin D (5 μg/mL; Sigma) to inhibit transcription. Cells were then harvested at the indicated time points following addition of inhibitor, and Rad51 protein and mRNA expression levels were determined by Western and Northern blot analyses, respectively. *RAD51* mRNA half-lives were deduced from the regression line based on mRNA degradation plots.

### *Luciferase Reporter Gene Assays*

For luciferase reporter gene analyses, a 1.8-kb fragment from the 5′-flanking region of the *RAD51* gene was isolated by genomic PCR and subcloned into the pGL3-basic vector (Promega, Madison, WI). RKO cells were transfected with 1 μg of each reporter construct using the Fugene 6 reagent (Roche Diagnostics Corporation). *Renilla* luciferase activity from a co-transfected pRL-SV40 control vector (5 ng/well) was used for normalization. *Firefly* and *Renilla* luciferase activities were measured using the Dual-luciferase Reporter Assay System kit (Promega) according to the manufacturer's instructions.

### *Cell Cycle and FACS Analysis*

Propidum iodide–based cell-cycle analyses were performed as described previously.[12] For FACS experiments, normoxic and hypoxic cells were incubated with 10 μg/mL Hoechst 33342 (Molecular Probes), followed by trypsinzation and three washes in 1X PBS. Cell sorting of specific G1- and S-phase cell populations was performed based on DNA content using a BD FACSvantage flow cytometer. RNA was extracted from the isolated cells using a TRIzol-based protocol. This technique has been recently reported to facilitate the recovery of intact mRNA from viable cells in specific phases of the cell cycle.[13]

### *Homologous Recombination Assay*

The shuttle vector plasmid pSupFG1/G144C, containing a *supFG1* gene with an inactivating G:C to C:G point mutation at position 144, has been described previously.[14] MCF-7 cells were transfected with 5 μg of pSupFG1/G144C plasmid DNA and 10 μg of a 1-kb homologous, double-stranded donor fragment containing the wild-type *supFG1* gene. After incubation for the indicated times in normoxia or hypoxia, plasmid DNA was then recovered using a modified Hirt lysate procedure.[14] The purified plasmid was subsequently used to transform *E. coli* SY302 cells by electroporation, followed by growth of the cells on indicator plates for genetic analysis of *supFG1* gene function as described previously.[14]

## RESULTS

To further elucidate the mechanism(s) by which hypoxia induces genetic instability in tumor cells, we examined patterns of DNA repair gene expression under hypoxia by transcriptome profiling.[15] These analyses suggested that *RAD51* gene expression may be decreased in response to hypoxic stress, a finding which was validated by quantitative PCR analysis (data not shown). These decreases were manifested at the protein level, as Western blot analyses revealed that prolonged exposure to severe hypoxia (48 h, 0.01% $O_2$) induced substantial decreases in Rad51 protein expression (FIG. 1A). The expression of HIF-1α and its downstream target, Glut1, are shown for comparison to confirm physiologically relevant levels of hypoxia. Levels of tubulin were unchanged and served as standards to confirm equal loading of cellular protein samples. Exposure of MCF-7 cells to the hypoxia-mimetic, desferrioxamine (DFX; 250 μM, 24 h), also resulted in decreased Rad51 protein expression (FIG. 1A). In addition, densitometry analysis was used to approximate hypoxia/normoxia (H/N) protein expression ratios for several cell lines evaluated in this study, based on triplicate hypoxia experiments and normalization to either β-actin or tubulin expression. As shown in FIGURE 1B, substantial hypoxia-mediated downregulation of Rad51 protein was observed in numerous human cell lines derived from a wide range of tissues, including A549 (lung), HeLa (cervix), RKO (colon), PC3 (prostate), and A431 (epidermis). Taken together, these data demonstrate that significant hypoxia-mediated downregulation of Rad51 protein is observed in numerous human cell lines derived from a wide range of tissues.

To determine whether the observed decreases in Rad51 protein expression could be accounted for by an increase in protein degradation, cycloheximide (CHX) chase experiments were performed in MCF-7 cells exposed to DFX. While a 24-h DFX exposure resulted in a threefold decrease in Rad51 protein expression as detected by Western blot analysis, Rad51 protein stability was not significantly altered in cells exposed to DFX versus no treatment following CHX addition (FIG. 1C). In contrast, HIF-1α expression was induced following DFX exposure, and then degraded rapidly

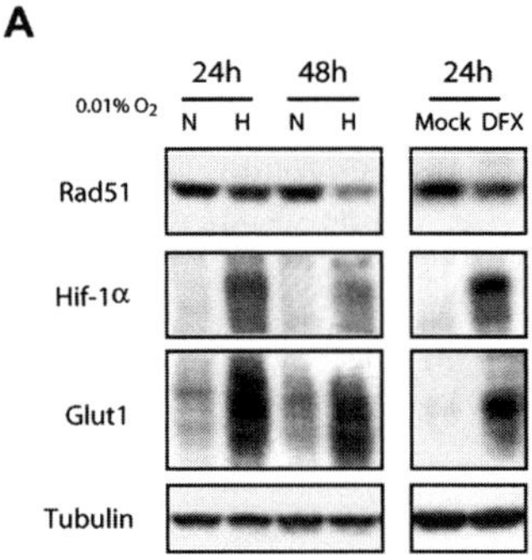


B

| Rad51 Protein Down-regulation in Selected Cell Lines | | | |
|---|---|---|---|
| Cell Line | Tissue | H/N Ratio | Error |
| MCF-7 | Breast | -6.0 | ±0.8 |
| A549 | Lung | -13.0 | ±1.7 |
| HeLa | Cervix | -2.9 | ±0.8 |
| SW480 | Colon | -2.3 | ±0.1 |
| A431 | Epidermis | -2.4 | ±0.2 |
| RKO | Colon | -6.3 | ±2.9 |
| PC3 | Prostate | -2.6 | ±0.1 |

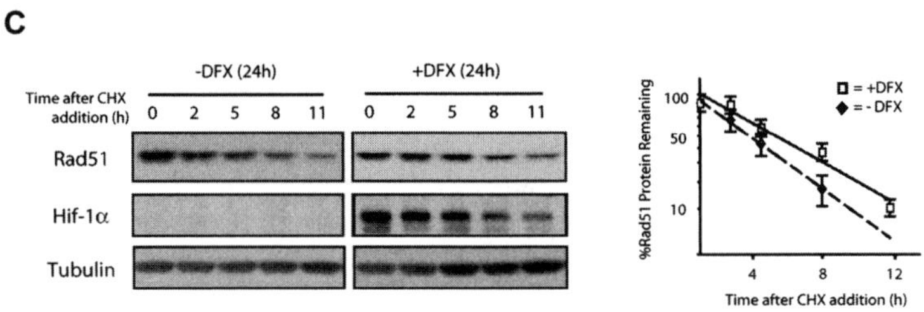


**FIGURE 1.** Decreased Rad51 protein expression in cell lines following exposure to hypoxia or the $Fe^{2+}$-chelator, desferrioxamine (DFX), and determination of Rad51 protein stability in DFX. **(A)** Western blot analyses were performed to determine the expression of Rad51 protein after exposure to normoxia (N lanes), hypoxia (0.01% $O_2$, H lanes), and DFX (250 μM, lane DFX) in MCF-7 cells. The expression of HIF-1α and Glut1 are shown for comparison to verify that physiologically relevant levels of hypoxia were present in the treated cells. Tubulin expression is also presented to confirm equal sample loading. **(B)** Average reduction in Rad51 protein induced by hypoxia (48h, 0.01% $O_2$) in selected cells, as determined by densitometry analysis of Western blots generated from duplicate or triplicate hypoxia experiments. The tissue of origin for each cell line is shown; reductions are expressed as H/N ratios normalized to the expression of β-actin or tubulin; and standard errors for each ratio are given. **(C)** To assess Rad51 protein stability, MCF-7 cells were exposed to DFX (250 μM) or to no treatment for 24 h followed by co-incubation with cycloheximide (CHX, 10 μg/mL) to block new protein synthesis. (*Left panel*) Cells were harvested at the indicated time points after the addition of CHX, and Rad51 protein expression was determined by Western blotting. The expression of HIF-1α is shown to confirm both the induction of chemical hypoxia and successful abrogation of new protein synthesis. (*Right panel*) Analysis of Rad51 protein expression at each time point after the addition of CHX in cells exposed to DFX or no treatment, quantified as described in **B**. Values in the graph indicate the percentage of Rad51 protein remaining in either DFX or untreated cells at each time point following normalization to tubulin.

after the addition of CHX, which confirms both the induction of chemical hypoxia and successful abrogation of new protein synthesis. These findings suggest that the hypoxia-mediated downregulation of the *RAD51* gene does not occur at the post-translational level.

In order to determine whether decreased *RAD51* expression persists during the post-hypoxic reoxygenation phase, Northern blot analyses were performed on total RNA extracted from MCF-7 cells after a 24- and 48-h exposure to 0.01% $O_2$, and also from cells that were returned to normoxic conditions for several days thereafter. Intriguingly, while *RAD51* mRNA levels were substantially decreased at both the 24-h and 48-h time points (approximately three- and eightfold, respectively), *RAD51* levels were lowest 24-h post-reoxygenation (approximately 12-fold, referred to as the 72-h time point; FIG. 2A). These levels did not return to normal, pre-hypoxia expression levels until after the 96-h time point, which represents a 48-h total period of post-hypoxia. The expression of *VEGF* is shown to verify the induction of physiologic levels of hypoxia, and *28S* rRNA is presented as a loading control. In addition, similar hypoxia-induced mRNA expression patterns were observed in the other human cell lines shown in FIGURE 1B, including A549, SiHa, and RKO (FIG. 2B and data not shown). These findings provide consistent evidence that hypoxia regulates the expression of the *RAD51* gene at the mRNA level in numerous cell lines and that this phenomenon persists during the post-hypoxic, reoxygenation period.

We next sought to determine whether hypoxia downregulates *RAD51* expression via a mechanism involving altered mRNA stability. To this end, actinomycin D (ActD) chase experiments were performed in MCF-7 cells exposed to DFX. While a 24-h DFX exposure resulted in a twofold decrease in *RAD51* mRNA expression (data not shown), mRNA stability was not significantly affected in cells exposed to DFX versus no treatment after the addition of ActD (FIG. 2C). *RAD51* mRNA half-lives were determined to be approximately 20 h and 15 h in DFX-exposed and untreated cells, respectively. In contrast, the expression of *VEGF* was induced following DFX exposure and degraded rapidly after the addition of ActD, which confirms both the induction of chemical hypoxia and the successful inhibition of transcription (data not shown). These data indicate that the hypoxia-induced downregulation of *RAD51* mRNA expression cannot be accounted for by decreases in the stability of the mRNA.

To test whether hypoxia-induced decreases in *RAD51* expression are associated with *RAD51* promoter repression, a *Firefly* luciferase reporter plasmid containing the *RAD51* promoter region (pGL3-Rad51p) was transiently transfected into RKO cells 4 h prior to normoxic or hypoxic exposure (0.01% $O_2$, 48 h), immediately followed by measurement of luciferase activity. Exposure to hypoxia resulted in substantial repression of pGL3-Rad51p reporter activity (fivefold; FIG. 2D). The activity of a hypoxia-inducible promoter (5X-HRE) increased approximately 50-fold under the same conditions (and thus served as a control to confirm physiologically relevant levels of hypoxia), and no change in activity was observed in the promoterless control plasmid, pGL3-Basic, in hypoxic cells. *Renilla* luciferase activity from a co-transfected pRL-SV40 control vector was used for normalization in these experiments. *RAD51* promoter activity was also repressed by hypoxia in MCF-7 and A549 cells (data not shown). Collectively, these findings suggest that hypoxia downregulates *RAD51* gene expression via a mechanism involving transcriptional repression.

We next sought to determine whether the hypoxia-inducible factors, HIF-1$\alpha$ and HIF-2$\alpha$, play a role in the repression of *RAD51* expression under hypoxia. While the

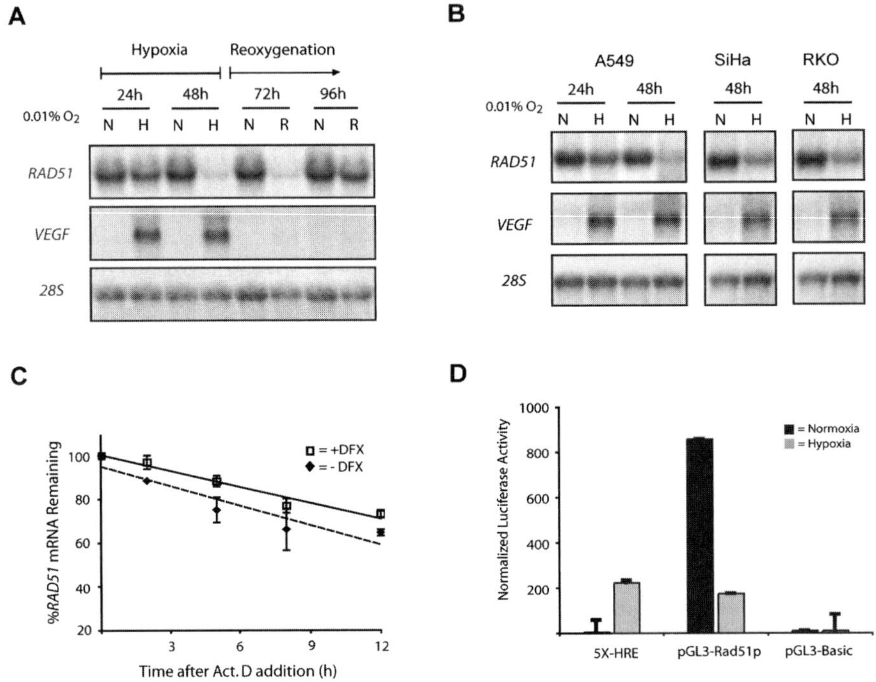


**FIGURE 2.** Transcriptional repression of the *RAD51* gene in hypoxic and post-hypoxic cells. **(A)** Northern blot analyses were performed to determine the expression patterns of *RAD51* mRNA in MCF-7 cells cultured under hypoxia for 48 h (0.01% $O_2$, lane H) and then following reoxygenation (R), or in normoxia only, as indicated by the timeline shown. Samples were obtained at 24 h intervals post-hypoxia (R lanes), with the 72- and 96-h time points representing 24 h and 48 h following reoxygenation (R), respectively. *VEGF* expression is shown for comparison to verify that physiologically relevant states of hypoxia and reoxygenation were obtained in the treated cells, and the expression of *28S* rRNA is also presented to confirm equal sample loading. **(B)** Northern blot analysis of *RAD51* mRNA expression following exposure to hypoxia (24 h and/or 48 h, 0.01% $O_2$) in A549, SiHa, and RKO cells. *VEGF* and *28S* expression are shown as in **A**. **(C)** To assess *RAD51* mRNA stability, MCF-7 cells were exposed to DFX or to no treatment for 24 h (250 μM), followed by co-incubation with actinomycin D (ActD, 5 μg/mL), to block transcription. Cells were harvested at the indicated time points after the addition of ActD, and *RAD51* mRNA expression was determined by Northern blot ting and further quantified by phosphoimager analysis of Northern blots. Values in the graph indicate the percentage of *RAD51* mRNA remaining in either DFX or untreated cells at each time point, and error bars are based on standard errors calculated from duplicate experiments. **(D)** Repression of *RAD51* promoter activity in hypoxia. *Firefly* luciferase activity represents *RAD51* promoter activity in normoxia and hypoxia following transient transfection of RKO cells with pGL3-Rad51p. The activities of a hypoxia-inducible promoter (5X-HRE) and a promoterless control plasmid (pGL3-Basic) are shown as controls for specificity and physiologically relevant levels of hypoxia. *Firefly* luciferase values were normalized to *Renilla* luciferase activity from a co-transfected pRL-SV40 control vector, and error bars are based on standard errors calculated from duplicate experiments.

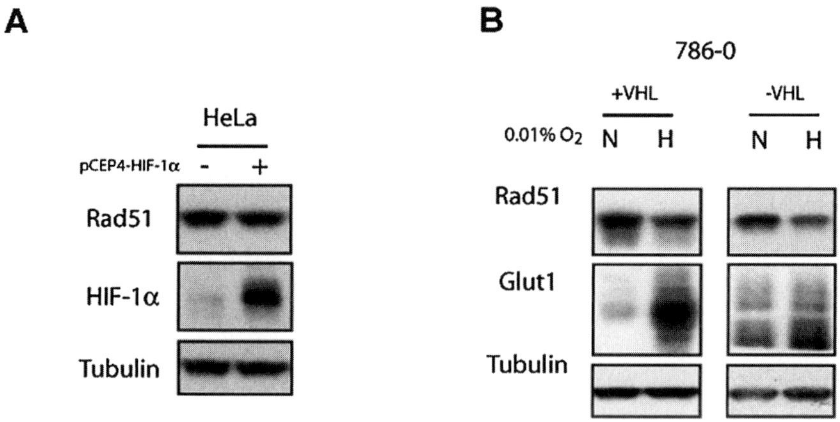


C

| G1-Shift and Rad51 Protein Levels | | |
|---|---|---|
| Cell Line | Fold Change (H/N) | |
| | G1-Shift | Rad51 |
| MCF-7 | 1.3 | -6.0 |
| A549 | 1.2 | -13.0 |
| HeLa | 1.2 | -2.9 |
| A431 | 1.0 | -2.4 |

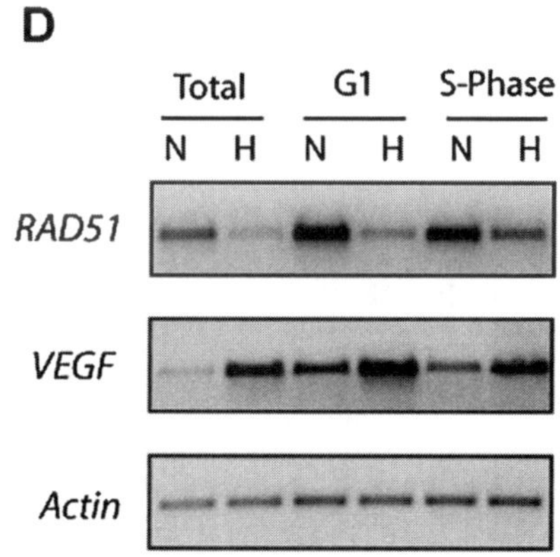


**FIGURE 3.** Decreased Rad51 expression is not associated with HIF expression or cell cycle profile. **(A)** Western blot analysis of Rad51 and HIF-1α expression levels in HeLa cells 48 h after transfection with the HIF-1α expression vector, pCEP4-HIF-1α. **(B)** Western blot analysis of Rad51 protein expression in 786-0 cells expressing either wild-type or mutant VHL following exposure to 48 h hypoxia (0.01% $O_2$). **(C)** Fold change in both the percentage of cells in G1-phase and Rad51 protein levels in hypoxia compared to normoxia, as calculated by flow cytometric analysis of propidium iodide (PI)-stained cells and from FIGURE 1B, respectively. **(D)** Semiquantitative RT-PCR analysis of *RAD51* mRNA expression in isolated G1- and S-phase populations of normoxic and hypoxic cells. Equal numbers of cell cycle-specific populations were obtained by DNA staining of cells with the vital fluorochrome, Hoechst 33342, followed by flow cytometric analysis and cell sorting. Unsorted cells processed in parallel are also shown for reference (Total). *VEGF* expression is shown for comparison to verify physiologically relevant states of hypoxia in normoxic and hypoxic cell populations, and the expression of β-actin is also presented to confirm equal sample loading.

role of HIF-1α as a transcriptional activator has been well established,[7] recent reports suggest that HIF-1α may also play a role in transcriptional repression either directly at the promoter level[16] or indirectly via the induction of transcriptional repressors such as DEC1.[17] As shown in FIGURE 3A, transient overexpression of a full-length HIF-1α cDNA (pCEP4-HIF-1α) in normoxic Hela cells was not associated with decreased expression of Rad51. To examine the role of HIF-2α in the regulation of *RAD51* expression, we used the 786-0 renal cell carcinoma cell line, which does not express VHL, a protein that targets multiple HIFs for ubiquitin-mediated proteolysis.[9] As a consequence, these cells overexpress HIF-2α (these cells do not express HIF-1α), and the expression of the VHL cDNA restores the normoxic regulation of HIF-2α.[9] As shown in FIGURE 3B, the expression of Rad51 protein was not significantly affected by VHL status or HIF-2α expression in normoxic cells, and exposure of both mutant and wild-type VHL 786-0 cells to hypoxia resulted in similar decreases in Rad51 expression. Northern blotting also revealed no differences in *RAD51* mRNA expression levels between the VHL mutant and wild-type cells in normoxia (data not shown). These data suggest that the hypoxia-mediated downregulation of *RAD51* expression occurs independently of HIF-2α. It also provides further evidence that the downregulation does not require the expression of HIF-1α, because the 786-0 cells lack HIF-1α expression.[9] Taken together, these data suggest hypoxia-induced decreases in *RAD51* gene expression are not mediated by HIF-dependent pathways.

It is possible that decreased *RAD51* expression in hypoxia could be attributed to cell-cycle profile changes, especially because *RAD51* mRNA expression levels have been shown to be substantially decreased during G0 and G1 in mammalian cells.[18] As shown in FIGURE 3C, no correlations were observed between hypoxia-induced G1-shifts and H/N ratios of Rad51 expression in the cell lines evaluated. For example, MCF7, A549, and HeLa cells all displayed small increases in the proportion of G1-phase cells upon exposure to hypoxia (1.3-, 1.2-. and 1.2-fold, respectively) and yet exhibited substantial (but variable) H/N ratios of Rad51 expression (–6.0, –13.0, and –2.9, respectively). In contrast, A431 cells displayed no detectable G1-shift under hypoxia and yet displayed H/N expression ratios similar to that observed in HeLa cells (–2.4-fold). Furthermore, substantial decreases in *RAD51* mRNA expression were observed both in G1- and S-phase–specific cell populations from normoxic versus hypoxic A549 cells (3.2- and 2.7-fold, respectively), as measured by semiquantitative reverse-transcriptase PCR (RT-PCR). These decreases were similar in magnitude to those observed in unsorted hypoxic cells that were processed in parallel (3.4-fold). Cell cycle phase–specific cell populations were obtained by DNA staining of cells with the vital fluorochrome, Hoechst 33342, followed by flow cytometric analysis and cell sorting. *VEGF* expression is shown for comparison to verify physiologically relevant states of hypoxia in the individual normoxic and hypoxic G1- and S-phase cell populations, and the expression of β-*actin* is also presented to confirm equal sample loading. Collectively, these findings provide strong evidence that decreased *RAD51* gene expression is more hypoxia-specific than cell cycle phase–dependent.

In order to determine whether hypoxia-induced reductions in Rad51 protein are associated with decreases in HR, we next measured HR activity in normoxic and hypoxic cells using a shuttle vector recombination assay. In this assay, cells are transfected with a plasmid containing a mutated *supF* reporter gene along with a wild-

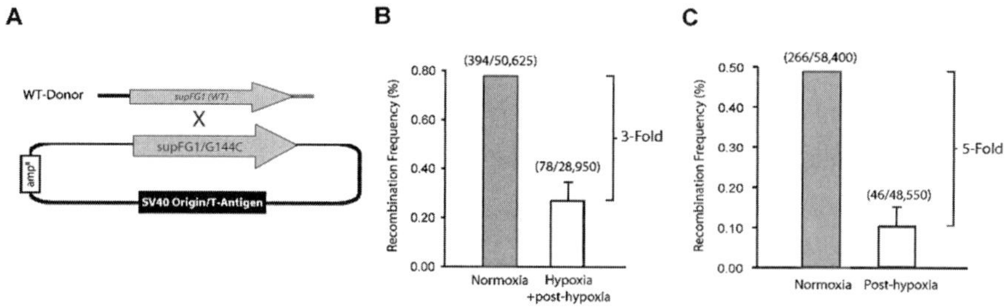


**FIGURE 4.** Decreased homologous recombination (HR) in hypoxic and post-hypoxic cells. (**A**) Schematic of the shuttle vector plasmid and donor DNA fragment used in the HR assays. The plasmid pSupFG1/G144C harbors a *supFG1* gene with an inactivating G:C to C:G point mutation at position 144; the donor is a homologous double-stranded DNA fragment that contains a portion of the wild-type *supFG1* gene. (**B**) Recombination frequencies in MCF-7 cells co-transfected with the shuttle vector and donor fragment followed by exposure either to 48 h hypoxia (0.01% $O_2$) immediately followed by reoxygenation and 24 h of normoxia (labeled Hypoxia + post-hypoxia), or to normoxia alone (labeled Normoxia). Figures in parentheses indicate total numbers of blue colonies over total number of colonies in each sample, and error bars are based on standard errors calculated from duplicate experiments. (**C**) Recombination frequencies in MCF-7 cells co-transfected with the shuttle vector and donor fragment in normoxia immediately following a 48-h exposure either to hypoxia (0.01% $O_2$, labeled Post-hypoxia) or normoxia alone (labeled Normoxia).

type (WT) recombination donor fragment into cells (schematic shown in FIG. 4A). The function of the *supFG1* gene can be assayed by recovery of the episomal shuttle vector plasmid from the cells under investigation with subsequent transformation into indicator bacteria. In this manner, the assay reports recombination events which revert the gene to the functional (WT) sequence as detected in a blue/white colony screen.[14] Co-transfection of the shuttle vector and WT donor fragment in MCF-7 cells immediately prior to hypoxic exposure (48 h, 0.01% $O_2$) followed by plasmid recovery 24 h post-hypoxia, revealed a threefold decrease in recombination frequency in hypoxic versus normoxic cells (FIG. 4B). Interestingly, we observed the most substantial decreases in HR frequencies when the cells were transfected during the post-hypoxic period (approximately fivefold; FIG. 4C), which thus paralleled the changes in expression of Rad51 protein under these conditions. These data provide evidence that decreased expression of Rad51 caused by hypoxia is associated with a substantial reduction in the capacity of cells to carry out HR both in hypoxia and during the post-hypoxic period.

## DISCUSSION

We have demonstrated that hypoxia specifically represses the expression of *RAD51*, a critical mediator of homologous recombination in mammalian cells. Downregulation of *RAD51* expression by hypoxia is not dependent on HIF expression or cell cycle profile, and the observed decreases in expression persist during the post-hypoxic period. We have also shown that these decreases are associated with functional impairments in HR repair in both hypoxic and post-hypoxic cells. Our analyses of protein half-life, mRNA stability, and promoter activity suggest that the downregulation of *RAD51* by hypoxia occurs primarily through a mechanism involving transcriptional repression. We have recently narrowed down the region in the *RAD51* promoter that mediates repression by hypoxia to an approximately 500-bp fragment within the core promoter of this gene by deletion studies with the promoter-luciferase construct described earlier (Bindra *et al.*, unpublished studies). *In silico* analysis of this region within the promoter reveals numerous putative transcription factor binding sites, including p53 and E2F binding sites. Studies are currently under way to determine whether these and other regulatory elements within this region mediate *RAD51* repression by hypoxia.

Substantial evidence now exists which suggests that tumor hypoxia plays a key role in the development of aggressive tumor phenotypes. We and others have shown that hypoxia induces alterations in DNA repair gene expression with functional consequences for DNA repair in tumor cells. In the present study, our findings suggest that hypoxia may induce genetic instability within the tumor microenvironment specifically via suppression of the HR pathway. Furthermore, downregulation of Rad51 expression may create heterogeneity in the DNA damage response among cells within tumors, with implications for the response to cancer therapies.

## ACKNOWLEDGMENTS

We thank Jianling Yuan, Shannon Gibson, Denise Hegan, and other members of the Glazer laboratory for insightful discussions regarding this manuscript.

## REFERENCES

1. Mihaylova, V.T. *et al.* 2003. Decreased expression of the DNA mismatch repair gene Mlh1 under hypoxic stress in mammalian cells. Mol. Cell. Biol. **23:** 3265–3273.
2. Reynolds, T.Y., S. Rockwell & P.M. Glazer. 1996. Genetic instability induced by the tumor microenvironment. Cancer Res. **56:** 5754–5757.
3. Young, S.D., R.S. Marshall & R.P. Hill 1988. Hypoxia induces DNA overreplication and enhances metastatic potential of murine tumor cells. Proc. Natl. Acad. Sci. USA **85:** 9533–9537.
4. Paquette, B. & J.B. Little. 1994. In vivo enhancement of genomic instability in minisatellite sequences of mouse C3H/10T1/2 cells transformed in vitro by X-rays. Cancer Res. **54:** 3173–3178.
5. Bindra, R.S. & P.M. Glazer. 2005. Genetic instability and the tumor microenvironment: towards the concept of microenvironment-induced mutagenesis. Mutat. Res. **569:** 75–85.
6. Denko, N.C. *et al.* 2003. Investigating hypoxic tumor physiology through gene expression patterns. Oncogene **22:** 5907–5914.
7. Harris, A.L. 2002. Hypoxia—a key regulatory factor in tumour growth. Nat. Rev. Cancer **2:** 38–47.
8. Koshiji, M. *et al.* 2005. HIF-1alpha induces genetic instability by transcriptionally downregulating MutSalpha expression. Mol. Cell **17:** 793–803.
9. Lonergan, K.M. *et al.* 1998. Regulation of hypoxia-inducible mRNAs by the von Hippel-Lindau tumor suppressor protein requires binding to complexes containing elongins B/C and Cul2. Mol. Cell. Biol. **18:** 732–741.
10. Shibata, T., A.J. Giaccia & J.M. Brown. 2000. Development of a hypoxia-responsive vector for tumor-specific gene therapy. Gene Ther. **7:** 493–498.

11. BROMFIELD, G.P. *et al.* 2003. Cell death in irradiated prostate epithelial cells: role of apoptotic and clonogenic cell kill. Prostate Cancer Prostatic Dis. **6:** 73–85.
12. BINDRA, R.S. *et al.* 2002. VHL-mediated hypoxia regulation of cyclin D1 in renal carcinoma cells. Cancer Res. **62:** 3014–3019.
13. JUAN, G., E. HERNANDO & C. CORDON-CARDO. 2002. Separation of live cells in different phases of the cell cycle for gene expression analysis. Cytometry **49:** 170–175.
14. CHAN, P.P. *et al.* 1999.Targeted correction of an episomal gene in mammalian cells by a short DNA fragment tethered to a triplex-forming oligonucleotide. J. Biol. Chem. **274:** 11541–11548.
15. BINDRA, R.S. *et al.* 2004. Down-regulation of Rad51 and decreased homologous recombination in hypoxic cancer cells. Mol. Cell. Biol. **24:** 8504–8518.
16. MAZURE, N.M. *et al.* 2002. Repression of alpha-fetoprotein gene expression under hypoxic conditions in human hepatoma cells: characterization of a negative hypoxia response element that mediates opposite effects of hypoxia inducible factor-1 and c-Myc. Cancer Res. **62:** 1158–1165.
17. IVANOVA, A.V. *et al.* 2001. Regulation of STRA13 by the von Hippel-Lindau tumor suppressor protein, hypoxia, and the UBC9/ubiquitin proteasome degradation pathway. J. Biol. Chem. **276:** 15306–15315.
18. FLYGARE, J., F. BENSON & D. HELLGREN. 1996. Expression of the human RAD51 gene during the cell cycle in primary human peripheral blood lymphocytes. Biochim. Biophys. Acta **1312:** 231–236.

# Index of Contributors